WORLDS OF AUTISM

Worlds of Autism

Across the Spectrum of Neurological Difference

Joyce Davidson and Michael Orsini EDITORS

University of Minnesota Press
Minneapolis • London

Published by the University of Minnesota Press
111 Third Avenue South, Suite 290
Minneapolis, MN 55401-2520
http://www.upress.umn.edu

Library of Congress Cataloging-in-Publication Data

Worlds of autism : across the spectrum of neurological difference /
Joyce Davidson and Michael Orsini, editors.
    Includes bibliographical references and index.
    ISBN 978-0-8166-8888-3 (hc)
    ISBN 978-0-8166-8889-0 (pb)
    1. Autism. 2. Autism spectrum disorders. I. Davidson, Joyce, editor.
 II. Orsini, Michael, 1967–, editor.
    RC553.A88W67 2013
    616.85'882—dc23

                                                        2013030442

Printed in the United States of America on acid-free paper

The University of Minnesota is an equal-opportunity educator and employer.

20 19 18 17 16 15 14 13   10 9 8 7 6 5 4 3 2 1

Contents

PART III. Diagnosis and Difference in Autism

PART IV. Cultural Productions
and Representations of Autism

Acknowledgments

We would like to acknowledge the generous financial support of the Social Sciences and Humanities Research Council of Canada. Many of the contributors to this volume presented drafts of their chapters at the 2010 Critical Autism Studies workshop at the University of Ottawa, and this event could not have taken place without the substantial funding provided through the SSHRC Aid to Research Workshop and Conferences Program. Thanks are also due Queen's University (Office of Research Services) and the University of Ottawa (Faculty of Social Sciences) for financial support.

We thank those workshop attendees whose work we could not include in this collection. Each contributed to our own understanding of critical autism studies, and we hope there are further opportunities to continue the important conversations that began at the Ottawa workshop.

At the University of Ottawa, Jenna Martinuzzi was an excellent conference organizer and Sarah Wiebe was a superb editorial assistant in the preparation of this book. Victoria Henderson from Queen's University provided invaluable assistance in the preparation of the grant application for funding the workshop.

Our sincere thanks to Danielle Kasprzak and Jason Weidemann, our editors at the University of Minnesota Press, for shepherding this project to the finishing line and for believing in a critical, interdisciplinary collection such as this. The University of Minnesota Press is a beacon for scholars at the intersections of disciplines and consistently produces remarkable publications. Thanks, too, to two anonymous reviewers of the manuscript; their thoughtful commentary was very much appreciated.

Joyce thanks Mick Smith, Katie Hemsworth, Sophie Edwards, and Victoria Henderson (again!). She dedicates this book to Emily Rain (our youngest workshop participant), her Gran and Grandad, and all her furred and feathered friends of the Hundred Acre Wood.

Michael acknowledges the support of friends, family, and colleagues who listened to his endless bellyaching, including Mary and Robert

Gordon, Dave and Carrie Longbottom, Shoshana Magnet, Francesca Scala, Miriam Smith, and Luc Turgeon. Most of all, he thanks Victoria, Emma, and Lucca for their consistent love and support, and his parents and Aunt Mary for "being there." Empathetic scholarship begins with the people who nourish us intellectually as well as emotionally.

INTRODUCTION. Critical Autism Studies
Notes on an Emerging Field

Michael Orsini and Joyce Davidson

It is difficult to think, much less write, about autism today without some reference to the statistics. Talk of "exploding" prevalence rates and a public health crisis of "epidemic proportions" dominates the landscape (see Nash 2002). The onward march of statistical knowledge about autism—from a prevalence rate of 1 in 150 in 2000, to 1 in 110 in 2006, and 1 in 88 in 2008 (Centers for Disease Control and Prevention 2012)—communicates a sense of undeniable urgency (Rice et al. 2007). Autism is depicted as unstoppable and difficult to contain. Failing to intervene early, parents are warned, can be disastrous. Although autism varies significantly in its effects on individuals, statistics aggregate the rich, qualitative experiences of life with autism into a language that is (too) easy to understand. The "objective" data about this complex condition homogenize the diversity of autistic experience and gloss over the situated knowledge of those most intimately affected by autism: autistic people themselves.

As the last few decades have shown, autistic people are increasingly determined to shape broader public discourses about this condition, either through artistic or cultural interventions or through direct engagement in political or social activities that communicate beyond autistic worlds the many varieties of being autistic. The Internet, for instance, provides an increasingly rich source of trenchant commentary about firsthand experience of what has come to be known as the autism spectrum, as well as interventions from parents and caregivers committed to sharing their own perspectives, insights, and challenges. One of the goals of this collection is to emphasize just how much *everyone*, whatever their relation to autism, still has to learn about—and from—autistic worlds. Although the insights that our variously positioned contributors provide here are not always of direct practical relevance—the book

cannot, for example, resolve the complex issues faced by parents struggling with school systems to accommodate their autistic child, or by
autistic adults facing stigma in the workplace—we do hope they prove
valuable to such directly affected individuals nonetheless, and in a number of different and important ways. We argue that empathetic academic
exploration of worlds of autism can help better contextualize a condition that can, after all, be read and indeed experienced only through
culture. As Roy Richard Grinker explains (2007, 11–12), autism "does
not exist outside of culture," and so we seek to understand it through
the cultural filters that bring it into focus, even as we are mindful of
overzealous efforts to read meaning into all things autistic. Sometimes,
so-called autistic behavior can be just as "random and casual, as open,
as any other behaviour" (Murray 2012, xii) and, of course, just as challenging to understand.

From its initial "discovery" in 1943, by Leo Kanner, as a distinct psychiatric disorder, to theories that it was caused by "refrigerator mothers"
and their cold, distant parenting (Bettelheim 1967), autism has been
steeped in contestation and controversy. Present-day skirmishes over
the place of Asperger Syndrome on the autism spectrum (Grinker 2010;
Ghaziuddin 2010) are the subject of intense debate in the research community, in the media, and among autistic people and the individuals
who care for them. Disagreements about autism's underlying causes and
how it should be treated (or whether it should be treated at all) continue
with an alarming regularity, especially in online forums dedicated to
autism research and advocacy. Even as parents, researchers, and autistic
people themselves work to confront and overcome some of these deep
divisions, the very notion of autism is in flux. The American Psychiatric
Association announced its intention to revise the definition of autism in
the fifth edition of its widely cited publication *Diagnostic and Statistical
Manual of Mental Disorders (DSM)*, which was released in May 2013. In
the preceding DSM, autism and Asperger Syndrome were identified
separately. Among other changes, the fifth edition folds autism and
Asperger Syndrome under the umbrella term "autism spectrum disorder," which encompasses deficits in two areas: social communication
and interaction, and restricted or repetitive behavior. In order to be
diagnosed under the first category, individuals must present deficits in
"social-emotion reciprocity, nonverbal communicative behaviors, and
in developing and maintaining relationships." As regards the second,

the repetitive patterns of behavior must meet at least two of five criteria, including repetitive speech or movements and "excessive adherence to routines" (American Psychiatric Association 2011).

The concept of an autism "spectrum," although intended to capture the diversity of the autism experience, can present challenges to systems or structures that depend upon clearly delineated definitions of disability in order for individuals to qualify for state support for programs or services (see Baker and Walsh, this volume). Moreover, this politics of naming—whether autism is a spectrum, a difference, or a disorder—has implications for how individuals who exhibit some of these characteristics or behaviors view themselves and interact with the world.

Policies and programs to deal with disability are often grounded in competing conceptions of how disability is produced and, correspondingly, what types of public action are required. Briefly, the dominant, medical model of disability locates disability in the individual and supports efforts to "cure" or help disabled people overcome difficulties thought to originate from their own problematic embodiment. In contrast, the social model views disability as the product of people's interactions with disabling and unsupportive environments. Rather than attempting to "fix" individuals, advocates of a social model support efforts to accommodate the diverse needs of disabled people in society through improvements to aspects of their social and material environments (see Pothier and Devlin 2006; Shakespeare 2006a, 2006b). As Chloe Silverman has argued in relation to the competing claims of advocates of medical and social models of disability, "The most successful studies are those that refuse to situate their claims firmly with one model or the other, but instead pay attention to the strategic uses of different models by various interested groups" (2008, 336). When it comes to resolving some of the "most crucial political questions surrounding autism," such as those concerning societal acceptance or accommodation, the distinctions advanced by these models of disability are not particularly helpful (336–37). Framing responses to autism in either/or terms—either it is a neurological difference to be celebrated or it is a disabling condition—can paralyze public discourses in ways that might ultimately be of little benefit to autistic people.

The last decade or so has seen a steady surge of literature from social scientists and humanities scholars concerned with autism and, in particular, with challenging dominant constructions of the condition that have been advanced in biomedical or therapeutic contexts. Philosophers such as Deborah Barnbaum (2008), Eva Kittay and Licia Carlson (2010), and Ronald Amundson (2000) have called attention to how cognitive disabilities confront notions embedded in moral philosophy. In *The Ethics of Autism* (2008), Barnbaum reflects on the boundaries of autistic personhood. For her part, Barnbaum argues for a form of "autistic integrity," which involves respect for autistic ways of being in the world that might be "incomprehensively different from the life led by those who are not autistic" (11). The scholar who has arguably done the most to advance our understanding of autism in the social sciences and humanities—in a way that has also had a significant impact on clinical understandings—is also a philosopher. Ian Hacking (2000) first advanced the idea of autism as an "interactive kind" and has been consistently cited in a wide variety of international and interdisciplinary contexts for his idea of "looping," which suggests that the classifications and categories we use to define populations—in this case, autistic people—transform not only the categories but also the populations so defined.

Majia Holmer Nadesan's *Constructing Autism* (2005) was one of the first book-length treatments of autism from a social-constructivist perspective, and it has influenced scholars interested in critiquing some of the assumptions that underpin autism research and policy. Cognizant that a social-constructivist perspective might be seen to obscure the "real" effects of autism on individuals and families, Nadesan is careful to link her theoretical interest in social construction with the way "the contemporary matrix of practices and institutions" that are used to identify or label autistic people contributes to "the production and interpretation of the behaviors, self awareness, and 'other' awareness of people understood as autistic" (5).

In her definitive cultural history of an alternative but similarly momentous health "crisis," Paula Treichler uses the term "epidemic of signification" to describe AIDS as both a "transmissible lethal disease and an epidemic of meanings or signification" (1999, 11). Emerging during particular historical periods and evoking specific political, social, cultural, and emotional responses, epidemics of signification reveal crises of meaning. In the 1980s, AIDS activists took great pains to communicate the urgency of action on AIDS, worried that fear of the then-mystery virus might immobilize decision makers to do nothing. Activists were also instrumental in sensitizing others to the need to separate the virus from the person, to resist the urge to mark the "other," as had been done in the early years of the epidemic. They worked tirelessly to frame AIDS in crisis terms but were careful to frame people with AIDS as vibrant actors with complex histories, people with much more than the virus in their blood system (see Epstein 1996; Gould 2009).

Although epidemic language makes autism "intelligible" to a range of actors affected by and invested in autism and provides a much-needed "discursive link" to justify policy intervention in the age of a scaled-back welfare state (see Bumiller, this volume), it does not communicate any fundamental truths about autism or about autistic experience. The fact that autism typically presents and tends to be diagnosed in young children adds to the drama of this unfolding narrative. In the current neoliberal context of state retrenchment and support for only the most deserving subjects, the idea of autism as "the thief of childhood" succeeds in striking a strong emotional chord. The "ransom notes" advertising campaign launched in 2007 by the New York University Child Study Center drew on a familiar trope of autism as an abductor of innocent children (Autistic Self Advocacy Network 2007). The billboard campaign featured simulations of ransom notes with scrawled or typed text, which included phrases such as "We have your son" and were signed "Autism" (Kras 2010). The campaign became a target of online efforts by activists associated with the Autistic Self Advocacy Network, which mobilized other disability groups to protest what they saw as outdated and stereotypical portraits of autistic people as doomed to lead unproductive, unfulfilled lives (Ne'eman 2007).

The narrative of an unfolding or looming epidemic is certainly not the only way in which autism has come to be known or understood. Autism fascinates researchers, scientists, the media, and the general public precisely because it communicates and reflects such a multiplicity of meanings. It is viewed as a scourge by some, a potent symbol of an environment gone awry by antivaccinationists, and as another way of being or interacting with the world by autistic self-advocates and others associated with the idea of neurodiversity. In the world of genetics, researchers have attached hope to the idea that they can unlock the mystery of autism through the identification of genetic markers (Bumiller 2009). The geneticization of autism, although criticized by autistic self-advocates as a new form of eugenics, has had other effects as well, including helping to shift the discourse of blame for autism away from "refrigerator mothers," whose parenting was once linked to autism.

Although it is difficult to ignore the conventional ways in which public-health discourses frame epidemics, we need to stop to ask how those epidemics are constituted and framed. What kinds of knowledge are mobilized to advance epidemic claims? In *The Autism Matrix* (2010), Gil Eyal and colleagues urge us to overturn existing dominant constructions that present autism in epidemic terms. As they argue, "It was not the epidemic that made autism visible, but the visibility of autism that made the epidemic" (2). The authors suggest that there are practical or pragmatic reasons for actors in the autism field to embrace the logic of a spiraling autism epidemic: these are "attempts to establish a discursive link, to throw an improvised rope bridge across from the autism social world to the worlds where decisions are made, resources allocated and actions taken—the worlds of politics, economics, medicine and science" (2–3). Although the authors are correct to call attention to the seemingly instrumental logic behind autism advocates' support for epidemic language, we would caution against a view of the social world of autism as being conceptually distinct from the worlds of politics, economics, medicine, and science. The "worlds of autism" that are explored in this collection lay claim to the fact that these worlds are themselves imbricated with other worlds such as to make them difficult to distinguish from one another. Autistic experience does not simply exist "out there" as a "voyeuristic freak show" to entertain the nonautistic masses, to use the words of prominent autistic self-advocate Amanda Baggs (2007). The social worlds of autism are revealing of nonautistic worlds, as well. Paying closer attention, for instance, to how nonverbal autistic individuals such as Baggs communicate their perspectives on autism challenges assumptions about what constitutes "normal" forms of communication.

When they are located in relation to individuals, depictions of autism have usually conformed to a narrative arc common to many stories about illnesses or challenging health conditions (Frank 1995). Arthur Frank classifies three types of narrative, although he is careful to note that they are not mutually exclusive: the restitution narrative, the chaos narrative, and the quest narrative (see Osteen, this volume). In contemporary culture, the most common is the restitution narrative, which clings to a belief in "restorable health." These narratives fulfill two important functions: "For the individual teller, the ending is a return to just before the beginning: 'good as new' or status quo ante. For the culture that prefers restitution stories, this narrative affirms that breakdowns can be fixed. The remedy, now secure in the family medicine cabinet, becomes a kind of talisman against future sickness" (Frank 1995, 90).

Autism can also be read through the two other narrative forms identified by Frank. The chaos narrative, often referred to as the antinarrative, is the least heard among the narratives, because the tellers are besieged by the disorder and cannot speak of or communicate their experience in a coherent fashion. The third form is the quest narrative, in which persons journey through and face the reality of their illness head-on in the belief that they were destined to learn something from this experience. In their search for alternative ways of experiencing illness, quest stories may include accounts of becoming politically active, forming a patients'-rights group, attending support-group meetings, and helping others who may be in a similar situation. Frank is clear that in many cases, all three narrative types are told. The three types are thus better viewed as "patterns in a kaleidoscope: for a moment, the colors are given one specific form, then the tube shifts and another one emerges" (76). The metaphor of the kaleidoscope is useful in thinking about the shifting patterns of autism that are reflected in discursive worlds, from the popular media, to public policy and scientific discourses. There are moments in which we might view the colors of autism in one specific form, but the picture can shift suddenly, kaleidoscopically, revealing another picture or pattern entirely.

Autism is far from settled, so it is perhaps not surprising that naming it, containing it, or diagnosing it is marked with controversy and deep disagreement. How do we make sense of the multiple and sometimes deeply contradictory depictions of autism? How is it possible to frame autism as "worse than cancer," as one Canadian advocate suggested in testimony before a Senate committee, because "the person with autism has a normal life span" (Standing Senate Committee on Social Affairs, Science, and Technology 2003, 9–13), but also to view it as the ideal "cognitive profile" to succeed in our information economy (Cowen 2009b)? An economist who has written extensively about autism, Tyler Cowen, argues that autistics might hold the key to surviving and thriving in our turbulent economic world. He suggests that some of the traits so derided in autistics—the tendency to perseverate or to systematize—are precisely the qualities that many nonautistics are trying to emulate in order to succeed in the brave new economy. Although autistics face challenges in adapting to some work environments, including, for example, those involving sustained social interaction (Davidson 2010; Shore 2001), they thrive in others. Universities, Cowen explains, are "especially conducive to autistics," because they allow them to "choose their own hours and work at home, and [foster] the ability to work on focused projects for long periods of time" (Cowen 2009a; see also Prince-Hughes 2002).

Whereas clinicians and other autism experts might focus our attention on the great strides being made in "treating" autism or isolating its possible genetic underpinnings (Silverman 2008a), critical autism scholars are interested in how different forms of expertise about autism become advanced and accepted in, for example, activist discourses or official government policy pronouncements (see Baker and Walsh, this volume) and in family settings. Stuart Murray's suggestion (2012) that we, in fact, know very little about autism should not be interpreted as an expression of pessimism, however. Rather, it is a potent reminder of how our knowledge is always in flux, provisional, subject to change. The subjectivities at the heart of our analyses do not exist a priori: they are shaped and constituted in processes of meaning making.

The current state of knowledge about autism is open to challenge and critique from various corners, including not only those from the scientific world but also those who are laypersons and nonacademic experts who bring different perspectives to the table. Although we seek to contribute to scholarly inquiry in understanding autism, academic debates must be integrated into broader discourses about autism that circulate in online autistic communities, among caregivers, and in a wide variety of other "nonacademic" contexts. Parents, for instance, have been in the vanguard of constructing knowledge about autism, pioneering approaches to care and treatment that are grounded in the experience of their everyday lives caring for their children (Silverman 2011). The general parental focus on treatment exists alongside first-person critiques by some autistic persons themselves who reject the need for any form of treatment, as well as antitreatment perspectives advanced by nonautistic parents of autistic children. Some of them have embraced the concept of neurodiversity, which was coined in the late 1990s by Australian advocate Judy Singer and journalist Harvey Blume. Advocates of neuro-diversity argue for greater recognition of what Kathleen Seidel terms the "variety of human wiring" on her popular Web site, neurodiversity .com (2013). Neurodiversity extends beyond autism to encompass other so-called brain-based differences, but in recent years it has become most closely associated with autistic self-advocacy (see Ortega 2009; Armstrong 2010; Baker 2011).

What's So "Critical" about Critical Autism Studies?

Culminating a collaborative and interdisciplinary effort that began with a workshop at the University of Ottawa in Canada, *Worlds of Autism* features contributors from Canada, the United States, the United Kingdom, Brazil, Australia, and France. We attempt to balance a range of perspectives by uniting researchers who are concerned, to a greater or lesser degree, with autistic subjectivities and the politics of cognitive difference. Although this book is geared primarily to an academic audience, we see its potential extending toward autistic individuals inside and outside academe, as well as policy makers and others involved in developing strategies and services with and for autistic people, including those in the burgeoning sector of autistic self-advocacy. Autistics and the individuals who love and care for them are the individuals who bring "critical" perspectives on autism into the social and political worlds that make a difference in the lives of people on the spectrum. Without these engagements, the autism spectrum would probably be a very different, more marginal, and arguably less emotionally accessible place. As Silverman explains in her recent book, *Understanding Autism* (2011), the role of parents as caregivers and as trailblazers in treatment models is marked by their feelings of attachment. Indeed, emotions and affect have begun to occupy their rightful place in the study of autism, in ways that move beyond more conventional understandings of autistic people as marked by an empathy deficit (see Davidson and Orsini 2010; McDonagh, this volume).

Contributors to this collection are cognizant of autism's complex history and take seriously the situated knowledge of autistic people themselves. But we should be clear that this unity is fragile, partial. Although the contributors might support approaches to autism that are destigmatizing and abilities-focused rather than deficit-based, there are competing interpretations of, for instance, the place of neurodiversity in the broader autism movement (see Ortega, this volume). For instance, in response to advocacy grounded in the idea of neurodiversity, Mark Osteen has warned of the danger of simply celebrating "disabilities as difference," as this might "work to eliminate the terms under which these differences become worthy of discussion" (2008, 3). Although contributors to this volume are generally united in moving beyond deficit-focused ways of thinking about autism, this unity is admittedly fragile (see Berg and Mol 1998). There is less unity, for instance, on how to view the autistic subject. At times, she or he is deeply politicized (Chamak and Bonniau, and Baker and Walsh, this volume), whereas at other times the subject is cast primarily as the object of biomedical or therapeutic intervention (Nadesan, this volume). These diverse framings of the autistic subject have consequences for how we view, analyze, and make sense of autistic experience. As Marc Berg and Annemarie Mol discuss in relation to the shattering of any notion of a unified medicine, thinking about diversity and difference calls our attention to both "unifying and disruptive forces; both continuities and discontinuities" (1998, 7).

These continuities and discontinuities reflect not only the shifting definitions of autism but also what it means to be autistic. Up until the last decade or so, it was not commonly known by nonautistics that autistic people might be interested in engaging politically in the field of autism, borrowing from the scripts of their social-movement forerunners in the disability movement. Although the emergence of the autistic self-advocacy movement bears similarities with the disability movements that preceded it (Davis 2002; Shakespeare 2006a, 2006b), we think there is something distinctive in the forms of autistic advocacy that have emerged in recent years. Autistic persons, by their very presence, help to confront the boundaries that separate autistic and non-autistic lifeworlds. We believe critical-autism-studies scholars are well positioned to contribute meaningfully to some of these debates about autistic personhood (see Barnbaum 2008; Hacking 2009b; Kittay and Carlson 2010; Ortega 2009; Wolff 2010), in much the same way that the work of disability-studies scholars more generally is informed by a deep understanding of the respective disability communities. Although autistic self-advocates have been influenced by their forerunners in the disability movement, the nature of autism means that for some autistic

people, unlike members of other disability communities, social interactions of any kind can be challenging. Indeed, for some, "the impetus
to engage in the public realm, to act politically, is perhaps motivated
by a desire to create the conditions where they have greater freedom to
express their individuality" (Bumiller 2008, 980).

Worlds of Autism consolidates and builds upon exciting scholarship
at the edges of the social sciences and the humanities, drawing insights
from a range of disciplines and subfields, including work in the area of
critical disability studies. Although scholars interested in autism have
been forced to tread some of the same ground that other disability activists and scholars walked before them, there are nonetheless some advantages in asking how or whether current disability-studies perspectives or approaches can provide sufficient context for our understanding
of the diversity of autistic experience. Disability-studies scholars have
illuminated the poverty of approaches to disability that treat disabled
people as defective or deficient, and have advanced instead views of
(dis)ability that foreground the ways in which societies collectively produce disabling conditions for individuals living with impairments. It is
equally incumbent on researchers interested in autism specifically to
question taken-for-granted assumptions about how autism might fit into
the models of disability that have been advanced and critiqued in the
disability-studies literature.

Although we coined the phrase "critical autism studies" as a title
for our workshop, we view the contours of this field as emergent and in
flux. Indeed, our goal in assembling this international, interdisciplinary
group of scholars was in part to interrogate rather than define or delimit
the boundaries of this emerging field of study. Of course, *Worlds of Autism*
cannot contain the depth or diversity of current work; for example, with
the exception of Francisco Ortega's chapter, it does not engage, to any
significant extent, with the work of critical neuroscientists (Choudhury
and Slaby 2011). Despite inevitable shortcomings and omissions in our
various discussions and writings since this collaborative project began,
we continue to question what exactly is "critical" about critical autism
studies, and attempt to keep the space open and accessible for new and
emerging scholars. Our collective response to date is far from exhaustive, yet we have identified three main elements of a critical approach to
the study of autism that shape the form and content of this collection:

1. Careful attention to the ways in which power relations shape the field of autism
2. Concern to advance new, enabling narratives of autism that challenge the predominant (deficit-focused and degrading) constructions that influence public opinion, policy, and popular culture
3. Commitment to develop new analytical frameworks using inclusive and nonreductive methodological and theoretical approaches to study the nature *and* culture of autism. The interdisciplinary research required (particularly in the social sciences and humanities) demands sensitivity to the kaleidoscopic complexity of this highly individualized, relational (dis)order.

We expand on each of these ideas in turn. First, a critical approach to autism entails an examination of how power relations operate in the autism field, whether in the research process (see Nadesan, and Raymaker and Nicolaidis, this volume), in attempts to "represent" autism in the media and popular culture (Osteen, this volume), or in policy deliberations (Baker and Walsh, this volume). What do government and policy responses to autism tell us about these unfolding power relations? How are attempts to reinvigorate the role of communities and civil society reshaping the roles and responsibilities of state actors in responding appropriately to autism? How are scientific interests in autism research negotiated, and how does the outcome reflect the kinds of research that are and are not funded? These are just some of the questions related to the circulations of power that motivate critical-autism-studies scholars.

Second, critical autism scholars interrogate dominant depictions of autism as a deficit disorder and challenge the often-uncritical distinction between so-called high- and low-functioning autism. This should not be confused with support for a celebratory approach to autism (see Armstrong 2010). Many autistic individuals, including self-advocates, accept the idea that autism can be disabling and that autistic people may require some assistance or support from the state or from caregivers. Like their predecessors in the disability movement, they largely reject, however, "outside naming" or definitions that might be imposed on them by experts. Yet, as Brigitte Chamak and Beatrice Bonniau's chapter explains with reference to advocacy in France, one must be careful not to assume that autistic advocates behave in uniform ways across different geographical contexts. Chamak and Bonniau have also been critical of the intense focus on diagnosing and "treating" autism in children and the relative societal and state neglect of the distinctive needs of adults on the spectrum, a theme that is addressed partly in Kristin Bumiller's critique of how autistic people fare under a neoliberal welfare state (this volume).

Challenging the deficit narrative of autism that is prevalent in literature that advocates a "cure" for neurodevelopmental difference (for example, Schopler 2001; Tidmarsh and Volkmar 2003; Zimmerman 2008), we see *Worlds of Autism* as part of a growing body of work that uses an abilities framework. This helps us to position autism as a complex relational (dis)order that challenges deeply rooted stereotypes of what has long been regarded as normal human experience. In contrast to the prevailing deficit narrative of autism, which individualizes and depoliticizes the autistic subject, an abilities framework not only respects the complex personhood of autistic individuals but also reveals how the negotiation of autistic identities holds important insights for how to view normalcy and (cognitive) difference (see Arneil 2009; Barnbaum 2008; Kittay and Carlson 2010; Wikler 2010). An abilities framework also reveals something of how we might imagine the potential of autistic political mobilization, in much the same way that Phil Brown and colleagues (2004) describe the emergence of "embodied health movements" of individuals whose shared biology can become the grounds for claims making (see also Orsini 2009; and Orsini and Smith 2010). Imagining autistic individuals as actors with agency helps to disrupt assumptions about legitimate forms of political expression, such as when autistic self-advocates counsel others to engage in "collective stimming" (*stimming* is shorthand for self-stimulation, meaning repetitive body movements such as rocking and hand flapping) as an act of resistance against professionals who view stimming as a behavior that should be discouraged.

Third, we think that these divergent understandings that have become attached to autism require us both to rethink the possibilities of what it means to do research on autism and to begin a sustained interdisciplinary conversation about what engaged scholarly enquiry into autism could or should entail (Solomon and Bagatell 2010). In their "Biocultures Manifesto" (2007), leading disability scholars Lennard Davis and David Morris call on researchers to trouble the strict separation between culture and biology: "The biological without the cultural, or the cultural without the biological, is doomed to be reductionist at best and inaccurate at worst." Social constructionism, they continue, is "self-limited and inaccurate if it implies that social facts may be entirely dissociated from biological facts" (411). Critical researchers must question the received wisdom about what constitutes knowledge, and must consistently and forcefully challenge the divide between science and humanities as well as other overly simplistic and harmful dichotomies, including that between fact and value, they argue. Although they do not discuss autism per se, Davis and Morris close their manifesto with a useful series of "provocative assaults" on received wisdom, some of which are reproduced here:

- It is untrue that the humanities are the realm of values and the sciences the realm of facts.
- Science isn't hard and the humanities aren't soft.
- You can't fully understand the results of a given data set without knowing the historical, social, cultural, and discursive fields surrounding the data. (418)

We situate *Worlds of Autism* in the spirit of radical inquiry proposed by Davis and Morris, recognizing, of course, that our contributors locate themselves, to varying degrees, at the intersection of biology and culture. Researchers working in the field of autism—not to mention scholars, activists, and other social science and humanities scholars of disability more broadly—can benefit from reframing their own approaches to research and inquiry in ways that do not reproduce the recurring difficulties associated with presumptions of a fact/value dichotomy. As contributors reveal throughout the book, what we (think we) know about autism—the so-called facts—are difficult to dislodge or disentangle from the social and discursive worlds in which they are embedded. Whether it is the "empathy deficit" that is supposedly characteristic of autism (see McDonagh, this volume) or the wisdom of dropping Asperger Syndrome from the *DSM* (Ghaziuddin 2010; Grinker 2010), what we understand and claim to know about autism is in constant flux, shaped profoundly by broader environments over which we have relatively little control. Thus, as neo-Foucauldian scholars have been at pains to argue, it is difficult to separate what we know about a given object from the various technologies that make it knowable or governable (Rose 2007; Rose and Novas 2005; Novas 2006).

The critical-autism-studies approach we advance here imagines the "academic" study of autism as a site of action and resistance, to be read in tandem with autistic and nonautistic forms of expression in literature, film, and other media. Some of the chapters explicitly tackle the challenges associated with frameworks that build upon existing approaches and attempt to refine them in order to take better account of the specificity of autism (for example, Raymaker and Nicolaidis, this volume, on community-based participatory research). Others interrogate the power relations embedded in genetically charged discourses related to autism (for example, Nadesan, this volume) or the problems associated with attempts to narrate autism in ways that are sufficiently reflective of its incredible diversity (Osteen, this volume). To that end, the "critical" in critical autism studies derives also from an active engagement with autistic communities. Whereas some of the contributors' work is based on research with autistics, others' work is informed by engagement with autism in their respective personal lives. Several of the contributors to this volume are either caregivers for autistic persons or self-identify as autistic themselves.

We view this collection as contributing to a form of "empathetic scholarship" (Osteen 2008, 297) that is concerned with inclusion and accommodation as well as autistic difference and personhood. Critical-autism-studies scholars are concerned with conducting research that respects the rules or principles of ethical conduct. As Michelle Dawson, a prominent Canadian autism researcher and Critical Autism Studies workshop participant, has argued, "I think it's very important that scientific and ethical standards not be lowered or discarded for autistics. . . . I am really hoping for advocacy which demands higher standards of science and ethics for autistics, but this hasn't happened yet" (Dawson 2012). We should stress, as well, that although many of the contributors approach the "scientific" study of autism in a critical manner, a "critical" approach to autism need not necessarily position itself squarely against approaches or findings associated with the "hard" sciences. Rather, we are critical of all reductive approaches to and representations of autism, regardless of their disciplinary origins, and particularly of those that are neglectful of the views and voices of the individuals and groups most intimately affected.

Thematic Overview

We have structured the book around four organizing themes that allow us to explore the emerging contours of critical autism studies: (1) approaching autism; (2) researching the politics and practice of care; (3) diagnosis and difference in autism; and (4) cultural productions and representations of autism.

Part I. Approaching Autism

The first part groups our interests in advancing a more nuanced understanding of personhood that makes space for the full spectrum of human experience, including a need to address fundamental issues related to what it means to be human. These chapters reveal that approaching autism critically involves intensive and extensive reflection on the myriad concepts and categories that have been used to shore up predominant and problematic constructions of autism, including the presence or absence of emotions such as empathy. Reflecting on these concepts and categories becomes critical to how we make sense of autism and its competing discourses.

In the first chapter, Patrick McDonagh examines a feature of personhood that has come to be much explored in recent years: empathy. As McDonagh explains, thanks to a raft of recent research, autism has become synonymous with an empathy deficit. Although *empathy* entered the English language only in the early twentieth century, recently it has been rebranded as a critical attribute for successful social functioning, both on the individual and the societal levels. Prominent Cambridge University researcher Simon Baron-Cohen (2003) has termed autism an "empathy disorder," so it is not surprising that the concepts of empathy and autism are enjoying similar attention in contemporary discourses of identity and pathology. McDonagh's chapter explores the growth of these concepts in tandem, arguing that autism's development as a spectrum disorder is closely connected to the increasing prominence of empathy as a marker of social success. He concludes that we should be suspicious of terms such as *empathy*, which are "ideologically loaded and culturally shaped" and can have negative effects on autistic people. Moreover, he says, the claim that empathy is a fundamental aspect of personhood is relatively weak.

Stuart Murray argues in his chapter that because of the various differences it embodies, autism offers a particular vantage point from which to ask questions about what constitutes "the human." Although such thinking can take the form of prejudicial discrimination, it also offers up a productive revision of ideas of self and agency. Murray explores such themes by drawing on Katherine Hayles's idea of the "posthuman condition" as being marked by "distributed cognition." Murray weighs the competing claims of the categories of human and posthuman in helping us to think more about autistic normality. Although it is potentially appealing to think of the posthuman category as opening a "radically productive space for autism," Murray is concerned that the realm of the posthuman might be a disembodied place where "the material links to the experience of a lived life, the day-to-day business of being autistic, could be lost." The area and tension between these two positions, and the possibilities of each, are the ground he covers by examining clinical conceptions of the condition, ideas of possible medical futures, and writings by those with autism.

In addition, Part I explores some of the fundamental tensions expressed in attempts to counter disability discrimination based on neurological differences. Some of the claims advanced by self-advocates and others associated with the neurodiversity movement draw on brain-based ideas to locate the "essential" features of autistic difference. Francisco Ortega's chapter explores how self-advocates draw on neuroscientific terms and metaphors to describe themselves and their relation to others. Neurodiversity challenges the notion that a neuroscientific basis for self-understanding is necessarily associated with an identity that is alienating or individualizing. Ortega argues that we should understand neurodiversity within the context of the diffusion of neuroscientific claims beyond the laboratory and their penetration in different domains of life. Favoring forms of neurological subjectivity, neuroscientific theories, practices, technologies, and therapies are, Ortega argues, reshaping how we think about ourselves and our relation to others.

Drawing on their qualitative research with individuals on the spectrum, Charlotte Brownlow and Lindsay O'Dell argue in their chapter that positioning people with autism (and equally importantly, those without a diagnosis who consider themselves neurotypical [NT]) as neurobiological citizens challenges the NT dominance of "the majority face-to-face world." Although a recourse to a biological discourse with which to

challenge mainstream disabling concepts of autism has gained some currency, Brownlow and O'Dell see this as a contingent and strategic alliance
between critical disability studies, people with autism, advocates, and a
biologized understanding of autism. In contrast to Ortega, who expresses
some concern about the essentialized categories produced by brain-based
identities, Brownlow and O'Dell suggest that this remains one of many
ways in which critical autism studies can move forward.

Part II. Researching the Politics and Practice of Care

The second part examines more closely how techniques of ordering
autistic experience—even the very notion of the autism "spectrum"—
can have a "looping effect" (see Hacking 2000, 2006) on autistics
themselves. Majia Nadesan's chapter explores the cultural and economic interests and frameworks that drive the increasing prevalence
of the narrative of genetic determinism, even in the context of new and
paradigm-destabilizing genomic findings. As she explains, contemporary public-health models utilizing problematic understandings of risk
seek to predict frequency of disease outbreaks. Autism risks are often
simply (and simplistically) calculated on the basis of population prevalence rates alone. Current prevalence rates sit at 11.3 per 1,000 (Centers
for Disease Control and Prevention 2012). Although prevalence rates
have increased over time, many epidemiologists and academics point to
the role of changing diagnostic criteria in shaping diagnostic outcomes.
This explanation presumes that actual autism rates are relatively stable,
because autism is regarded as a fundamentally gene-based disorder.
New research points to the role of gene mutations and alleles in increasing autism susceptibility, but Nadesan argues that a closer examination
of this research suggests that genetic contributions are usually mediated
by environmental inputs.

Kristin Bumiller focuses on how autism is reshaping the U.S. welfare state, and on the corresponding privatization of responsibilities.
Despite its much-vaunted promise, Bumiller argues that the shift toward a model of community-based care, coupled with neoliberal social
policies, is leading to a form of privatized care for autistic children. This
has brought community integration in name only, where the location of
care has moved from public institutions to the isolation of the household. Under this new system, the state effectively downloads a range of

responsibilities for the care of autistic persons onto the backs of those working inside private homes. The state's narrowed responsibility for children with disabilities resides mainly with the public-school system, which depends upon an adequate individualized education plan for parents of autistic children. Although community-based care for children with disabilities and deinstitutionalization held out the promise of greater autonomy and decision-making power for parents, this devolution of authority has had deleterious effects on families and children affected by autism. This focus on the family deflects much-needed attention away from the failure of many U.S. public institutions—including schools, Social Security, disability and employment services, and housing programs—to cope with the immediate care challenges associated with autism, particularly in adulthood.

Dora Raymaker and Christina Nicolaidis's chapter implores us to rethink conventional ways of classifying the researcher–participant relationship and positions the interactions between autistic persons and scientists or researchers as complex and interconnected. These interactions can have profound effects on how society views, treats, and funds both community projects and academic research. Traditional approaches to science, they argue, typically have a history of failing minority communities, leading to a legacy of mistrust among minority communities vis-à-vis researchers. The failure to include minorities in the research process often creates a feedback loop that further widens the gap between research participants and researchers. Drawing on the tools and practice of community-based participatory research, Raymaker and Nicolaidis explore the potential of a shift to participatory modes of knowledge production, drawing on a case study involving a project with autistic adults that they themselves led.

Part III. Diagnosis and Difference in Autism

The third part challenges common assumptions about the relationship between diagnoses and identity and explores how public policy and activism are both fraught with tensions and subject to jurisdictional considerations. Sara Ryan's chapter explores the accounts of nineteen people diagnosed with autism during adulthood in the United Kingdom. Participants describe problematic childhoods and identify the reasons they sought a diagnosis of autism at that particular stage in their lives. The analysis highlights how, for the majority of participants, not getting a diagnosis would signify a problem to them; they worried that they might *not* have autism. Receiving the diagnosis was, therefore, largely a relief to participants, who were able to reflect on some of their actions and behaviors in light of the diagnosis and make changes to improve their lives and the lives of those around them. The diagnosis provided access to support, allowing two participants, for example, to return to university after unsuccessful experiences in the past. The main consequence of the diagnostic journey for most participants was an acceptance of their own difference and official recognition resulting from what they described as "formal diagnosis." This raises questions about the often-negative connotations and use of the term *diagnosis* and about the processes and structures surrounding the "identification" of people with autism.

Drawing on the tools of public policy and political science, Dana Lee Baker and Lila Walsh's chapter explores how political and public discourses surrounding neurodiversity and neurological difference incorporate assumptions about the relationship between a so-called level of functioning and the relevance of rights-based movements to individuals on the autism spectrum. It is often asserted that neurodiversity perspectives reflect the needs and goals of those considered higher-functioning while shortchanging those experiencing a higher degree of disability. In particular, their chapter examines the degree to which this argument has been employed as a way of effectively managing healthy political conflict through the construction of a loyal opposition rather than as a tool used to divide and conquer proponents of autism-related policy.

Brigitte Chamak and Beatrice Bonniau's chapter shifts the focus to the distinctive characteristics of autism advocacy in France, which reveals a series of sharp and intriguing distinctions from activism in the North American context. In contrast to the dominant model of mobilization in North America, in which groups reject the framing of autism as a disease, the main aims of the key French-speaking autism-advocacy association, Satedi, are to shed light on autistic functioning, to help autistic persons and their families, and to influence the orientation of the research on autism and political decisions. Chamak and Bonniau argue that the French system, which is characterized by opposition to communitarian ideas as well as by a partnership between the state and

parents' associations, has been successful in muting the development
of radical demands from autism advocates. Their chapter forces us to
confront how the politicization of demands made by autistic persons
does not operate in a political vacuum, and points to the need to adapt
our understanding of mobilization strategies to the particular political-
institutional context. The French case challenges any generalizable trends
we might glean from autism advocacy, especially the dominance of the
Western conception of social-movement interaction with the state in
the area of disability more broadly (see Chamak 2008).

Part IV. Cultural Productions and Representations of Autism

The increasing availability of narratives by autistic people provides us
with an opportunity to see the world from an autistic perspective, or
at least to "travel in parallel" with autistic persons (see Davidson and
Henderson 2010; Singer 2003) as they reveal something of what the world
looks and feels like for them (Grandin 1986, 1995, 2005; Mukhopadhyay
2000; Williams 1992, 1994). Of course, we must avoid sweeping generalizations about autistic persons on the basis of the experiences of any
one individual; Ian Hacking suggests instead that we view each person as
"helping to create a language about what was hitherto unknown" (2009a,
1467). He is quick, however, to distance himself from mainstream depictions of autism as a puzzle or mystery to be solved, as the U.S. autism-
advocacy group Autism Speaks is wont to do (the organization's logo represents a piece from a jigsaw puzzle). Autobiographical narratives do not
reflect or represent what life on the spectrum is like for everyone, nor can
they be judged "according to some pre-existing criteria for describing experiences and sensibilities." Rather, Hacking continues, they "constitute"
what it means to be autistic for those who are on the spectrum and also
for those who are not (1467).

As Mark Osteen explains in his chapter, autism presents peculiar
challenges to narrative representation. Many autistic persons have difficulties with the associative processes essential for narrative thought.
In addition, because autistic persons crave routine, life with autism
often seems relentlessly repetitive; yet at other times autism manifests
itself as constant chaos or disruption, recalling one of the three narrative types identified earlier by Arthur Frank. Each of these experiences
resists being narrated: How does one tell a story in which events don't

change? How does an author do representational justice to chaos without irrevocably changing its nature? Is it even possible to render chaotic experience and nonlinear consciousness through linear narrative? These factors partly explain the prevalence of "cure" stories in autism literature, whereby authors evade autism's narrative challenges by crafting tales in which autism itself is eliminated. Osteen analyzes the methods that authors—both autistic and neurotypical, in both fiction and nonfiction—employ to cope with autism's narrative challenges, including harnessing genre conventions (mystery, the bildungsroman), using tropes of repetition (echoes, mirrors, interior monologue), and inserting nonnarrative elements (graphs, comic panels, drawings). Although Osteen suggests that cinema has largely failed to depict autism successfully, it nonetheless possesses the greatest potential for representing autism authentically through its capacity to blend narrative and nonnarrative elements.

Next, our own coauthored contribution asks whether firsthand accounts of online activities and experiences suggest that they expand or contract the social and emotional horizons of autistic lifeworlds. Although the potential importance of the Internet for autistic persons has been acknowledged in previous research, little empirical research exists on the uses and meanings of the Internet by people on the spectrum. We highlight the dangers of narratives that generalize inappropriately across radically different embodied and emotional experiences, a theme raised by other critical autism scholars who challenge universalizing accounts of what it means to be on the spectrum (for example, Ortega, this volume). In tackling such questions, the chapter is particularly concerned to explore what Internet use means for the geographies of some autistic persons' lives, asking how it affects, for example, their daily mobility; their sense of social, spatial, and emotional connection; and what this in turn means for their sense and "story" of self.

Drawing on her experience with her son Charlie, Kristina Chew's chapter explores the challenges of communicating with and for "nonverbal" or "minimally verbal" autistic persons. Normally, she explains, these communications are perceived as so difficult to decode that they verge on the untranslatable and unknowable. This (mis)perception invites nonautistics to displace autistic voices with their own. But, she asks, what if we presume that there is always something meaningful being communicated? Opening with a brief examination of current conventional approaches to speaking for and about autism and autistic persons, Chew turns to examining her own representational practice with Charlie, drawing on Walter Benjamin's understanding of translation as a framework for recentering people with autism as makers of meaning. In order to "help" autistic persons, Chew argues, "we need to know both what autism is and what autism means; otherwise, our definitions risk being accurate but insignificant and risk erasing the autistic others for whom we ostensibly speak."

Finally, Dawn Eddings Prince's chapter provides a distinctive and compelling perspective on her journey from being an undiagnosed autistic child caught in a web of sensory sensitivities, to her unfolding life as a student, a dropout, a primatologist, a professor, and eventually also a writer of her own and others' experience of autism. Throughout her chapter, Prince draws on her own intimate experience and nature-infused language to bridge communication gaps between those on and off the spectrum and between those inside and outside the academy. It becomes clear that Prince occupies an unusual and often uncomfortable position in relation to the academic world, and despite her declared passion for her discipline of anthropology, she demonstrates very powerfully her sense that academic language—including and perhaps especially that which "represents" the lives of autistic persons—can cut when it should strive to connect; academic language is, she explains, an intensely "violent activity" in which the realities of autistic lives are often "lost in translation." Our final contributions, from both Chew and Prince, thus sound a cautionary note about the potential dangers associated with the project of critical autism studies, and serve as a powerful reminder of the profound responsibilities that researching and writing about the lives of others entail.

Conclusion

In this introduction, we have sought to chart a rich, complex terrain for the critical study of autism. Although we eschewed any rigid demarcation of the boundaries of critical autism studies, we did outline and elaborate some of the main preoccupations of the scholars whose work is featured in this volume, including the role of power relations in shaping the experience of autism; the advancement of new, more enabling narratives of autism that challenge the predominant (deficit-focused and degrading) constructions that currently influence public opinion, policy, and popular culture; and, finally, the creation of new analytical frameworks that highlight the contributions of social science and humanities research to understanding autism as a complex relational (dis)order. The purpose of such a critical and informed study of autism is not merely to attack "science" or to use autism as an opportunity to vault one academic discipline or approach to the summit of critical autism studies. This collection derives much of its strength from contributions from and—perhaps especially—collaborations between a broad range of disciplinary perspectives, including anthropology, English literature, sociology, systems science, geography, gender studies, philosophy, political studies, and medicine. It also benefits immeasurably from the involvement of contributors with more intimate experience (as caregivers and autistics) of life on the spectrum.

As we explained, what we know about autism is deeply embedded in a series of historical, social, cultural, and discursive contexts. Moreover, we echo Stuart Murray's important reminder that although we indeed know much about autism, "if we we're honest, the foundational observation we might make, the 'central fact' about autism with which we should probably start, is that we don't know very much about it at all" (2012, 3). It might seem somewhat strange to conclude with such a robust disclaimer an introduction to a collection that claims to advance new frameworks for thinking about the study of autism. Our undeniable ignorance should not, however, be cause for collective dismay. Rather, we view it as motivation to ask tough questions about what we do and do not (but might come to) know, using an innovative combination of methodological and theoretical tools, approaches, and frameworks, some of which might be situated outside of our respective fields of competence and comfort.

Moreover, what we *do* know about autism needs to be informed by a deep appreciation for what individuals living on the spectrum have to say about what it means to be autistic, all the while being mindful that our attempts to speak about the rich diversity of "autistic presence" should not be misconstrued as a form of charity bestowed upon those who do not or cannot communicate in typical ways. Autistic persons obviously do communicate without the aid of nonautistic persons, even if these forms of communication are not always recognized, accepted, or supported in academic or policy settings (much as they are neglected in many typical everyday and social settings, too). Nonautistics and researchers purporting to reflect or even represent autistic experience need to bring all possible humility to the task of speaking for and about autistic persons. In her important account of social science perspectives on autism, Silverman reminds researchers that autistic persons have been "vulnerable to enrolment in the theoretical programs of ambitious researchers, without even being consulted" (2008b, 337). We hope this book enacts some movement beyond this unacceptable (and not entirely) past position and toward a more ethically informed present, as we collaboratively chart and elaborate the many dynamic and significant forms of autistic presence. Autistic presence "is here and always will be so. Such presence is the final yardstick by which all the various attempts to understand or interpret it, whether made through science or metaphor, are to be measured" (Murray 2012, 105). We hope that *Worlds of Autism* can contribute to understandings of the many varieties of autistic presence, and that it resonates with many of those who intervene in and partially shape the worlds of autism, including scholars, community advocates and activists, parents and caregivers, and, ultimately and most significantly, autistic persons themselves.

REFERENCES

American Psychiatric Association. 2011. "Autism Spectrum Disorder." *DSM-5 Development*, revised January 26. Accessed October 31, 2012, http://www.dsm5 .org/ProposedRevisions/Pages/proposedrevision.aspx?rid=94#.

Amundson, R. 2000. "Against Normal Function." *Studies in History and Philosophy of Biological and Biomedical Sciences* 31 (1): 33–53.

Armstrong, T. 2010. *Neurodiversity: Discovering the Extraordinary Gifts of Autism, ADHD, Dyslexia, and Other Brain Differences.* Cambridge, Mass.: Da Capo Press.

Arneil, B. 2009. "Disability, Self-Image, and Modern Political Theory." *Political Theory* 37 (2): 218–42.

Autistic Self Advocacy Network. 2007. "An Urgent Call to Action: Tell NYU Child Study Center to Abandon Stereotypes against People with Disabilities," December 8. Accessed May 6, 2013, http://autisticadvocacy.org/2007/12/ tell-nyu-child-study-center-to-abandon-stereotypes/.

Baggs, A. 2007. *In My Language.* Accessed February 7, 2012, http://www.youtube .com/watch?v=JnylM1hI2jc.

Baker, D. L. 2011. *The Politics of Neurodiversity: Why Public Policy Matters.* Boulder, Co.: Lynne Rienner.

Barnbaum, D. 2008. *The Ethics of Autism: Among Them, but Not of Them.* Bloomington: Indiana University Press.

Baron-Cohen, S. 2003. *The Essential Difference: Male and Female Brains and the Truth about Autism.* New York: Basic Books.

Berg, M., and A. Mol, eds. 1998. *Differences in Medicine: Unravelling Practices, Techniques, and Bodies*. Durham, N.C.: Duke University Press.

Bettelheim, B. 1967. *The Empty Fortress: Infantile Autism and the Birth of the Self*. New York: Free Press.

Brown, P., et al. 2004. "Embodied Health Movements: New Approaches to Social Movements in Health." *Sociology of Health and Illness* 26 (1): 50–80.

Bumiller, K. 2008. "Quirky Citizens: Autism, Gender, and Reimagining Disability." *Signs: Journal of Women in Culture and Society* 33 (4): 967–91.

———. 2009. "The Geneticization of Autism: From New Reproductive Technologies to the Conception of Genetic Normalcy." *Signs: Journal of Women in Culture and Society* 34 (4): 875–98.

Centers for Disease Control and Prevention. 2012. "Prevalence of Autism Spectrum Disorders—Autism and Developmental Disabilities Monitoring Network, 14 sites, United States, 2008." *Morbidity and Mortality Weekly Report* 61 (31): 1–19.

Chamak, B. 2008. "Autism and Social Movements: French Parents' Associations and International Autistic Individuals' Organizations." *Sociology of Health and Illness* 30 (1): 76–96.

Choudhury, S., and J. Slaby, eds. 2011. *Critical Neuroscience: A Handbook of the Social and Cultural Contexts of Neuroscience*. London: Wiley-Blackwell.

Cowen, T. 2009a. "Autism as Academic Paradigm." *Chronicle of Higher Education*, July 13.

———. 2009b. *Create Your Own Economy: The Path to Prosperity in a Disordered World*. New York: Dutton.

Davidson, J. 2010. "It Cuts Both Ways: A Relational Approach to Access and Accommodation for Autism." *Social Science and Medicine* 70 (2): 305–12.

Davidson, J., and V. L. Henderson. 2010. "'Travel in Parallel with Us for a While': Sensory Geographies of Autism." *Canadian Geographer* 54 (4): 462–75.

Davidson, J., and M. Orsini. 2010. "The Place of Emotions in Critical Autism Studies." *Emotion, Space, and Society* 3 (2): 131–33.

Davis, L. J. 2002. *Bending Over Backwards: Disability, Dismodernism, and Other Difficult Positions*. New York: New York University Press.

Davis, L. J., and D. Morris. 2007. "Biocultures Manifesto." *New Literary History* 38 (3): 411–18.

Dawson, M. 2012. "Autistic in the UK," April 12. Autism Crisis: Science and Ethics in the Era of Autism Politics. Accessed July 12, 2013, http://autismcrisis .blogspot.com/.

Epstein, S. 1996. *Impure Science: AIDS, Activism, and the Politics of Knowledge*. Berkeley: University of California Press.

Eyal, G., et al. 2010. *The Autism Matrix: The Social Origins of the Autism Epidemic*. Cambridge: Polity.

Frank, A. W. 1995. *The Wounded Storyteller: Body, Illness, and Ethics*. Chicago: University of Chicago Press.

Ghaziuddin, M. 2010. "Brief Report: Should the DSM V Drop Asperger Syndrome?" *Journal of Autism and Developmental Disorders* 40 (9): 1146–48.

Gould, D. 2009. *Moving Politics: Emotion and ACT UP's Fight against AIDS*. Chicago: University of Chicago Press.

Grandin, T. 1986. *Emergence: Labeled Autistic.* Novato, Calif.: Arena Press.

———. 1995. *Thinking in Pictures: And Other Reports from My Life with Autism.* New York: Doubleday.

———. 2005. *Emergence: Labeled Autistic; A True Story, with a Supplement.* New York: Grand Central.

Grinker, R. R. 2007. *Unstrange Minds: Remapping the World of Autism.* New York: Basic Books.

———. 2010. "Disorder out of Chaos." *New York Times,* February 10.

Hacking, I. 2000. *The Social Construction of What?* Cambridge, Mass.: Harvard University Press.

———. 2006. "Making Up People." *London Review of Books* 28 (16): 23–26.

———. 2009a. "Autistic Autobiography." *Philosophical Transactions of the Royal Society* (B) 364: 1467–73.

———. 2009b. "Humans, Aliens, and Autism." *Daedalus* 138 (3): 44–59.

Kittay, E. F., and L. Carlson, eds. 2010. *Cognitive Disability and Its Challenge to Moral Philosophy.* London: Wiley-Blackwell.

Kras, J. F. 2010. "The 'Ransom Notes' Affair: When the Neurodiversity Movement Came of Age." *Disability Studies Quarterly* 30 (1). Accessed May 6, 2013, http://www.dsq-sds.org/article/view/1065/1254.

Mukhopadhyay, T. R. 2000. *How Can I Talk If My Lips Don't Move? Inside My Autistic Mind.* New York: Arcade.

Murray, S. 2012. *Autism.* New York: Routledge.

Nadesan, M. H. 2005. *Constructing Autism: Unravelling the "Truth" and Understanding the Social.* New York: Routledge.

Nash, J. M. 2002. "The Secrets of Autism: The Number of Children Diagnosed with Autism and Asperger's in the US Is Exploding. Why?" *Time,* May 2, 47–56. Accessed February 7, 2012, http://www.time.com/time/magazine/article/0,9171,1002364,00.html.

Ne'eman, A. 2007. "An Open Letter on the NYU Ransom Notes Campaign." PetitionOnline.com. Accessed October 29, 2012, http://www.petitiononline.com/ransom/petition.html.

Neurodiversity.com. 2013. Accessed May 6, http://www.neurodiversity.com.

Novas, C. 2006. "The Political Economy of Hope: Patients' Organizations, Science, and Biovalue." *BioSocieties* 1 (3): 289–305.

Orsini, M. 2009. "Contesting the Autistic Subject: Biological Citizenship and the Autism/Autistic Movement." In *Critical Interventions in the Ethics of Health Care,* edited by S. Murray and D. Holmes. London: Ashgate.

Orsini, M., and M. Smith. 2010. "Social Movements, Knowledge, and Public Policy: The Case of Autism Activism in Canada and the U.S." *Critical Policy Studies* 4 (1): 38–57.

Ortega, F. 2009. "The Cerebral Subject and the Challenge of Neurodiversity." *BioSocieties* 4 (4): 425–45.

Osteen, M., ed. 2008. *Autism and Representation.* New York: Routledge.

Pothier, D., and R. Devlin. 2006. "Toward a Critical Theory of Dis-citizenship." Introduction to *Critical Disability Theory: Essays in Philosophy, Politics, Policy, and Law,* edited by D. Pothier and R. Devlin, 1–24. Vancouver: University of British Columbia Press.

Prince-Hughes, D. 2002. *Aquamarine Blue 5: Personal Stories of College Students with Autism.* Athens, Ohio: Swallow Press.

Rice, C. E., et al. 2007. "A Public Health Collaboration for the Surveillance of Autism Spectrum Disorders." *Paediatric and Perinatal Epidemiology* 21 (2): 179–90.

Rose, N. 2007. *The Politics of Life Itself: Biomedicine, Power, and Subjectivity in the Twenty-First Century.* Princeton, N.J.: Princeton University Press.

Rose, N., and C. Novas. 2005. "Biological Citizenship." In *Global Assemblages: Technology, Politics, and Ethics as Anthropological Problems,* edited by A. Ong and S. J. Collier, 439–63. London: Blackwell.

Schopler, E. 2001. *The Research Basis for Autism Intervention.* New York: Kluwer.

Shakespeare, T. 2006a. *Disability Rights and Wrongs.* New York: Routledge.

———. 2006b. "The Social Model of Disability." In *The Disability Studies Reader,* edited by L. J. Davis, 2nd ed., 197–204. New York: Routledge.

Shore, S. 2001. *Beyond the Wall: Personal Experiences with Autism and Asperger Syndrome.* 2nd ed. Shawnee Mission, Kans.: Autism Asperger Publishing.

Silverman, C. 2008a. "Brains, Pedigrees, and Promises: Lessons from the Politics of Autism Genetics." In *Biosocialities, Genetics, and the Social Sciences: Making Biologies and Identities,* edited by S. Gibbon and C. Novas, 38–54. New York: Routledge.

———. 2008b. "Fieldwork on Another Planet: Social Science Perspectives on the Autism Spectrum." *BioSocieties* 3 (3): 325–41.

———. 2011. *Understanding Autism: Parents, Doctors, and the History of a Disorder.* Princeton, N.J.: Princeton University Press.

Singer, J. 2003. "Travels in a Parallel Space: An Invitation." Foreword to *Women from Another Planet? Our Lives in the Universe of Autism,* edited by J. Kearns Miller, xi–xiii. Bloomington, Ind.: Dancing Minds.

Solomon, O., and N. Bagatell. 2010. "Autism: Rethinking the Possibilities." *Ethos* 38 (1): 1–7.

Standing Senate Committee on Social Affairs, Science, and Technology. 2003. *First Meeting on Mental Health and Mental Illness, Proceedings,* February 26.

Tidmarsh, L., and F. R. Volkmar. 2003. "Diagnosis and Epidemiology of Autism Spectrum Disorders." *Canadian Journal of Psychiatry* 48 (8): 517–25.

Treichler, P. 1999. *How to Have Theory in an Epidemic.* Durham, N.C.: Duke University Press.

Wikler, D. 2010. "Cognitive Disability, Paternalism, and the Global Burden of Disease." In Kittay and Carlson 2010, 183–200.

Williams, D. 1992. *Nobody Nowhere: The Extraordinary Autobiography of an Autistic.* New York: Times Books.

———. 1994. *Somebody Somewhere: Breaking Free from the World of Autism.* New York: Times Books.

Wolff, J. 2010. "Cognitive Disability in a Society of Equals." In Kittay and Carlson 2010, 147–60.

Zimmerman, A., ed. 2008. *Autism: Current Theories and Evidence.* Totowa, N.J.: Human Press / Springer Science.

PART I. Approaching Autism

Autism in an Age of Empathy

A Cautionary Critique

Patrick McDonagh

"**E**mpathy is among the most important of human characteristics," writes Simon Baron-Cohen. "It enables not just social relationships and communication, but is a major basis for our moral code and for the inhibition of aggression. And whilst empathy may have some simpler equivalents in non-human species, its remarkable flowering in the human case is unique" (2006, 536). Baron-Cohen is not alone in his belief in empathy's fundamental importance to human identity. "Empathy," says philosopher Lou Agosta, "puts the human in human being," whereas "the loss of empathy is equivalent to the loss of the individual's being human" (2010, xiii–xiv). Recent years have seen a boom of empathy-related publications and projects, including Jeremy Rifkin's best-selling *The Empathic Civilization* (2009) and a torrent of books on emotional and social intelligence by writers following the trail blazed by Daniel Goleman (1995, 2006), all stressing the importance of empathy for both the social and professional success of individuals and, increasingly, the economic success of societies. Empathy's status has never been higher.

If we are to believe that the capacity for empathy is humanity's great gift, the lack of empathy must also be a source of concern. A recent and highly publicized study from the University of Michigan found that today's college students are 40 percent less empathetic than those of thirty years ago and are more materialistic and narcissistic (Bielski 2010). Rifkin, working in a similar vein, posits the existence of contemporary "unadulterated narcissists," also nurtured by overindulgent parents and the Internet, and, borrowing a term from sixteenth-century theologians, tags them "monsters" (2009, 585). How, he asks, can they hope to achieve full human consciousness without this element most integral to common humanity?

This question is especially compelling for autistic people, as well as for our understanding of autism. "Autism is an empathy disorder," writes Baron-Cohen (2003, 137), and although this position remains controversial, there is no doubt that the condition is increasingly represented as an inability to empathize, just as empathy itself is growing its cultural capital. But if autism is a disorder of empathy, as Baron-Cohen and others suggest, and if empathy is fundamental to human identity, how are we to conceptualize the idea of autism? Where, in this schema, would an abstracted "autistic population" fit? Such a formulation positions "autistic people," broadly understood, as a contrast group, something less than fully human, who occupy a space outside the empathic society where their presence assures the majority of their capacity for empathy (just as, at the start of the twentieth century, the presence of people segregated in institutions for the "feeble-minded" assured those outside these institutions of their own status as rational and intelligent beings).

Given the apparent importance of empathy, we need a clear definition of the concept. But this, too, presents some challenges. Just what is empathy, and how do we know when we have it—or the capacity to use it? Baron-Cohen and Sally Wheelwright write that, even though empathy is probably "as old as Homo sapiens itself" and "despite [its] obvious importance . . . , it is a difficult concept to define" (2004, 163), and they are not alone in puzzling over this problem. Lou Agosta laments our "radical Socratic ignorance" of a "neglected and under-theorized" empathy, but notes that we are witnessing "the start of a proliferation of psychological, neurological and philosophical research on empathy"; however, he concedes, "the inconvenient truth remains: We do not know what empathy is" (2010, xiii). If empathy is as old as humanity, we might well wonder where it has been hiding for so many years and why it remains so difficult to define.

These questions should also prompt us to ask why the relatively recent concept of empathy is now being positioned as central to human identity. What follows is a preliminary critique of the autism/empathy dichotomy. I propose that empathy, such as it is, takes form and is understood within specific cultures, with its meaning shifting across time and geography. I support this idea by tracking the parallel rise of the concepts of empathy and autism up to their recent locations as the two poles of an opposition and by exploring their historical precedents. My goal is to flesh out the connection between autism and empathy and to suggest how the conceptualization of these two categories may affect those people identified as autistic. But first let us start by attending to the relationship between autism and empathy as hypothesized by Simon Baron-Cohen and others.

The Autism-and-Empathy Connection

The paths of autism and empathy have intersected only recently. A lack of empathy does not appear among the first observations in early descriptions of autism by Leo Kanner (1943), who instead focuses on problems of affective contact—arguably a related concern, but undeniably distinct; nor does Hans Asperger ([1944] 1991) concern himself with questions of empathy. Uta Frith's *Autism* (1989) refers to empathy in passing, noting that "the most general description of social impairment in Autism is lack of empathy" (154), and, in an early "theory of mind" reference, saying that "if autistic people cannot conceptualize mental states very well, then they cannot empathize with mental states of others, such as their feelings" (167). This is a hint of things to come, but she offers no more on the topic. Lorna Wing's seminal 1981 article notes that people with Asperger Syndrome share certain characteristics with people with schizoid personalities, notably "lack of empathy, single-mindedness, odd communication, social isolation and oversensitivity" (121), but a failure to empathize is hardly the condition's defining feature.

In a 1991 lecture, though, Christopher Gilberg refers to autism as a "disorder of empathy," arguing that the theory-of-mind deficits that were being associated with autistic children in studies by Simon Baron-Cohen inevitably imply a problem with empathy, as well (Gilberg 1992). Indeed, Baron-Cohen is the most prominent researcher to make the apparent lack of empathy in autism into the condition's defining characteristic, and his theories seem to be driving not only research into this area but also the connection of the two in popular culture. In some of his earlier writings, Baron-Cohen seems hesitant to discuss empathy, noting in *Mindblindness* (1995) that this reluctance "in part reflects [his] own view that we are still a long way from having a good theory of emotion" (136). However, he overcomes these qualms in developing the "extreme male brain" theory of autism presented in *The Essential Difference: Male and Female Brains and the Truth about Autism* (2003), where empathy plays a prominent role as an "essential difference" between what he identifies as "systematizing" male and "empathizing" female brains. This built on the gendered distinction that he had proposed earlier in "The Extreme Male Brain Theory of Autism" (2002), in which he attempted to explain the apparent higher ratio of males to females with autism. In this influential model of autism, often cited by autism professionals and popular media alike, an empathy deficit becomes the defining characteristic of autism.

Empathizing, as presented by Baron-Cohen, is "the drive to identify another person's emotions and thoughts, and to respond to them with an appropriate emotion. Empathy does not just entail the cold calculation of what someone else thinks and feels (or what is sometimes called mind reading). . . . Empathizing occurs when we feel an appropriate emotional reaction, an emotion triggered by the other person's emotion, and it is done in order to understand another person, to predict their behavior, and to connect or resonate with them emotionally" (2003, 2). One thing to stress here is what empathy isn't: it is not a calculation (cold or otherwise). Empathizing, Baron-Cohen asserts, "is about *naturally and spontaneously* tuning into the other person's thoughts and feelings, whatever these might be" (21; emphasis added). Further, he notes, "you do it [i.e., empathize] because you can't help doing it, because you care about the other person's thoughts and feelings, because it matters." He concedes that people "less skilled at empathizing" may do it "only when reminded, or if they discover that they are included more often when they do or say the right thing, and they may even rehearse how to empathize in order to get the benefits." This sort of faux empathy is enacted to smooth experiences in the social world, but it is not, he stresses, "natural" or spontaneous empathy. Of such individuals, he notes, "other people's feelings matter less to them, and it takes an effort to maintain empathic appearances." By contrast, "It's easy for the natural empathizer. It requires no effort at all. They can keep going for hours" (24). Notably, unnatural empathizers are not truly empathizing at all, no matter how much effort they may put into it; they are only maintaining an appearance, creating the illusion of empathy.

The distinction between imitation and the real thing is that empathy "ensures that you see a person as a person, with feelings, rather than a thing to be used to satisfy your own needs and desires" (24). Further, this has profound social consequences: "People build moral codes from natural empathy, fellow feeling and compassion. It would be marvelous if systematizing, the pure process of logic, could give us a sense of justice and injustice, but, as history has shown us, logic and legal systems can be used to defend autocratic, even genocidal regimes—Nazism is one of the clearest recent examples of this" (25). So when Baron-Cohen posits empathy as a natural and spontaneous characteristic of what he calls the "female" empathic brain, as opposed to a "male" systematizing brain, there are values assigned to the different categories, along with a profound reliance on gender stereotypes (Karafyllis 2008). According to this model, autistic people are neurologically incapable of "putting themselves in someone else's shoes, imagining the world through someone else's eyes and responding appropriately to someone else's feelings" (Baron-Cohen 2003, 137).

The sum of Baron-Cohen's theories is that human brains fall between a "female" empathizing type and a "male" systemizing one, in what he has designated the empathizing-systematizing (E-S) theory of the brain. Individual brains can be placed along this spectrum through "empathy quotient" tests. If one lies too far to the "systematizing" end of the scale, one has an "extreme male brain," likely caused by an excess of testosterone in the mother during pregnancy. This extreme male brain, he argues, is the cause of autism and explains why males are much more prevalent along the autistic spectrum than females (2009). The "theory of mind" module and "extreme male brain" frameworks have been greeted with much skepticism (Blackburn, Gottschewski, and Niki 2000; Gallagher 2004a, 2004b; Karafyllis 2008; Leudar and Costall 2009). At the same time, though, other researchers have developed Baron-Cohen's gendered brain theories. Christopher Badcock and Bernard Crespi, building on the notion of the "selfish gene," have argued that the male-/female-brain phenomenon is the consequence of the paternal or maternal expression or suppression of genes—that is, the "imprinting" of these genes—rather than an excess of testosterone (2006, 2008b). They propose that "some cases of autism may be the result of the paternally biased expression of genes involved with brain development." Instead of placing autism in polar relation to empathy, they argue that "autism can be considered as the diametric opposite of paranoia and the full spectrum of related psychotic and mood disorders, which include schizophrenia, bipolar disorder and major depression" (2008a, 1054).

But although researchers like Badcock and Crespi have proposed alternative, sex-based theories of autism, Baron-Cohen's arguments are the ones that have acquired an influence well beyond academia, with his books being published as mass-market paperbacks and Baron-Cohen himself appearing regularly on the BBC and other media outlets to discuss autism-related issues. His most recent work at publication, *The Science of Evil* (2011), posits an empathy deficit as fundamental to certain forms of evil. However, he differentiates those who sit at one extreme of the empathy spectrum with "zero degrees of empathy" (15): there are "zero-negative" empathy deficits, found in psychopaths, narcissists, and those with borderline personality disorders; and "zero-positive" deficits, characteristic of autistics and those with Asperger Syndrome, who, although they may have "abnormalities in the empathy circuit in their brain" (122), do not usually act cruelly toward others.

Of course, not everyone agrees that people with autism suffer from an "empathy deficit"; many autistic people assert that they do experience empathy. It could be, as some have suggested, that autistic people work to understand others through different processes—they may not empathize according to a specific notion of the idea structured to exclude them, but they can still find ways of comprehending others in a manner that suggests a capacity for empathy (Jurecic 2006; Rogers et al. 2007). The autistic writer Donna Williams has described experiencing an "intense, uncontrollable empathy" for others (1998, 59). Temple Grandin, in *Animals in Translation* (2005), and Dawn Prince-Hughes, in *Songs of the Gorilla Nation* (2004), argue that autistic experience enables a particular kind of engagement—one might call it empathic—with members of other species, and significant relationships with animals recur in many other autistic autobiographical narratives; these interactions may express empathic concerns while avoiding the intense social complications of human relations (Davidson and Smith 2009). Grandin also recounts the role of tactile sensations in helping her develop an empathic awareness of others and explains that "for me to have empathy I have to visually put myself in the other person's place" (2006, 99). She summarizes her approach to developing empathy by noting that she "empathize[s] through [her] senses rather than in a more emotional abstract manner" (2008, 136). We should ask whether this "empathizing through one's senses" might count as a form of empathy even though it is not the process defined by Baron-Cohen. The contemporary psychologist Adam Smith, drawing on a number of autism narratives, posits a distinction between cognitive and emotional empathy and proposes that most autistic people are quite capable of emotional empathy but have a difficult time developing a cognitive empathy rooted in theory-of-mind deficiency; he concludes hesitantly that although "the study of autism is probably the study of an empathy disorder," Baron-Cohen's "definition of empathizing seems tailored to the extreme-male-brain theory of autism" (Smith 2008, 289). To further explore the connection—or disconnection, as the case may be—between autism and empathy, we should delve into the history of these notions.

The Shaping of Empathy and Autism

The terms *empathy* and *autism* both made their debut in psychological theory in German writings at the start of the twentieth century. In 1873, the German philosopher and art historian Robert Vischer, under the influence of German romanticism, borrowed the term *Einfühlung*, which had been circulating in literary criticism, to designate the psychological "emotional projection" of the self onto an object of beauty or aesthetic contemplation. The notion was eventually taken up by psychologists, most notably Theodor Lipps, who in 1903 developed *Einfühlung* to identify the psychological process at play when a viewer contemplates and fuses with an art object: "*Einfühlung* is the fact described here that the object is ego and thereby the ego object. It is the fact that the contrast between myself and the object disappears" (translated and quoted in Jahoda 2005, 155). In 1905, Lipps extended the concept beyond a process concerned with how we engage with works of art to explain how we know other people, as well (Jahoda 2005; Wispé 1987).

Einfühlung was translated into English as "empathy" by the American psychologist Edward Titchener in his 1909 work *Experimental Psychology of the Thought Processes*, in which he wrote of the way an onlooker's "mind's muscle" reacted internally to the qualities of an object being observed: "Not only do I see gravity and modesty and pride and courtesy and stateliness, but I feel or act them in the mind's muscle. That is, I suppose, a simple case of empathy, if we may coin that term as a rendering of *Einfühlung*." He took the new term from the Greek *empatheia*—literally, "in" *(em)* + "suffering or passion" *(pathos)*. In 1915, Titchener elaborated further on empathy: "We are told of a shocking accident, and we gasp and shrink and feel nauseated as we imagine it; we are told of some new delightful fruit, and our mouth waters as if we were about to taste it. This tendency to feel oneself into a situation is called EMPATHY;—on the analogy with sympathy, which is feeling together with another" (quoted in Wispé 1987, 22).

Thus *empathy* entered the English language, to be used in psychology as well as in aesthetic and literary criticism (following *Einfühlung*'s original application). Despite its relatively common use, though, its precise definition has remained unstable, its meaning varying as theorists and practitioners apply the term according to their own notions (Jahoda 2005). All the same, the idea of empathy has gained status in the popular consciousness over the past two decades, often being linked with the social and emotional skills whose importance is proclaimed in such books as Daniel Goleman's best-selling *Emotional Intelligence* (1995) and *Social Intelligence* (2006).

Autism follows a comparable trajectory, appearing in German-language writings before eventually moving into English (and other languages). The term made its debut in a 1908 speech by the Swiss psychiatrist Eugen Bleuler (Murray 2008), who later used the term in print in his 1911 work *Dementia Praecox*, writing that "autistic schizophrenics" are "the most severe schizophrenics . . . [who] live in a world of their own" (1950, 63). Bleuler's neologism enjoyed a limited circulation but did not take firm root (Nadesan 2005). Not until Leo Kanner's "Autistic Disturbances of Affective Contact" (1943) and Hans Asperger's "Die 'Autistichen Psychopathen' im Kindesalter" (published in Austria in 1944 and translated in 1991 by Uta Frith as "'Autistic Psychopathy' in Childhood") did the term appear in its more currently recognizable forms: these works described children with very similar conditions, each using Bleuler's coinage. From these first clinical observations and into the 1960s and 1970s, autism remained a rare condition, with the Kannerian version appearing in somewhere between 4.5 and 10 in 10,000 people (Frith 1989, 52). The changes in prevalence rates paralleled a series of seminal works in the 1980s and 1990s: Lorna Wing's 1981 article "Asperger's Syndrome: A Clinical Account," in which she introduced Asperger's ideas to an English-speaking professional audience and hinted at an autistic spectrum that encompassed many more people than did classic Kannerian autism; Frith's 1991 translation of Asperger's article into English; and the subsequent positioning of Asperger Syndrome at the "high-functioning" end of the new autistic spectrum in the *DSM-IV*, in 1994. (However, the *DSM-V*—still unreleased at the time of writing—has, among its proposed changes, the deletion of Asperger Syndrome as a form of autism, to be replaced by a diagnosis of "mild autism spectrum disorder." It remains to be seen what impact the *DSM-V*'s new categorizations of mild, moderate, and severe "autism spectrum disorder" may have on the number of diagnoses.) So, from 10 or fewer cases in 10,000 people back in the 1960s, numbers have jumped almost tenfold; according to an Autism Society press release, American rates are as high as 1 in 110, or almost 1 percent of the population (2011), with Autism Society Canada citing prevalence rates in children as being 1 in 165 (2011). These numbers remain uncertain and contested, yet the momentum behind them is clear. Diagnoses of autism have been on the rise, and, as with empathy, the concept's higher profile and increasing significance in cultural discourses are clear to all.

Before questioning what makes the ideas of empathy and autism so compelling at this moment in history, though, we should look even further back at precursor notions for these concepts. What did we have before we had empathy?

The Prehistory of Empathy

In English, the term most closely associated with *empathy* is *sympathy*, which entered the language in the 1560s and was quickly adopted, enjoying status as a "quasi-technical term" from the seventeenth to the early twentieth centuries, when, as Gustav Jahoda writes, empathy "gradually conquered much of the ground previously occupied by sympathy, especially, but not only, in the psychological literature" (2005, 151). To understand empathy and how it functions in the structuring of ideas used to organize society, it might be useful to consider its precursor, sympathy, especially as formulated by two of its most prominent early theorists, David Hume and Adam Smith.

David Hume writes in his *Treatise of Human Nature*, composed in 1739–40, "No human quality is more remarkable, both in itself and in its consequences, than that propensity we have to sympathize with others, and to receive by communication their inclinations and sentiments, however different from or even contrary to our own" (1978, 316). In a passage interesting for its economic subtext, Hume writes:

Upon the whole, there remains nothing, which can give us an esteem for power and riches, and a contempt for meanness and poverty, except the principle of *sympathy*, by which we enter into the sentiments of the rich and poor, and partake of their pleasure and meanness. Riches give satisfaction to their possessor; and this satisfaction is conveyed to the beholder by the imagination, which produces an idea resembling the original impression in force and vivacity. This agreeable idea or impression is connected with love, which is an agreeable passion. (362)

Wealth is a test case for Hume's notion of the sympathetic process; we can sympathize with both wealthy and poor, but we admire, esteem, or even love the condition of wealth, whereas we must feel contempt for poverty and pity for those who find themselves in it. Both of these responses, Hume argues, stem from the workings of sympathy. He elaborates further:

In general we may remark, that the minds of men are mirrors to one another, not only because they reflect each others' emotions, but also because those rays or passions, sentiments and opinions may often be reverberated, and may decay away by insensible degrees. Thus the pleasure, which a rich man receives from his possessions, being thrown upon the beholder, causes a pleasure and esteem; which sentiments again, being perceiv'd and sympathiz'd with, encrease the pleasure of the possessor; and being once more reflected, become a new foundation for pleasure and esteem in the beholder. (365)

Hume's sympathy involves an interaction between the observed and the beholder, in which (in this example) both experience the pleasure of the wealth of the one being observed. It is an economy of sentiments, an exchange that benefits both participants.

Smith's formulation of sympathy in his *Theory of Moral Sentiments* (first published in 1759 and then revised for a further five editions before Smith's death, in 1790) develops Hume's notions. Smith thought of sympathy in precise functional terms, and in those terms it is fundamental to his analyses of human relations and societies. "As we have no immediate experience of what other men feel, we can form no idea of

the manner in which they are affected, but by conceiving what we ourselves should feel in the like situation," he writes (1982, 9). Describing
what we might experience seeing "our brother" upon the rack, Smith
says that, through the sympathetic imagination, "we place ourselves in
his situation, we conceive ourselves enduring all the same torments, we
enter as it were into his body, and become in some measure the same
person with him, and even feel something which, though weaker in
degree, is not altogether unlike them" (9). In this passage, Smith's notions of sympathy recall very closely our current definitions of empathy. Smith goes on to claim that sympathy is a form of "fellow-feeling,"
which, though perhaps originally allied with compassion and pity, can
now, "without much impropriety, be made use of to denote our fellow-
feeling with any passion whatever" (10). It is the means by which people
can come to understand another's opinions or sentiments, even if one
does not approve of them. Our judgment of "propriety" or "impropriety"
is thus dependent upon the exercise of our sympathy (17). Sympathy, he
argues, is necessary for enabling social interactions, as it allows us to
judge the moral validity or desirability of a particular course of action,
thought, or exchange. This assessment is facilitated by his notion of the
impartial spectator, an internalization of social judgments that creates
the conscience; for Smith, "conscience is a social product, a mirror of
social feeling" that functions because "we are all anxious to stand well
with our fellows" (Raphael 2007, 35). Smith's sympathy is fundamental: without it, social interactions, and thus society itself, would not be
possible. With this in mind, we can follow a couple of other important
points: the connection between these ideas and Smith's more famous
economic theories, and the way Smith's integrated philosophy functions
in relation to one prominent autism precursor group, those people identified by contemporaries as "idiots." (At this point we are leaving aside
another of autism's important precursor concepts, the idea of "private
reason" [Goodey 2006, 2011], which, within Smith's framework, need
not have a disabling impact comparable to "idiocy.")

     Much has been written about the relationship between *The Theory of
Moral Sentiments* and Smith's more famous work, *The Wealth of Nations*,
first published in 1776. In the latter, Smith describes what he sees as a
fundamental disposition of humans: "the propensity to truck, barter, and
exchange one thing for another" (1986, 117), a propensity, he stresses,
that is guided entirely by self-interest. Readers have long been perturbed

by "the Adam Smith problem": the apparent contradiction between the notion in *The Theory of Moral Sentiments* that "man is a sympathetic animal" and the idea from *The Wealth of Nations* that "man is a selfish animal who acts for his own benefit." However, these two notions are not mutually incompatible. Although "benevolence" may spring from "sympathy," Smith never equates the two; as Leonidas Montes points out, "Sympathy . . . pertains to both the origin of moral judgment and to the process of attaining it," and as such, "the sympathetic process . . . entails a motivational force that is shaped by a continuous process of transformation inherent in human interaction" (2004, 52–53). The sympathetic process is a force motivating and directing social behavior, and it becomes the means by which one acquires moral autonomy; it is, as Montes summarizes, "part of a complex social phenomenon in which human beings take part in a continuous reciprocal interplay" (55), and, as such, is fundamental to the disposition "to truck, barter and exchange" that underlies Smith's economic analysis in *The Wealth of Nations*. The point to stress here is that Smith's economic theory grows out of his theory that moral sentiments, fundamentally "sympathy," enable society to function as it does. The two are not in opposition; in fact, his theory of economic activities relies upon his ideas about sympathy and moral sentiments.

Smith also identifies a number of outlier groups, including those who are somehow incapable of benefiting from the sympathetic processes. In some instances, one's "impartial spectator" may judge one harshly because of an apparent "impropriety" of one's being. In an intriguing passage in *The Theory of Moral Sentiments*, he notes that this judgment may even be an exacerbating factor in cases of "idiocy":

> Those unfortunate persons whom nature has formed a good deal below the common level, seem sometimes to rate themselves still more below it than they really are. This humility appears sometimes to sink them into idiotism. . . . The idiot feels himself below every company into which you can introduce him . . . [and is] always stamped with a distinct consciousness of his own great inferiority. He seems to shrink and, as it were, to retire from your look and conversation; and to feel, when he places himself in your situation, that, notwithstanding your apparent condescension, you cannot help considering him as immensely below you. . . . That instinct

of pride, necessary to support them upon an equality with their
brethren, seems totally wanting. (1982, 260–61)

Smith contemplates the possibility that some forms of social identity,
including devalued identities like that of the "idiot," are amplified, if not
actually created, through the dynamics of social interactions and the
internal judgments of one's impartial spectator. The "idiots" described
here form part of a contrast group of individuals who cannot prosper by
sympathy, in this instance because they recognize an "impropriety" in
their own being and hence turn their disgust inward upon themselves.

Sympathy, for Smith, is no passive emotion; it is a motivating force
that enables social and economic interactions (Fontaine 1997; Montes
2004). These interactions also played a role in how "idiocy" was expressed and understood in his schema; in the capacity to "truck, barter
and exchange," people identified as "idiots," whose "self-interest" is devalued along with their notion of "self," would also be disadvantaged.
Smith's use of the idea of sympathy sets an interesting precedent and
leads us to ask whether similar concerns might be clustered around empathy, especially as it performs similar functions to sympathy in terms
of social cohesion and community building. If, in Smith's analysis, a
well-developed sympathy is critical for economic activities, might not a
comparable association exist between empathy and economics? And how
does this matter to the way we see autism? This leads to another fundamental question: Could autism be perceived as problematic not because
people with autism are diminished in humanity because of their apparent empathy deficit, but rather because their particular qualities may be
seen as disadvantageous in an economy that demands empathy?

Autism, Empathy, and Economics

Smith's notion of sympathy underpinned a theory of market capitalism
motivated by self-interest; what role, we should ask, does empathy play
in contemporary global economics? We can easily imagine economic
advantages in being able to empathize with the other—to get into the
heads of others, to feel their pain, understand their motivations, anticipate their choices, and perhaps, through a form of economic therapy
(funding for mutually beneficial projects, say), redirect their actions to
suit our own interests.

Certainly, the *idea* of autism seems counter to such activity. When a group of young French economists rebelled against the notion of a *Homo economicus* guided by mathematical principles—that figure presumed to exist by generations of economists—they founded a movement critical of the rationalist dogmatism of neoclassical economics and labeled it "post-autistic economics"; the movement sought to "liberate economics from its autistic obsession with formal models that have no obvious empirical reference" (Fullbrook 2000, 1). (The critical journal arising out of these debates, the *Post-autistic Economics Review*, was published online from 2000 to 2008, when the name was changed to *Real World Economics Review*; it remains available online.) According to the "postautistic" economists, a pluralist approach, incorporating insights from sociology, psychology, and other disciplines, is necessary for proper economic analysis, and previous theoretical approaches that did not consider the social, cultural, and environmental contexts of economic activities were engaged in behavior that was metaphorically autistic. This choice of metaphor is telling: postautistic economists identify autism as a defining feature of a neoclassical economics that proves insufficient to deal with the complexity of exchanges across different cultures, within heterogeneous societies, and during periods of social and environmental change. In short, "autistic" economics fail to engage with human complexities, supplanting them with a reductive model of a nonexistent creature, the rational *Homo economicus*. It is an economics without empathy.

The actual experience (economic and otherwise) of autistic people may belie this metaphor, though. Tyler Cowen, an economist who also identifies as autistic, presents an alternative version of autistic economics in his *Create Your Own Economy* (2009). Like Adam Smith, Cowen presents an expansive notion of the economic realm, one embracing social psychology, and argues that the autistic capacity to learn by organizing and ordering rather than through narrative explication offers autistic people a unique ability to make sense of information (again, economic and otherwise) and also provides a useful model for nonautistics.

Cowen's model prioritizing organized over narrative learning does not make a concerted case for the role of empathy in economic understanding. Like Adam Smith, however, Cowen emphasizes the social context of economic activity and the role of interpersonal relations and judgments in determining economic choices. But increasingly, many economists, even those without direct affiliation with the postautistic-economics movement, draw explicitly upon the concept of empathy. Jeremy Rifkin, a trained economist, writes in his popular work *The Empathic Civilization* (2009) that empathy provides the key to "the meaning of life," which is "to enter into relationships with others in order to deeply experience, as much as one can, the reality of existence" (156). Indeed, he notes, "empathy [is] at the very core of what it means to be a fully aware and responsible human being" (401)—a claim repeated elsewhere in the literature on empathy (Agosta 2010; Baron-Cohen 2006). Rifkin deals with the problem of an evident lack of empathy in many historical cultures by hypothesizing that societies pass through stages of mythological, theological, and ideological consciousness to arrive at a psychological consciousness, which characterizes contemporary occidental cultures. Closely akin to this psychological consciousness is an even higher level, that of empathic consciousness, which in Rifkin's narrative has been reached by a small but significant minority of humans across the globe. So only now, Rifkin insists, have we reached a critical mass capable of leading our fellows to the "Age of Empathy" (2009, 472).

In Rifkin's account, empathy's current cultural capital is closely linked to economic issues, especially the growing realization that communities across the globe are bound by shared economic and environmental concerns. In North America and Europe, urban communities continue to develop local economies heavily dependent upon service industries, which require a capacity to connect with—that is, to empathize with—the client. These communities are also culturally heterogeneous, marking a relatively recent demographic shift that requires a willingness to accept other ideas and other ways of living. Throughout his argument, Rifkin establishes a series of contrast groups of those lacking an empathic consciousness, which include those societies (mainly non-occidental) whose most powerful members remain mired in an ideological or theological consciousness, and more localized contrast groups, including "narcissists, sociopaths or autistically challenged individuals" (42). Rifkin cites Baron-Cohen's autistic nonempaths to support his argument that the roots of empathy are neurological; noting the breakdown of "mirror neurons" in autistic people, Rifkin informs his readers that "autistic children are characterized by the inability to read other people's intentions, express emotions, learn languages and exhibit pro-social behavior. They are unable to empathize" (85–86). Later, he reinforces the point: "Severely autistic children who have an impoverished mirror neuron system are unable to learn language because they don't have the potential empathic building blocks—mirror neurons—and therefore are unable to learn about and from others" (104). Of course, much recent work on neuroplasticity argues that the brain is a flexible and adaptive organ (Doidge 2007). This research challenges the notion that we require a specific neurological "tool" (such as mirror neurons) to carry out a specific task (such as making us empathetic), rendering premature any definite pronouncements about the centrality of mirror neurons to the development of connections (empathetic or otherwise) between people. However, such reservations do not enter into Rifkin's account, because autism is not central to his argument. In his formulation, autistic people are simply a convenient contrast group used to assert the existence and the importance of empathy: his people with autism are without empathy so that we can see how important empathy truly is.

Empathy has truly come of age in the realm of realpolitik. Not only is it being defined as the capacity to understand the experiences of others but increasingly it is being presented as a means of using this understanding to direct the behaviors of the object of empathy. "Emotional labor," a concept first articulated by Arlie Hochschild in her 1983 book *The Managed Heart,* now characterizes an approach to working that involves the "performance" of empathy (or at least of signs of empathy), not only in service positions but also across different levels of management and civil service, as well as in such fields as health care and education. Today, the concepts of empathy and "emotional intelligence" resonate within the business world as tools for leaders to ensure productive workforces and the consequent ongoing viability of corporations (Karafyllis and Ulshöfer 2008). Not surprisingly, a number of writers on empathy also work as high-level business or economics consultants: Rifkin, for example, is founder and president of the Foundation on Economic Trends, founder and chair of the Third Industrial Revolution Global CEO Business Roundtable, and adviser to the European Parliament, as well as to the governments of Spain and Germany; psychologist Daniel Goleman—who followed *Emotional Intelligence* (1996) with the coauthored 2002 work *Primal Leadership: Realizing the Power of Emotional Intelligence* (with Boyatzis and McKee)—also speaks to business leaders on the benefits of emotional and social intelligence, setting the pace for numerous other consultants who teach empathic leadership in corporate settings.

Empathy, clearly, is not simply the capacity to put oneself in the skin of the other but also a tool to anticipate, modify, and benefit from the actions of these others. As such, it is a tool useful for the exercise of power.

Conclusion

Despite the many recent and prominent formulations of "empathy," we still do not have a firm sense of what precisely defines this quality. Nor are we likely to. Empathy is an abstraction, a reification; any definition is bound to be the sum of a cluster of responses that someone (or some culture) decides a priori are "empathetic." Consequently, the claim that empathy is a fundamental human trait seems particularly weak, and furthermore risks excluding from "humanity" those figured to be lacking in empathy, just as those judged deficient in rationality or intelligence were (and largely remain) excluded from contemporary society. The notion of empathy, like that of intelligence, seems to require a contrast group of outsiders whose exclusion from "empathic consciousness" can assure the rest of us that we are acceptably empathic (even if we have mainly "male" brains). Hence, it is convenient that some people—like those with autism—are allegedly without empathy and can, in these accounts, serve as models of life devoid of empathy. But although difficulties in interpersonal relationships may remain a component of autism, this is not necessarily the same thing as a lack of empathy; nor does it signal such a condition, unless we are to define empathy narrowly to exclude various ways of trying to understand and (apparently) empathize, or even sympathize, with others.

In creating a space for exploring the idea of autism and its relation to parallel and intersecting discourses (such as that of empathy), a critical autism studies has the potential to alert us to the ideological functions that can be performed when we try to define autism and its relation to notions put forth as "fundamental human characteristics." Although my short critique is intended primarily as a preliminary sketch of one aspect of a complex issue, it does offer certain observations—most notably that the idea of empathy is ideologically loaded and culturally shaped, and so is its inverse relationship with autism. It also raises questions and enables further hypotheses. For instance, could the current cultural anxiety about autism be a response fed in part by a sense of cultural alienation, disengagement, or disempowerment—feelings that are anything but empathic? Perhaps most important, it points to a disturbing movement in writings that use autism as a test case for validating the concept of empathy. This strategy succeeds only at the cost of creating new exiles. If empathy is seen as fundamental to humanity, those who are not particularly empathic (according to whatever definition of the term is dominant) thus acquire identities defined by this lack and pathologized by their resistance to therapy. Like the Age of Meritocratic Intelligence before it, the Age of Empathy will strive to create its barbarians to be placed outside the gates.

ACKNOWLEDGMENTS

Thanks to Michael Orsini, Joyce Davidson, and the participants at the Critical Autism Studies workshop in Ottawa, September 2010, as well as to Lynne Peters, Chris Goodey, Tim Stainton, Rachelle Hole, Lynn Rose, Ernie Baatz, Susan Stanfield, Aaron Johannes, and Sheldon Goldfarb for helping me to shape the ideas in this chapter.

REFERENCES

Agosta, L. 2010. *Empathy in the Context of Philosophy*. New York: Palgrave Macmillan.
American Psychiatric Association. 1994. *Diagnostic and Statistical Manual of Mental Disorders*. 4th ed. Washington, D.C.: American Psychiatric Association.
Asperger, H. (1944) 1991. "'Autistic Psychopathy' in Childhood." In *Autism and Asperger Syndrome*, edited and translated by U. Frith, 76–136. Cambridge: Cambridge University Press.
Autism Society. 2011. "U.S. Autism Prevalence Rises to 1 in 110." Accessed January 3, http://www.autismsociety.org/site/News2?news_iv_ctrl=1&page=NewsArticle&id=15481.
Autism Society Canada. 2011. "Prevalence." Accessed January 3, http://www.autismsocietycanada.ca/asd_research/research_prevalence/index_e.html.
Badcock, C., and B. Crespi. 2006. "Imbalanced Genomic Printing in Brain Development: An Evolutionary Basis for the Aetiology of Autism." *Journal of Evolutionary Biology* 19 (4): 1007–32.
———. 2008a. "Battle of the Sexes May Set the Brain." *Nature*, August 28, 1054–55.
———. 2008b. "Psychosis and Autism as Diametrical Disorders of the Social Brain." *Behavioral and Brain Sciences* 31 (3): 241–61.
Baron-Cohen, S. 1995. *Mindblindness: An Essay on Autism and Theory of Mind*. Cambridge, Mass.: MIT Press.
———. 2002. "The Extreme Male Brain Theory of Autism." *Trends in Cognitive Sciences* 6 (6): 248–54.
———. 2003. *The Essential Difference: Male and Female Brains and the Truth about Autism*. New York: Basic Books.
———. 2006. "Empathy: Freudian Origins and Twenty-First-Century Neuroscience." *Psychologist* 19 (9): 536–37.

———. 2009. "Autism: The Empathizing-Systemizing (E-S) Theory." In *The Year in Cognitive Neuroscience, 2009* (annual), 68–80. New York: New York Academy of Sciences.

———. 2011. *The Science of Evil: On Empathy and the Origins of Cruelty.* New York: Basic Books.

Baron-Cohen, S., and S. Wheelwright. 2004. "The Empathy Quotient: An Investigation of Adults with Asperger Syndrome or High Functioning Autism, and Normal Sex Differences." *Journal of Autism and Developmental Disorders* 34 (2): 163–75.

Bielski, Z. 2010. "Today's College Kids Are 40-Per-Cent Less Empathic, Study Finds." *Globe and Mail,* June 1. Accessed May 1, 2013, http://www.theglobeandmail .com/life/work/todays-college-kids-are-40-per-cent-less-empathetic-study-finds/article1587609/.

Blackburn, J. K., E. G. Gottschewski, and L. Niki. 2000. "A Discussion about Theory of Mind: From an Autistic Perspective." Paper presented at the Sixth Annual Conference of Autism Europe, Glasgow, Scotland, May 19–21. Available at http://www.autistics.org/library/AE2000-ToM.html.

Bleuler, E. (1911) 1950. *Dementia Praecox; or, The Group of Schizophrenias.* Translated by J. Zinkin. New York: International Universities Press.

Cowen, T. 2009. *Create Your Own Economy: The Path to Prosperity in a Disordered World.* New York: Dutton.

Davidson, J., and M. Smith. 2009. "Autistic Autobiographies and More-Than-Human Emotional Geographies." *Environment and Planning D: Society and Space* 27 (5): 898–916.

Doidge, N. 2007. *The Brain That Changes Itself.* New York: Viking.

Fontaine, P. 1997. "Identification and Economic Behavior: Sympathy and Empathy in Historical Perspective." *Economics and Philosophy* 13 (2): 261–80.

Frith, U. 1989. *Autism: Explaining the Enigma.* Oxford: Blackwell.

Fullbrook, E. 2000. "Amartya Sen Enters the Debate." *Post-autistic Economics Newsletter,* no. 3: 1–3. Accessed May 1, 2013, http://www.paecon.net/PAEReview/wholeissues/issue3.htm.

Gallagher, S. 2004a. "Situational Understanding: A Gurwitschian Critique of Theory of Mind." *Contributions to Phenomenology* 52: 25–44.

———. 2004b. "Understanding Interpersonal Problems in Autism: Interaction Theory as an Alternative to Theory of Mind." *Philosophy, Psychiatry, and Psychology* 11 (3): 199–217.

Gilberg, C. 1992. "Autism and Autistic-Like Conditions: Subclasses among Disorders of Empathy." *Journal of Child Psychology and Psychiatry* 33 (5): 813–42.

Goleman, D. 1995. *Emotional Intelligence: Why It Can Matter More Than IQ.* New York: Bantam.

———. 2006. *Social Intelligence: The New Science of Social Relationships.* New York: Bantam.

Goleman, D., R. Boyatzis, and A. McKee. 2002. *Primal Leadership: Realizing the Power of Emotional Intelligence.* Boston: Harvard Business School Press.

Goodey, C. 2006. "Heterodoxy and Private Reason: Autism's Historical Companions." Paper presented at "Autism and Representation," Liverpool John Morris University, Liverpool, England, February 24–25.

———. 2011. *A History of Intelligence and "Intellectual Disability": The Shaping of Psychology in Early Modern Europe.* Farnham, U.K.: Ashgate.

Grandin, T. 2005. *Animals in Translation: Using the Mysteries of Autism to Decode Animal Behavior.* Orlando, Fla.: Harcourt.

———. 2006. *Thinking in Pictures: And Other Reports from My Life with Autism.* 2nd ed. New York: Vintage.

———. 2008. *The Way I See It: A Personal Look at Autism and Asperger's.* Arlington, Tex.: Future Horizons.

Hochschild, A. R. 1983. *The Managed Heart: Commercialization of Human Feeling.* Berkeley: University of California Press.

Hume, D. (1739–40) 1978. *A Treatise of Human Nature.* Oxford: Clarendon.

Jahoda, G. 2005. "Theodor Lipps and the Shift from 'Sympathy' to 'Empathy.'" *Journal of the History of the Behavioral Sciences* 41 (2): 151–63.

Jurecic, A. 2006. "Mindblindness: Autism, Writing, and the Problem of Empathy." *Literature and Medicine* 25 (1): 1–23.

Kanner, L. 1943. "Autistic Disturbances of Affective Contact." *Nervous Child* 2: 217–50.

Karafyllis, N. C. 2008. "Oneself as Other? Autism and Emotional Intelligence as Pop Science, and the Establishment of 'Essential' Differences." In Karafyllis and Ulshöfer, *Sexualized Brains,* 1–49.

Karafyllis, N. C., and G. Ulshöfer. 2008. "Intelligent Emotions and Sexualized Brains: Discourses, Scientific Models, and Their Interdependencies." In Karafyllis and Ulshöfer, *Sexualized Brains,* 237–316.

———, eds. 2008. *Sexualized Brains: Scientific Modelling of Emotional Intelligence from a Cultural Perspective.* Cambridge, Mass.: MIT Press.

Leudar, I., and A. Costall, eds. 2009. *Against Theory of Mind.* Basingstoke, U.K.: Palgrave Macmillan.

Montes, L. 2004. *Adam Smith in Context: A Critical Reassessment of Some Central Components of His Thought.* Basingstoke, U.K.: Palgrave Macmillan.

Murray, S. 2008. *Representing Autism: Culture, Narrative, Fascination.* Liverpool, U.K.: Liverpool University Press.

Nadesan, M. H. 2005. *Constructing Autism: Unravelling the "Truth" and Understanding the Social.* New York: Routledge.

Prince-Hughes, D. 2004. *Songs of the Gorilla Nation: My Journey through Autism.* New York: Harmony.

Raphael, D. D. 2007. *The Impartial Spectator: Adam Smith's Moral Philosophy.* Oxford: Clarendon.

Rifkin, J. 2009. *The Empathic Civilization: The Race to Global Consciousness in a World in Crisis.* New York: Tarcher/Penguin.

Rogers, K., et al. 2007. "Who Cares? Revisiting Empathy in Asperger Syndrome." *Journal of Autism and Developmental Disorders* 37 (4): 709–15.

Smith, A. (1759–74) 1982. *The Theory of Moral Sentiments.* Edited by D. D. Raphael and A. L. Macfie. Indianapolis, Ind.: Liberty Classics.

———. (1776) 1986. *The Wealth of Nations.* London: Penguin.

Smith, A. 2008. "The Empathy Imbalance Hypothesis of Autism: A Theoretical Approach to Cognitive and Emotional Empathy in Autistic Development." *Psychological Record* 59 (2): 273–94.

Williams, D. 1998. *Autism and Sensing: The Unlost Instinct.* London: Kingsley.
Wing, L. 1981. "Asperger's Syndrome: A Clinical Account." *Psychological Medicine* 11 (1): 115–29.
Wispé, L. 1987. "History of the Concept of Empathy." In *Empathy and Its Development,* edited by N. Eisenberg and J. Strayer, 17–37. Cambridge: Cambridge University Press.

Autism and the Posthuman

Stuart Murray

Outhumaning the Human

In *Not Even Wrong* (2004), his book on the history of autism inspired by his relationship with his autistic son Morgan, Paul Collins pauses for a moment during his wider argument to note a particular way in which the condition interacts with an idea of the human:

> Autists are described by others—and by themselves—as aliens among humans. But there's an irony to this, for precisely the opposite is true. They are us, and to understand them is to begin to understand what it means to be human. Think of it: a disability is usually defined in terms of what is missing. . . . But autism is *an ability and a disability*: it is as much about what is abundant as what is missing, an overexpression of the very traits that make our species unique. Other animals are social, but only humans are capable of abstract logic. The autistic outhumans the humans, and we can scarcely recognize the result. (161; emphasis in original)

What might seem like a straightforward statement here in fact contains a number of complexities. The autism-alien association is, as Collins observes, one that has become standard when discussing the condition. Inspired in large measure by Temple Grandin's comment to Oliver Sacks that having autism made her "feel like an anthropologist on Mars" (Sacks 1995, 295) and Sacks's subsequent use of the phrase as the title for his 1995 collection of case studies, the idea of a "natural" link between autism and alien, as an account of the experience of life, has developed to a point where the combination of the words can appear to offer a straightforward description of the condition. As such, a text such as Jasmine Lee O'Neill's *Through the Eyes of Aliens: A Book about Autistic People* (1998) offers O'Neill's understanding of verisimilitude and is not a title that conveys, say, prejudice through its idea of autism as

"otherworldly." Neil Badmington has referred to contemporary fascination with aliens, in relation to questions of the spectrum of humanity,
as "alien chic" (2004), and Ian Hacking, who has written on autism and
the idea of the alien, notes that as a culture "we seem to hold up aliens as
mirrors to teach what is best or worst in us or in the human condition"
(2009, 45). Hacking's insight here catches the idea of range in Collins's
other observations: that those with autism "are us" and form the platform for an "understanding" of nonautistic humanity, but also that, in
the processes of "outhumaning" ideas of a human norm, they move beyond core categories of humanity to suggest wider possibilities.

Collins's idea that autism is absence, supplement and excess, or humanity and nonhumanity, all at the same time, is one that is increasingly gaining purchase in critical thinking on the condition that stems
from disability studies, bioethics, and philosophy. The idea that "we can
scarcely recognize the result" of such thinking works subsequently as a
signpost toward an unformed future in which autism might further be
discussed and theorized. In part, the fact that discussion of the condition has arrived at this point is the culmination of efforts to achieve a
more subtle and nuanced understanding of autism; knowing that we no
longer routinely label those who are autistic as "subhuman" and do not
automatically deem them of no worth and consign them to lives of bru-
tal institutionalization is a tribute to processes of education about the
disabled that have sought to develop a language of rights and inclusion
understood by all. Such productive measures can only be welcomed.
Nevertheless, it should not be denied that Collins's positioning of autism in relation to a broader category of humanity is not without its
problems. In its desire to capture a sense of full engagement with the
nondisabled majority, it threatens to render autism diffuse to a point
where it loses any specificity in its interaction with the notion of "the
human." If autism is somehow less, more, *and* something else when discussed in the context of the ways in which we think about the broader
category of humanity, then where exactly does it stand, and how precisely is it constituted?

This essay makes a specific intervention into this debate through a
concentration on autism and the posthuman, and aims to think through
the multiple and often confusing arguments that come with the juxtapo-
sition of the two terms. In so doing, it picks up on Collins's idea that the
condition "outhumans the humans," that it gestures toward a beyond,

or a "post-," that represents a space of cultural enactment, and possibly agency, separate from any configuration of a human norm. Such a posthuman position is one that, on the surface, appears to engage with a number of the metaphors that circulate about autistic subjectivity, especially those connected to technology and the digital flow of information, the by-now-somewhat-clichéd idea that the autistic brain is a "hard drive" that has been incorrectly "wired." The link, then, is not only one that might seem appealing to those involved in philosophy and posthumanism generally, in that it opens up new spaces for the consideration of core categories such as "self" and "being"; it also talks to a generally articulated language used increasingly in descriptions of the condition. On the one hand, it appears that posthumanism offers a potentially radically productive space for autism, a beyond where disability is not an issue because ideas of normative biological humanity itself have been transformed, and (to be autism-specific) where that transformation has taken place in areas, such as the flow of information, in which we might feel that the condition, because of its nature, has a specific relevance. On the other hand, a posthuman conception of autism might involve languages and structures that are dangerous precisely because, in that move to a space of beyond, the material links to the experience of a lived life, the day-to-day business of being autistic, could be lost. The area and tension between these two positions, and the possibilities of each, are the territories I will seek to cover here through an examination of theory, clinical conceptions of the condition, ideas of possible medical futures, and writings by those with autism.

On one level, the productive idea of a posthuman autistic humanity could also be thought of in terms of a "radical humanism." The damage done to those with disabilities in the name of humanism is, of course, long-standing, especially the associations between modernity and eugenics that emerged from the end of the nineteenth century into the twentieth. In spite of this, the contemporary moment still contains what Badmington has referred to as "the persistence of humanism" (2004, 34–63), and a number of attempts have been made to promote a radical humanism that keeps positive aspects of the idea's history while practicing a critique of its negative aspects. Pauline Johnson's 1994 study *Feminism as Radical Humanism*, with its advocacy of plurality, diversity, and autonomy under the banner of a new conception of humanism, is one such study, as is the idea advanced by Martin Halliwell and Andy

Mousley that humanist thought is "both a pluralistic and self-critical tradition that folds in and over itself, provoking a series of questions and problems rather than necessarily providing consolation or edification" (2003, 16). The idea is given great range and force in the late work of Edward Said, including the notion of a "democratic criticism" advanced in his last book, *Humanism and Democratic Criticism* (2004). Central to his idea of humanism in this text, Said develops what he terms an idea of "participatory citizenship." He observes that there is

> no contradiction at all between the practice of humanism and the practice of participatory citizenship. Humanism is not about withdrawal and exclusion. Quite the reverse; its purpose is to make things more available to critical scrutiny as the product of human labor, human energies for emancipation and enlightenment, and, just as importantly, human misreadings of and misinterpretations of the collective past and present. . . .
>
> . . . In my understanding of its relevance today, humanism is not a way of consolidating and affirming what "we" have always known and felt, but rather a means of questioning, upsetting, and reformulating so much of what is presented to us as commodified, packaged, uncontroversial, and uncritically codified certainties. (22, 28)

Although they are general, the kinds of revisionist processes Said outlines here offer the prospect of a humanism radicalized by an understanding of difference, where a category like disability (and, for our purposes, specifically autism) can be understood to provide an idea of the human changed by the material consequences of what Deborah Barnbaum has termed, in the context of a discussion of ethics, "autistic integrity" (2008, 204). What individual in a position of autism advocacy or care would not want to embrace an idea of citizenship conceived of in such terms? And the "uncritically codified certainties" that surround the assumed normative position of ableism, and that continue to resort to outdated concepts of "retardation," are surely ripe for the manner of critique suggested here.

Yet the question still remains whether humanism can escape its history, or whether the prejudices it enacts even in its most recent formations are, at heart, a part of its very structure. It is still very much the case that the clinical language surrounding autism, especially that connected to diagnosis, reinforces the link between the condition and an idea of the human constituted in terms of the "working" mind. To read over the relevant guidance on diagnosing autism provided in the American Psychiatric Association's *Diagnostic and Statistical Manual of Mental Disorders* (*DSM* [2000]) and the World Health Organization's *International Classification of Mental and Behavioural Disorders* (*ICD* [2009]), the two manuals used globally, is to be struck by the force with which the language of impairment is almost endlessly repeated. The examples, in *DSM-IV* alone, of "failure," "lack," and "delay," as well as "stereotyped," "repetitive," "restricted," "inflexible," "non-functional," "disturbance," and "abnormal" behaviors all deemed relevant to recognizing autism (*DSM-IV-TR* 2000, 75), point to the instrumental use of a deficit model that constructs the condition continually as a problem. The perspective on autism that conceives of it in such terms stems clearly from notions of human wholeness which, in turn, have their roots in those strands of humanist thinking, whether romantic, existential, or civic, that stress the value of perfectionist notions of "human" or "self" (Halliwell and Mousley 2003, 19–58, 79–98). If it seems a touch dualistic to say that the promise of a radical or critical humanism is betrayed by the ways in which a working method of "the human" is put into action, the biases of such clinical terminology do make the argument plausible. And it is a process replicated in the media, where discussions of autism and disability more generally often return to an idea of "function," displayed, for example, in the excitement of news organizations over developments in prenatal genetic testing and consequent ideas of the "worth" of a disabled life. Such suggestions of the working value of the person with disability always have, as their shadow, the seemingly straightforward notion of the fully functional, "natural," nondisabled body or mind (see Murray 2010).

If the desire to radicalize humanism is laudable for its concerns with a situated sense of political agency (Said's "citizenship"), it is still the case that the majority of the spaces in which an idea of "the human" is made to work display hierarchies of mind and body that continue to label a condition such as autism a "disorder." Mark Osteen has observed that commentators from all disciplines come to discuss autism "carrying too much clinical baggage," a point of engagement that all too often produces "preconceived conclusions" concerning ideas of exactly how human the individual with autism might be (2008, 12–13). Equally, the desire for narratives of "recovery" or "overcoming" with regard to the condition illustrate the power of a wide social and cultural desire for those who are autistic to somehow "regain" a full humanity they supposedly lack; and the drift toward affective language, with questions of empathy, for example, consolidates a type of cultural approach to the condition that is worryingly prescriptive. As James T. Fisher notes in his discussion of the many "conversion narratives" that surround autism, the condition "is widely understood as a disorder of selfhood in which persons fail by virtue of their condition to fulfil the birthright of developing, disclosing and searching for an individual identity. The presence of autistic persons thus constitutes a kind of scandal in a culture where the subject in search of self is virtually equated with what makes us human" (2008, 51). Given that the kinds of representations described by Fisher and Osteen are all too common, what might be the outline of a posthuman autism, seen in terms of both the individual and, possibly more problematically, the collective? If the category of "the human" is too frequently reductive when placed in dialogue with autism, what may be possible in theorizing the condition within thinking that seeks to leave human embodiment behind?

Contexts of the Posthuman

The posthuman critique of humanism is relentless in its characterization of the limitations of a concentration on "the human" as a category. In *How We Became Posthuman* (1999), N. Katherine Hayles charts the dismantling of the liberal-humanist subject and the "emergence of the posthuman as an informational-material entity" (11), where a concern with patterns of information is central to the idea of extending notions of consciousness and embodiment. A consequence of this is, as Hayles goes on to observe, that "becoming a posthuman means much more than having prosthetic devices grafted onto one's body. It means envisioning humans as information-processing machines with fundamental similarities to other kinds of information-processing machines, especially intelligent computers" (246). Within such environments, disability perhaps need not be seen as the kind of absence and lack that is so familiar from humanist rhetoric, and a number of disability scholars have embraced this kind of space as one fertile for the development of productive models of disabled presence. Rosemarie Garland-Thomson, for example, has declared that postmodern writing is "the most congenial cultural mode in which disability is represented," because it "no longer mourns unity, even though it grapples with multiplicity" (1997, 166). Lennard J. Davis goes even further, arguing that "postmodernism is still based on a humanistic model" and coining a new term, *dismodernism*, to act as a more precise label for the place disability might occupy beyond humanist categories (2002, 30). Davis's dismodernism is a wide category, but it interacts with the ideas of information-processing that Hayles identifies as being at the core of posthuman identities: "The dismodernist subject is in fact disabled, only completed by technology and by interventions. Rather than the idea of the complete, independent subject, endowed with rights (which are in actuality conferred by privilege), the dismodernist subject sees that metanarratives are only 'socially created' and accepts them as that, gaining help and relying on legislation, law and technology" (Davis 2002, 30). If some scholars of the posthuman might still query the idea of a subject within legislation and law, Davis makes explicit the position of disability within a world "completed by technology," in which the technological is not the gas chamber or a statistically enabled mode of measure and institutional prejudice, but rather a process of enablement allowing the fulfilled figure of a disabled life. Such a location catches a flavor of the optimism of some posthuman theorizing.

The latest thinking within disability studies to consider the relationship between posthumanism and disability strikes a more cautious note. Fiona Kumari Campbell's 2009 book *Contours of Ableism* considers both the posthuman and the transhuman (she says "both words are often used interchangeably") in the context of the production of abled and disabled identities (67). Campbell acknowledges that "there is little debate about the potential merits of certain enhancement technologies in 'bettering' the lives of those individuals that in today's circumstances we consider 'impaired'" (72), but her conclusion on the relationship is less optimistic: "Possibilities of post-humanism developed within the context of technologies of ableism may provide a 'new deal' for some— but on closer examination the tentacles of ableism reassert itself [*sic*] through a dominant trend in the literature and research to propose a virile style of transhumanism that despises vulnerability" (75). The idea of the "vulnerable" certainly stands in opposition to the more utopian

and celebratory aspects of posthuman thinking and also serves as a reminder of those nineteenth- and twentieth-century eugenic processes
that saw those who were vulnerable, autistics among them, fall into the
category of the subhuman. For Campbell, the fear is that the disabled
will again be left behind in any posthuman world governed by a "virile,"
and therefore generated, desire for technological progress.

Other writers without a specific disability focus are equally suspicious about the proposed promises of posthumanism. In his 2002 study
Our Posthuman Future, Francis Fukuyama considers what he terms the
"consequences of the biotechnology revolution," in which "the most significant threat posed by contemporary biotechnology is the possibility
that it will alter human nature and thereby move us into a 'posthuman'
stage of history" (7). For Fukuyama, categories like "human nature,"
"common humanity," and "natural rights" (11, 13) are stable concepts
that have been proved as such over historical time. Biotechnological
science, especially neuropharmacology and prenatal genetic screening,
threaten these core concepts of "the human" because of their potential
to alter the accepted categories of human behavior. Fukuyama criticizes
the American pharmaceutical industry, for example, for suggesting that
it "can provide self-esteem in a bottle," and worries over the "creation" of
such conditions as ADD and ADHD, the latter quite possibly, as he puts
it, not "a disease at all but rather just the tail of the bell curve describing
the distribution of perfectly normal human behavior" (46–49). More
pertinent to a discussion of autism is Fukuyama's assertion that genetic
screening and engineering suggest "the prospect of a new kind of eugenics, with all the moral implications with which that word is fraught,
and ultimately the ability to change human nature" (72). Moreover, pre-
implantation genetic diagnosis offers the possibility to create genetic
profiles. All of these are steps on the path toward "the ultimate prize of
modern genetic technology," namely, "the designer baby" and the ultimate genetically modified being (2002, 76).

These last points about genetics catch the complexities and contra-
dictions of Fukuyama's thinking. His concerns surrounding the potential use of prenatal genetic testing mirror those of autism advocates
such as Ari Ne'eman and Amanda Baggs, who see the threat of such
biotechnology in its capacity to provide a means to eradicate the condition (see Baggs 2010a). But whereas Ne'eman and Baggs oppose genetic intervention on the grounds of the validity of human variation and

neurobehavioral difference that autism indicates, Fukuyama's concept of human nature displays no awareness of neurodiversity whatsoever. His static concept of "the human" is the product of a pure humanism, one that extends into a "natural" celebration of other humanist categories, such as liberal democracy ("the only viable and legitimate political system for modern societies" [2002, 14]), without any consideration of groups, like those with disabilities, for whom such an idea of humanity can itself be a threat and who are frequently pushed to the bottom of any liberal democratic system. Fukuyama's analysis of the potential perils of a posthuman future may be subtle in its sense of the interplay between science and politics, but it is utterly ignorant of the ways in which disability complicates such questions. As David Mitchell has written of disability representation generally, it does not always promote a "search for a more positive story of disability," but frequently outlines the "thoroughgoing challenge that disability invites of the undergirding authorization to interpret" (2002, 24). Fukuyama's simplistic conception of "the human" is exactly the kind of "undergirding" of which Mitchell speaks here, and the interpretive authority he derives from it in his subsequent theorizing means he works from a fatally flawed critical position as he tries to outline possible human futures.

In his 2009 study *Digimodernism: How New Technologies Dismantle the Postmodern and Reconfigure Our Culture*, Alan Kirby is, as his subtitle implies, more positive than Fukuyama about how the technological, and especially digital technology, might influence the future. Calling an end to a period of postmodernism that he deems to be elitist and now out of date, Kirby cautiously celebrates the democratic nature of much digital technology. While putting forward his thesis, however, he makes a sudden detour to draw an intriguing parallel with autism that moves beyond the obvious linkage of the condition with technology. Kirby may feel that a digimodern age is our new reality, but he views the argument that contemporary culture's fixation with technology has somehow made society "more autistic" to be false, claiming instead that this actually speaks to what he terms "pseudoautism," or "characteristics deriving locally from particular experiences and lacking the neurological basis of clinical autism" (230). In fact, Kirby asserts, autism constitutes the *opposite* to the emerging digital and posthuman world his study maps out: "The perfectly shaped excluded other of contemporary society: the model of 'sickness' generated by the ways in which orthodox social values define health and the 'normal,'" as he puts it. He goes on: "Autism, I would argue, is the ready-made antithesis of the peculiarities of today's world; it is the mark of that which our society despises, marginalizes, and makes impossible, and is produced as the exact contrary of hegemonic forces in a variety of contexts" (230–31). In outlining the most "decisive" of those contexts, he identifies "a pseudo-philosophical or antiscientific drift toward the denigration of knowledge and cleverness, increasingly objects of contempt and derision," as well as "a consumerist hatred of nonutilitarian information, and the new social orthodox of instrumentalist learning," and "a society which sneers at high levels of literacy or numeracy as though symptoms of personal inadequacy, [and] which fetishizes the superstitions of New Ageism, conspiracy theories, and pseudomedical quackery" (232–33). In opposition to this, Kirby argues, "autism's contrasting embrace of exhaustive knowledge, its love and recall of facts, its rich and grammatically correct use of language, its insistence on rationality, truth and rigor; all of this constructs autism as an incapacity to accept the sub-intellectual barbarism of its age" (233).

Kirby admits that he is largely representing Asperger Syndrome here, and so is not discussing the majority of autistic experiences, but the claim (especially in its near-vitriolic passion) is extraordinary nonetheless. His even more extreme conclusion, that "a society whose values produce autism so perfectly as its excluded other does not deserve to survive; nor will it" (233), positions autism as an arguably heroic humanist antidote to the nexus of posthuman technological concerns, particularly in the notion of the condition as some form of beacon of "truth."

It might be possible to see how Kirby's argument about autism's status as an "excluded other" illuminates the extent to which Fukuyama's ignorance of neurodiversity does indeed exclude disability in discussions of biotechnology. But even if this is the case, the characterization of the condition as a rearguard action against the "barbarism" of a contemporary digital age throws up a number of challenging, and potentially contradictory, complexities. It is arresting to see Kirby's thesis as a marker of autistic integrity and the value of the life lived with the condition, but it creates a unity of autistic subjectivity that misjudges the condition to the point of indulging in stereotypes about autistic "rationality," where the person with autism is always immersed in systems, always free from emotion, and always engaged in some kind of mental empiricism—the autistic as automaton. And, of course, we should not forget that a belief in the rational, and especially an uninterrogated idea of the rational—a position Kirby's analysis suggests here implicitly—is one of the abiding core values of humanism.

Posthumanism emerges from all this theorizing as a complex and contested space. For some, it is exciting and productive precisely because of its desire to move beyond, and redefine, the human, whereas for others, this redefinition threatens exclusionary practices that will limit the real nature of human variation. A posthuman future is, thus, amenable to disability but also carries the potential to destroy it; it is neurodiversity but also eugenics, depending on which version one might subscribe to. If, to quote Badmington, the posthuman "sets its sights upon the moments at which humanism begins to deconstruct itself" (2004, 12), then the space of such "moments" is one of both disjuncture and potential continuity when it comes to representing the disabled. It is fair enough to ask, again, where this leaves autism.

Back to the Future

In responding to this question, and in seeking to secure a path through these complexities, we might note some factors that help to provide clarity. First, it should be recognized that the place of autism within the idea of the technological imagined in a posthuman world is not a clear one. For many commentators (both Campbell and Fukuyama fall into this category), technology in such contexts is intrinsically connected to notions of technological *advancement*, the production of engineered and pharmaceutical prosthetics, for example, or the development of implants, voice machines, and surgical techniques. What such thinking misses, of course, is the inherent nature of neurodiversity and the possibility that a condition such as autism might not exist in a relationship with technology defined by ideas of "improvement." Rather, there could be a *parallel* between the workings of the autistic brain and the characterization of information, or representation of technological bodies, as they exist in posthuman thinking. This position counters Kirby's argument, given that it complicates the relationship between ideas of autistic "processing" and digital technology; but although it is essential to be aware of the automaton stereotype, autism's own associations with such technology, particularly systems of computing or processing, and with objects does invite connections in such a parallel fashion. For example, a preference for objects rather than people, a not-uncommon autistic trait, echoes ideas of a posthuman revision of embodiment (see Badmington 2004, 93–98), and the relationship between computing and human intelligence goes at least as far back as Alan Turing's classic 1950 essay "Computing Machinery and Intelligence." (The perils of retrospective diagnosis notwithstanding, placing Turing on the autistic spectrum is now not especially controversial, given what we know of his life.)

Second, the fascination with the cyborg (a classic posthuman figure in the wake of Donna Haraway's writings [1991, 2000]) might suggest a kind of autistic-being-in-the-world. If, to pick up again on Hacking's work on the subject, the alien and the human are not held apart in contemporary thinking but actually inform each other, the resulting hybrid figure—whether cyborg or some other form of posthuman subject—can provocatively be read in terms of autism (2009, 45). Here, some autistic traits are potentially positive and desirable, and within the various ongoing bioethical debates surrounding human enhancement, there are echoes of a productive posthuman position in which skills surrounding intelligence and processing are valued (Murray and Holmes 2009, 1–11). Taken out of the context of disability, certain autistic characteristics offer a "best version" of the condition in which selective human capacities are honed and developed for the betterment of humankind as a whole.

We can recognize in the work of a number of writers with, and about, autism the signs of posthumanism's concentration on the centrality of systems and information flow, its preoccupation with cybernetics and technology, and its suggestion of the limitations of the human as a coherent category. Temple Grandin's articulation, in her autobiographical writing, of her visual thinking and information processing (2006) fits this idea; the ways in which such topics are fictionalized in Elizabeth Moon's 2002 near-future novel, *Speed of Dark*, and are present in Moon's essays on autism (e.g., 2003), do likewise. Moon's ideas about questions of the role of cognition in understanding autism, for example, are expressed entirely in terms of computer processing:

> Why am I so sure that the central aspects of cognition are not the problem in autism? Observation, both of autistic children and (through their writing) of adult autistic individuals, combined with a knowledge of how information processing works in complex

systems like computers and humans. Where autistic individuals are presented with correct data in a sensory format they can use (such as math), they reason clearly and well; they understand cause and effect in physical (nonsocial) situations very well. Many if not most autistic children have no trouble learning letters, numbers, and they may pick up reading (simple decoding) even faster than the average child. But letters and numbers hold still on the page. Where they clearly fall behind is in situations where the necessary data require sensory processing in multiple channels—which all social interaction definitely does. (2003)

When social interaction is seen in terms of data processing, as it is here, then the parallels with posthumanism and a disembodied consciousness seem clear.

Dawn Prince-Hughes's anthropological overstepping of the boundaries between the human and nonhuman in *Songs of the Gorilla Nation* (2004) takes a posthuman argument even further, seeing clear boundaries to the human and connections between autism and animals. These kinds of links are present in Grandin's groundbreaking work on cattle management as well (2005). All of these, and other loose cultural and media-driven ideas—about Asperger Syndrome especially—fit with the idea of "distributed cognition" that Hayles puts forward in *How We Became Posthuman* as being constitutive of posthuman neurology (1999, ix). Equally, the idea of reflexivity, central to notions of posthuman thinking on the way information produces the very consequences that a system presupposes, fits with the idea of "looping" that Hacking has identified in the processes of diagnosing autism (1999). "Looping" here means that the processes of diagnosing autism *create* the condition as one of deficit, because the foundational systems and languages that are used are set up to produce such an end product. Posthuman theorizing on the virtual and on information patterning has clear interactions here both with how autism works and how it is perceived within diagnostic criteria. It is an illuminating dialogue.

Posthuman thought also includes theories taken from evolutionary biology, especially a call to understand the long history of biological evolution, that offer the potential to be specific about how we might see autism within the frame of neurodiversity. As Hayles puts it, "The post-human view considers consciousness, regarded as the seat of human identity in the Western tradition long before Descartes thought he was a mind thinking, as an epiphenomenon, as an evolutionary upstart trying to claim that it is the whole show when in actuality it is a minor sideshow," while "the posthuman view thinks of the body as the original prosthesis we all learn to manipulate, so that extending or replacing the body with other prostheses becomes a continuation of a process that began before we were born" (1999, 2–3). If the current state of being human is seen in these terms, as only a single point in a potentially infinite continuum, then the differences that constitute autism, especially cognitive exceptionality and the sensory experiences of the body, can be seen as modes of being that offer new perspectives through which the human state might be conceived. Here, in an echo of the human-enhancement debate mentioned earlier, what autism can teach a non-autistic majority about *potential* humans of the future is highly suggestive in the ways in which it offers opportunities to understand broad human variation.

Although such thinking is provocative, we need to admit to its limits, and here we return to the questions of embodiment. As a number of theorists have shown, a driving concern of much posthuman thinking has been to outline the ways in which information has come to be conceptualized in terms that stress its distance from the material forms in which it might appear to be carried; in a provocative phrase, Hayles calls this "how *information lost its body*" (2; emphasis in original). Such an expression forms part of the more general posthumanist relegation of the importance of embodiment in its concentration on information patterning. Even given the suggestive points about evolution made earlier, this is a situation that leaves autism in a complex position. For all that might be gained by a focus on lived experience as understood through the lens of systems or information processes, how much might we lose if we take the body out of our thinking about autism? In their autobiographical writings, both Donna Williams (1992) and Tito Rajarshi Mukhopadhyay (2000) have stressed the importance of sensory reactions to the environment in establishing their autistic identities—reactions that convey a strong sense of a physical and embodied relationship with the surrounding environment. Equally, in "In My Language," her 2007 YouTube phenomenon, Amanda Baggs begins the "untranslated" section of her video with a series of images of her body interacting with its surroundings—a hand in running water, her face experiencing textures, or her voice creating soundscapes—that rely on physical, embodied sensations in the production of proprioceptive feedback. In her essays, Baggs is very specific about how such sensory experiences not only constitute a vital part of her interiority but also shape her attitudes toward comprehending her surroundings and the language through which these issues are expressed:

> My first memories involve sensations of all kinds. Colors. Sounds. Textures. Flavors. Smells. Shapes. Tones. These are short words, but the meaning of them is long, involved, and complex. Some things caught my attention, others did not, but all of them were absorbed into my mind. . . . These sensory impressions were re-peated long enough for me to become deeply familiar with them. This familiarity resolved into patterns that formed the basis for more patterns, and—to this day—all of this continues to form the basis for how I understand things. When I say patterns, however, most people think I mean categories. I don't mean categories in any usual sense. I mean things fitting together in certain ways, outside of me. I mean perceiving connections without force-fitting a set of thoughts on top of them. This is how I handle not only sensory impressions but language itself. This is why I was able to work out which words go with which responses long before I was able to work out the meaning of the words and why—to this day—my ability to fit words into familiar patterns outstrips my ability to understand the words themselves. (2010b)

The body here is not something to be transcended or forgotten; rather, it is a formative and integral element in Baggs's conception of her autistic self. And although her sense of patterning does not conform to ortho-dox modes of information gathering or retention (in terms of not being "categories"), neither is it obviously about the kind of flow recognizable from posthuman theorizing on pattern construction and dissemination. It is best to see her idea of patterning as a process enacted from within a particular formation of autism, the logic of which may well be immune to nonautistic representation.

There is a further issue to be considered. Hayles notes that some work-ing in the field of posthumanism possess an overcelebratory sense of its transformational possibilities, "as if it were a universal human condition," when in fact, "it affects only a small fraction of the world's population" (1999, 6). History has taught us that the kinds of communities routinely excluded from the celebratory rhetoric of human possibility are the poor, the marginalized, and the disabled (this last category often including both poor and marginalized as well, of course). Whatever we might learn from autism about the ways in which we might download human consciousness, it is unlikely that those who have the condition will be at the front of the queue at some utopian moment when such downloading takes place. What if posthumanism simply becomes the next grand theory that finds ways to dispossess those with autism from the rights of citizenship to which they are entitled (a move that presents an extended and condition-specific version of Fukuyama's thesis)? The worry here is that such thinking will evacuate the material status of an autistic-being-in-the-world. In previous work, I have suggested that it is exactly a consideration of the material, or what I call "presence," that is central to any understanding of the condition:

> It is autistic presence, in all its many forms, that is the core of all attempts to discuss agency and legitimacy in those subjects for whom autism is in some way part of their representational existence. It is also autistic presence that resists the many discourses that would simplify or ignore the condition. The material nature of such presence, the excess it creates when confronted with any idea of what "normal" human activity or behaviour might be, stubbornly refuses to be reduced to any narrative—medical, social or cultural—that might seek to contain it without reference to its own terms. (Murray 2008, xviii)

In relation to this, it is revealing that posthuman theories of information suggest, according to Hayles, that information is "a pattern, not a presence" (1999, 18), a phrase that obviously suggests a very different sense of being than the one I outline.

In stressing the necessity of concentrating on material embodiment and presence when discussing autism, I am not indulging in some form of unimaginative humanism or nostalgic desire for unity and fixed notions of identity. Equally, in choosing to worry about the limits of posthumanism rather than to emphasize its promise, such an argument does not subscribe to Fukuyama's fears about technology or, conversely, dismiss a scientific future that illuminates the condition. Rather, it is fair to assert that the present moment in our thinking about autism is one in which we grasp at various forms of understanding, from scientific and ethical to legal and individual. At such a foundational time, excluding the material presence of the condition as it manifests itself in its multiple varieties is a dangerous act. There is surely no reason not to work toward a future in which a productive sense of autism, complete with the positive dimensions discussed here, cannot be outlined in tandem with conversations in which those who have the condition play a paramount role, and through which the twin aspects of a material ordinary and yet exceptional life with autism can be respected. To return to Paul Collins's observation with which we started, it is precisely because autism does "outhuman the human" that considering it as embodied and material does not return us to a simplistic humanism. The condition revises the terms of what any idea of "the human" can mean.

In trying to contextualize and explain the manner in which the multiple intersections of autism and the posthuman come together, we might return to an appropriately flexible sense of history, for all that "the historical" is a category some posthuman theorists conceive as invariably associated with ideas of "human progress." Developments in genetic and neurobiological research, along with further conversations with those with autism, may well produce a future from which any historian of the condition looking back on the start of the twenty-first century from the vantage point of a hundred years will see it as a period marked by ignorance, in which vaccine scares and cure therapies proliferated in the vacuum created by a lack of adequate understanding; we are perhaps unavoidably in the prehistory of autism in terms of the narratives of the future—scientific, social, and cultural—in which it will come to be written. Indeed, in addressing the cultural, we need to admit to the fact that the ways in which autism is characterized in the contemporary moment are frequently culturally specific. As Brigitte Chamak and Beatrice Bonniau outline in this volume in their discussion of autism in France, where ideas of neurodiversity are seen as problematic both within and without autism communities, the detail of the social and medical conceptions of the condition within a national institutional framework can dominate how autism is understood. With so little clinical consensus on autism, national and geocultural differences will only continue to provide revisions to our thinking about the condition.

Donna Williams, in dialogue with Adam Feinstein in his 2010 history of autism, asserts, "At present, we are merely the fools of tomorrow, no more enlightened than those who diagnosed 2-year-olds as psychotic, brain-damaged or emotionally disturbed in the 1940s through to the 1970s" (Feinstein 2010, 294). We do not want to characterize the present in this manner, of course, but admitting the limits of current thinking is not necessarily the worst way to face the future. The history of autism—from Bruno Bettleheim to Andrew Wakefield and the others that Paul Offit has termed "false prophets" (2008)—is littered with the claims of those who proclaimed that they knew in what ways autism and "the human" interact, and the promise of the posthuman has to be tempered by this knowledge of the past. It may well be that a posthuman future will signal an enlightened attitude toward the condition, and this essay has suggested some of the possible forms this might take; equally, there is no doubt that an escape from reductive humanist terms and frames of reference is to be welcomed. But the limits of the posthuman are, as we have seen, not simply questions of the creative imagination or philosophical boundary crossing; they speak to real concerns about the place of those with disabilities in a world centered on information exchange and technology. Maybe less celebration and more critique, an ongoing commitment to what this volume recognizes as a necessary "critical autism studies," are the best course of action for now.

ACKNOWLEDGMENTS

My thanks to Clare Barker and Richard Ashcroft for their comments on an earlier draft of this chapter.

REFERENCES

American Psychiatric Association. 2000. *DSM-IV-TR: Diagnostic and Statistical Manual of Mental Disorders*. 4th ed., text revision. Arlington, Va.: American Psychiatric Association.

Badmington, N. 2004. *Alien Chic: Posthumanism and the Other Within*. London: Routledge.

Baggs, A. 2007. "In My Language." YouTube. Accessed March 19, 2011, http://www.youtube.com/watch?v=JnylM1hI2jc.

———. 2010a. "Love, Devotion, Hope, Prevention, and Cure." Autistics.org. Accessed August 23, 2010, http://www.autistics.org/library/love.html.

———. 2010b. "Up in the Clouds and Down in the Valley: My Richness and Yours." *Disability Studies Quarterly* 30 (1). Accessed April 4, 2010, http://www.dsq-sds.org/article/view/1052/1238.

Barnbaum, D. R. 2008. *The Ethics of Autism: Among Them, but Not of Them*. Bloomington: Indiana University Press.

Campbell, F. K. 2009. *Contours of Ableism: The Production of Disability and Abledness*. Basingstoke, U.K.: Palgrave Macmillan.

Collins, P. 2004. *Not Even Wrong: A Father's Journey into the Lost History of Autism*. New York: Bloomsbury.

Davis, L. J. 2002. *Bending Over Backwards: Disability, Dismodernism, and Other Difficult Positions*. New York: New York University Press.

Feinstein, A. 2010. *A History of Autism: Conversations with the Pioneers*. Chichester, U.K.: Wiley-Blackwell.

Fisher, J. T. 2008. "No Search, No Subject? Autism and the American Conversion Narrative." In Osteen, *Autism and Representation*, 51–64.

Fukuyama, F. 2002. *Our Posthuman Future: Consequences of the Biotechnology Revolution*. London: Profile.

Garland-Thomson, R. 1997. *Extraordinary Bodies: Figuring Physical Disability in American Culture and Literature*. New York: Columbia University Press.

Grandin, T. 2005. *Animals in Translation: Using the Mysteries of Autism to Decode Animal Behavior*. London: Bloomsbury.

———. 2006. *Thinking in Pictures: And Other Reports from My Life with Autism*. London: Bloomsbury.

Hacking, I. 1999. *The Social Construction of What?* Cambridge, Mass.: Harvard University Press.

———. 2009. "Humans, Aliens, and Autism." *Daedalus*, Summer, 44–59.

Halliwell, M., and A. Mousley. 2003. *Critical Humanisms: Humanist/Anti-humanist Dialogues*. Edinburgh, U.K.: Edinburgh University Press.

Haraway, D. J. 1991. *Simians, Cyborgs, and Women: The Reinvention of Nature*. London: Free Association.

———. 2000. "A Cyborg Manifesto: Science, Technology, and Socialist-Feminism in the Late Twentieth Century." In *Posthumanism*, edited by N. Badmington, 69–84. Basingstoke, U.K.: Palgrave.

Hayles, N. K. 1999. *How We Became Posthuman. Virtual Bodies in Cybernetics, Literature, and Informatics*. Chicago: University of Chicago Press.

Johnson, P. 1994. *Feminism as Radical Humanism*. Boulder: Westview.

Kirby, A. 2009. *Digimodernism: How New Technologies Dismantle the Postmodern and Reconfigure Our Culture*. New York: Continuum.

Mitchell, D. 2002. "Narrative Prosthesis and the Materiality of Metaphor." In *Disability Studies: Enabling the Humanities*, edited by S. L. Snyder, B. J. Brueggemann, and R. Garland-Thomson, 15–30. New York: Modern Language Association of America.

Moon, E. 2002. *Speed of Dark*. London: Orbit.

———. 2003. "Autism: Past, Future, Speculative." *MoonScape: Elizabeth Moon, Science Fiction and Fantasy Writer*. Accessed April 8, 2011, http://www.elizabethmoon.com/autism-general.html.

Mukhopadhyay, T. R. 2000. *Beyond the Silence: My Life, the World, and Autism*. London: National Autistic Society.

Murray, S. 2008. *Representing Autism*. Liverpool, U.K.: Liverpool University Press.

———. 2010. "Autism Functions / The Function of Autism." *Disability Studies Quarterly* 30 (1). Accessed April 4, 2010, http://www.dsq-sds.org/article/view/1048/1229.

Murray, S. J., and D. Holmes, eds. 2009. *Critical Interventions in the Ethics of Health-care: Challenging the Principle of Autonomy in Bioethics.* London: Ashgate.

Offit, P. 2008. *Autism's False Prophets: Bad Science, Risky Medicine, and the Search for a Cure.* New York: Columbia University Press.

O'Neill, J. L. 1998. *Through the Eyes of Aliens: A Book about Autistic People.* London: Kingsley.

Osteen, M., ed. 2008. *Autism and Representation.* New York: Routledge.

———. 2008. "Autism and Representation: A Comprehensive Introduction." In Osteen, *Autism and Representation,* 1–47.

Prince-Hughes, D. 2004. *Songs of the Gorilla Nation: My Journey through Autism.* New York: Harmony.

Sacks, O. 1995. "An Anthropologist on Mars." In *An Anthropologist on Mars: Seven Paradoxical Tales.* New York: Knopf. Originally published in the *New Yorker,* December 27, 1993.

Said, E. W. 2004. *Humanism and Democratic Criticism.* London: Palgrave Macmillan.

Turing, A. M. 1950. "Computing Machinery and Intelligence." *Mind: A Quarterly Review of Psychology and Philosophy* 59: 433–60.

Williams, D. 1992. *Nobody Nowhere: The Extraordinary Autobiography of an Autistic.* New York: Times Books.

World Health Organization. 2009. *ICD-10: International Statistical Classification of Diseases and Related Health Problems.* 10th rev., vol. 1. Geneva: World Health Organization.

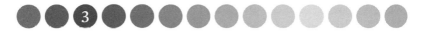

Cerebralizing Autism within the Neurodiversity Movement

Francisco Ortega

We are a world of funny brains, and neuroscience will help us to understand and appreciate the new mix.

—*Larry Welkowitz, creator of the audio post* Asperger's Conversations

Cerebral Subjectivization

The 1990s were officially launched by then–U.S. president George H. W. Bush as the "Decade of the Brain" (Bush 1990), and some believe that the first hundred years of the new millennium will be its century (Dowling 2007). Such gestures support the drive to solve the puzzle of human consciousness and unravel the secrets of an organ described as the most complex of the universe. But proclaiming a decade or a century of the brain also signals the omnipresence of the brain as a major icon of contemporary culture—from literature and the plastic arts to medicine and the human sciences, theology and spirituality, politics and marketing; from emerging research areas such as neuroeconomics, neurotheology, neurolaw, neuropsychoanalysis, or neuroeducation to an expanding universe of neuropractices.

Since the Decade of the Brain, there has been a steady increase in the hybridization of neuroscience with education, marketing, and psychiatry. Coupled with the wide circulation of portrayals of the brain in the media and health literature, popularized versions of neuroscientific "facts" about mental processes, human diversity, and clinical conditions have in this way begun to reach a number of audiences. Recently, several scholars have suggested that the resultant incorporation of neuroscientific language into popular self-understanding reflects the "impact" of neuroscience on society (Illes 2005; Martin 2000, 2007, 2010; Ortega and Vidal 2011; Rees and Rose 2004; Vrecko 2006). This effect has been deemed likely due to the authority of neuroscientific facts in contemporary biomedicalized societies (McCabe and Castel 2008; Weisberg et al. 2008). Much recent research has pointed to a growing "neurorealism," a belief in the truth of the visual images of the brain and, linked to this, an increasing "neuroessentialism," that is, the equation of subjectivity with the brain (Racine 2010).

Contemporary cognitive neuroscience research has been attempting to unravel "brain-based evidence" of hardwired human capacities to make rational choices, understand other minds, and achieve goals. More recently, research in cognitive neuroscience has been characterized by an increasing preoccupation with the study of human differences. Brain-imaging studies, for example, are used to detect structural and functional differences in the brain between genders, cultures, and sexual orientations, and increasingly they strive to differentiate people diagnosed with mental disorders as well (Hyman 2007). With the constant popularization of these theories in the media, and not least the strongly encouraged public-engagement work of neuroscientists and neuroethicists (Illes et al. 2010; Morein-Zamir and Sahakian 2010), individuals find increasing opportunities to come into contact with versions of "brain stories" and to fashion themselves with and through such cerebral vocabularies. Neuroscientific theories, or their popular representations, as a consequence, have begun to be incorporated into people's commonsense ways of understanding themselves and others.

As cognitive neuroscience steps up its focus on neurological distinctions between different "kinds of people," researchers in the social sciences and humanities have begun to investigate the role of neurological vocabulary in the constitution of identities. Metaphors such as the "neurochemical self" (Rose 2007) and the "cerebral subject" (Ehrenberg 2004; Ortega and Vidal 2007, 2011; Vidal 2009) have been used to capture the "anthropological figure" underlying the neuroscientific theories that have diffused into popular culture and that continue to fuel the expanding genres of brain-based practices, technologies, and therapies.[1] When I speak of the "cerebral subject," I do not mean to reify the notion. It obviously differs from the transcendental subject of Kantian philosophy and Husserlian phenomenology, as well as from the subject that, from Descartes to Husserl and beyond, has been understood mainly as self-awareness and self-consciousness. The cerebral subject is an "anthropological figure" that has no reality prior to its performative embodiments (Ortega and Vidal 2011). In other words, the process of subjectivization has ontological preeminence, and that is why, to analyze the cerebral subject, one should focus on its formation and the practices of self-constitution through which individuals fashion themselves in cerebral terms.

This process can be understood as involving "technologies of the self" (Foucault 1988) and the diffusion of expert knowledge in popular culture. "Making up people," as Ian Hacking calls it (2002, 111), involves the creation of descriptive or diagnostic categories through expert knowledge; individuals assimilate these categories into their descriptions and practices of the self, and thereby transform them and bring about realities that experts must in turn confront. Such co-construction of categorical and personal identity is what Hacking has characterized as the "looping effect of human kinds" (1995).

The psychiatric label of autism or Asperger Syndrome affects the persons so labeled and/or their families and caregivers, and potentially changes their behavior and hence the meaning of the label itself. The label has undergone transformations because of changing neurobiological and genetic theories. The looping effect encompasses not only scientific and diagnostic developments but also parent and self-advocacy groups, as well as general images of autism and Asperger Syndrome in popular movies, TV programs, personal testimonials, novels, blogs, and other Internet resources (Murray 2008; Osteen 2008).

Some autistic persons and groups draw on neuroscientific terms and metaphors in their self-definition, in their claims to neurodiversity and to rights and other social compensations, as well as in the practices consistent with those claims. Although autism advocacy and neurodiversity have been the object of several studies,[2] the cerebralization of autistic culture has only recently begun to be examined (Ortega 2009; Brownlow and O'Dell, this volume). The analysis of the cerebralization of autism within the neurodiversity movement intends to contribute to the emerging field of "critical autism studies," which, unlike the individualizing and depoliticizing prevailing deficit narrative of autism, challenges the ways in which we think about notions of diversity, justice, normalcy, and identity and discloses how the negotiation of autistic identities holds important insights concerning the normalcy of (cognitive) difference and the potential for transnational collective action. Contributing to the field of critical autism studies implies not only challenging predominant (degrading and deficit-focused) constructions of autism discourses and subjectivities; criticism within the field of autism studies demands that we critique the so-called critical discourses, as well. It should also reflect on the shortcomings of emancipatory ways of self-fashioning and identity politics within the autistic self-advocacy movement. Although, on the one hand, seeing oneself as neurodiverse (that is, cerebralizing autism) strengthens one's sense of identity and helps erase the social stigma often associated with predominant constructions of autism, it may, on the other hand, solipsistically constrict what it means to be human. The search for new and nonpathologized forms of identity and community stands in tension with reductionist forms of identity politics.

In what follows, I sketch some preliminary insights from ongoing ethnographic research investigating the relationship that people with autism forge with their brains.[3] My aim is to explore the forms of brain-based subjectivization among autistic self-advocates. I also want to challenge the suggestion that neuroscience is transforming the way we understand ourselves. Finally, I would like to call into question the assumption that solipsistic and reductionist ways of being and sociality necessarily result from cerebral descriptions of personhood and community. This has important implications for the emerging field of critical autism studies, because brain-related terms are mobilized by autistic self-advocates to destabilize prevailing (and often degrading) constructions of autism narratives and identities and notions of diversity, justice, and normalcy. If, on the one hand, the cerebralization of autism leads to a search for nonpathologized forms of identity and community, it may, on the other hand, lead to a form of identity politics that narrows important aspects of personhood. Critical autism studies should therefore take account of the possible shortcomings of so-called emancipatory discourse within the autistic self-advocacy movement.

Developing Neurological Identities

Biological bases of mental phenomena are contested for a number of reasons. This is most clearly demonstrated in the case of psychiatric diagnoses. Conflicts around the medical, social, epistemic, and ontological status of mental disorders, as well as discussions about etiology, diagnosis, and therapeutics have been present in the history of psychiatry for the last 150 years (Rosenberg 2002, 2006). Although there is no consensus about many psychiatric disorders, several material and identitarian implications follow from the simple fact of considering a certain physical-mental state as a disease or disorder. Nosological entities— especially psychiatric disorders—need to negotiate their existence as a social fact that provides or withdraws a certain amount of power to the individuals affected by the diagnosis.

Patients and their families, for example, may use a diagnosis as a way of creating self-help groups and/or steering public policies favorable to the research and treatment of diseases.[4] Individuals organize these groups to legitimize health-related issues whose reality may be disputed as uncontested nosological categories, as in the cases of chronic fatigue syndrome (Bülow 2008) and excessive daytime sleepiness (Clarke and Amerom 2007). These constitute what Joseph Dumit has called "illnesses you have to fight to get" (2006). The goals of the "fight" are diverse, ranging from attaining social legitimacy to more concrete objectives, such as obtaining full insurance coverage and other forms of compensation that depend on the acceptance by the specialist's community, the medical establishment, and other stakeholders engaged in the process of determining whether the "disorder" justifies the pleaded reparation. This recognition usually involves the search for a somatic or material cause of the disorder, for "social legitimacy presupposes somatic identity," as historian Charles Rosenberg has observed (2006, 414).

Autism constitutes a psychiatric category exposed to public negotiation by both medical and nonmedical actors (Orsini 2009, Silverman 2008b). The ontological status of autism, a "problematic category" (Rosenberg 2006), is being disputed. For some people it is a disorder, and for others it is an example of the brain's natural diversity. Research about the neurodiversity movement reiterates this heterogeneity. Neurological identities for these people enable the formation of biosocialities, as well as forms of biological citizenship (Brownlow and O'Dell, this volume; Orsini 2009).[5] I use the phrase "neurological identities" (like the phrase "cerebral subject") to draw attention to how people frequently draw upon neuroscientific language to describe themselves and their relation to others. This does not mean they talk of themselves exclusively or self-consciously in this way, but that implicitly or explicitly they draw on vocabulary or metaphors that imply an equivalence between their self-concept and the brain. This may happen as a means for self-understanding and/or as a public rhetoric to gain rights and other compensation, as well as political recognition, given the present prestige of brain discourses and their social pervasiveness. Depending on the context, cerebral vocabularies can be advanced for individuals' self-understanding or for political goals. Frequently, both aspirations are related, and/or autistic people shift from one aim to the other. Yet self-understanding and political goals rely on the notion of the brain as a major cultural icon in contemporary societies.

Analysis of the ways in which people appropriate neuroscientific vocabulary provides insights into the extent to which autistic individuals are being understood, and are understanding themselves, as "kinds of brains" through neurological descriptions. Such neurological categories may contribute to "making up people." These "kinds of people" are frequently identified with "kinds of brains" (Dumit 2003, 2004), whether or not the descriptions are contested or embraced by those defined. In his recent work on autism, Hacking refers to autistics as a "kind of people"—a kind that has historically been medicalized, normalized, and administered—both in antiessentialist terms and as a way that autistics might experience themselves and interact with others (2006, 2007, 2009a, 2009b, 2010a, 2010b). The label of autism or Asperger Syndrome affects the persons so labeled and their families and caretakers, and can potentially modify their behavior. Hacking insists that recent autism activism and the publication of personal testimonies and autistic autobiographies can produce the "looping effect" of deconstructing the trope of the "alien" commonly used in popular culture to refer to the reciprocal relation between autistic people and the neurotypical universe. Autobiographies, blogs, and other resources both help autistic people to understand neurotypical behavior and vice versa.

Autistic Identities

Emerging in the 1990s, the neurodiversity movement was organized with the goal of redefining autism as a human specificity not to be treated but instead to be respected in the same way as other human differences, such as gender, race, and sexuality (Singer 1999). For autistic self-advocates, atypical neurological wiring forms the basis of these differences and the construction of an identity. By drawing on neuroscientific language and metaphors, several self-advocates construe autism as a positive attribute, emphasizing the natural differences from nonautistic, or "neurotypical" (NT), people and their brains.

Although some autistics do not see their condition as a pervading part of their selves (Brownlow 2007), others argue that it is "pervasive, it colors every experience, every sensation, perception, thought, emotion, and encounter, every aspect of existence" (Sinclair 1993). These latter people emphasize the positively constitutive function of the category of autism by calling themselves "autistics" or "aspies"; autism thus appears as an integral part of their identity (Silverman 2008a, 2008b). For example, autism-rights activist Jim Sinclair explains that the expression "person with autism"—compared with "autistic person," where autism is an integral part of personhood—suggests that autism "is something had—so bad," he says, "that it isn't even consistent with being a person" (1999). Michelle Dawson comments that characterizing someone as a "person with autism" is as inadequate as defining a woman as a "person with femaleness" (quoted in Harmon 2004).

Among such neurodiversity advocates, autistic identity is a source of pride; some go as far as seeing it as a "gift" (Antonetta 2005). Whatever the exact worth attributed to autistic identity, the diagnosis tends to bring comfort: "Finally an explanation," said a man diagnosed at age thirty-six, "finally a sense of why and how" (quoted in Shapiro 2006). Ian Hacking has noted that "many misfit adults now recognize themselves as autistics, or so they say. It really helps to be able to put a label to your oddities. It brings a kind of peace: so that is what I am" (2006). Judy Singer, who is widely credited with having coined the term *neurodiversity* in 1999, expounds on the "benefits of a clear identity" (62), and self-advocate Jane Meyerding describes the advantages of adopting autism as an explanatory system; the labeling, she explains, generates "signposts" and "shorthands" that help autistics position themselves with respect to the surrounding culture (2003).

One function of embracing the vocabulary of the brain, what Singer described as "neurological self-awareness" (1999), is to remove the stigmatizing weight of psychotherapeutic discourses on autism. Turning to the brain-based explanation as an alternative, however, does not lead to the adoption of the deficit model underlying the neurocognitive theories such as "mindblindness" (Baron-Cohen 1995), "weak central coherence" (Pellicano et al. 2006), and "executive dysfunction" (Hill 2004). Rather, autistic self-advocates draw on these theories involving the brain (often imprecisely) to substantiate the notion of a natural difference instead of evidence for pathology.

The neurologization of one's condition deflects attention from subjective, contextual, and interpersonal processes (Luhrmann 2000). In the predominant diathesis-stress model, such processes are involved in the onset and course of the disease; but the ultimate cause is in the brain. This may have positive consequences. Talking about her own experience of manic depression, anthropologist Emily Martin remembers, "I often heard from my psychiatrist that my problem was related to my neurotransmitters, and I always found this comforting" (2007, 13). It seems, as Martin observes, that "if something is in the mind, it can be controlled and mastered, and a person who fails to do so is morally at fault" (8). Thus, the intrinsic innocence of the body powerfully contributes to elevating neurodiversity to the rank of value.

This value works beyond the individual level. Lawrence Kirmayer has described how objectifying distress and shifting it away from interpersonal concerns displace it toward a realm of impersonal causes (1988, 72). Yet biological explanations also facilitate new ways of bringing together patients, families, and scientists (Gibbon and Novas 2008; Rose 2007); etiological impersonality becomes the ground for the establishment of communities of people who see themselves as autistics (rather than as having autism) because their brains are "wired" in a certain way. At work here is what Ian Hacking has described as "labeling from below" (1995, 2002). The neurologization of autism opens the way to redefining the condition in terms of cerebral *difference*. But it is important to remember, again, that this emphasis on the brain is shared by the parents, families, and doctors, who see the patients in their care as suffering from a terrible disease rather than benefiting from a different neural wiring. It is not that those patients aren't perceived as different, but that the difference is pathological and therefore lacks the positive valence of diversity.

Pro- and antineurodiversity advocates share the view that autism is a neurological condition. From the point of view of assessing the condition as positive or negative, its neurological nature is secondary. In contrast, for neurodiversity activists, the prestige of the neurosciences helps support their positive judgment about their condition; neuroscientific research, largely taking the form of the "wiring" metaphor, seems to legitimize their attitudes toward their diagnosis.

Neurodiversity and the Politics of Neurological Differences

Whether superficial or well informed, neurodiversity advocates' engagement with the neurosciences has become a major vehicle for fashioning their personal identity. Self-advocates draw on neuroscientific terms and metaphors to describe themselves and their relation to others, as well as to establish a venue for securing social rights and gaining political recognition. The process began about fifteen years ago. In her emblematically entitled "Thoughts on Finding Myself Differently Brained" (1998), Meyerding relates how she was "surprised" to find herself "moving into the realm of neurology." Now, as a growing corpus of social science research has been showing, the move into the realm of neurology was largely embodied by movement into the blogosphere (Miller and Slater 2000; Wilson and Peterson 2002). The phenomenon is not restricted to autism and neurodiversity but concerns other groups as well, including deaf and blind bloggers (Goggin and Newell 2003; Goggin and Noonan 2006). Nonetheless, autistic blogs, chats, and Web sites stand out for the place they give to the neurosciences, or at least to a way of speaking saturated with "neuro" terminology, in connection with the development of a positive sense of identity.

Muskie, creator of a satirical Web site called Institute for the Study of the Neurologically Typical, writes, "My brain is a jewel," and he considers his "experience of life" possibly superior to that of neurotypical persons. "I love the way my brain works," declares another writer. "I always have and it's one of the things I can now admit to myself. . . . No, I am not changing anything" (quoted in Shapiro 2006). Meyerding reports that her boss and friends "think they have conveyed what it is they expect me to do, but they have been speaking in a language my brain doesn't understand" (1998).

Note how these testimonies slide without warning from "my brain" to "I" and "me": "I love the way my brain works"; "those people speak to me in ways my brain doesn't understand." Individuals are brains, and brains are personified. The creator of the audio post *Asperger's Conversations* says that "we're a world of funny brains" and that "neuroscience will help us to understand and appreciate the new mix" (Welkowitz 2009). Another self-advocate speaks of repeating a test "when my brain is working better" and comments, "It can be hard when my brain is hating me and I'm struggling to keep calm" (Matzk 2008). One could give many other examples of this kind of language, which suggests that the elevation of neurodiversity to the rank of value presupposes that we are essentially our brains. But we need to ask what this identification of self and brain means and how it works.

Sometimes "brain" and "mind" are interchangeable. Muskie simply juxtaposes "My brain is a jewel" with "I am in awe of the mind that I have" (2002). He is obviously talking about the same thing. The brain sometimes stands metonymically for the person or "I," as when self-advocates write "my brain doesn't understand" or refer to "whatever phrase th[e] non-voluntary portion of my brain happens to be using" (Meyerding 1998) or claim "we are a world of funny brains." On other occasions, the state of the brain represents a state or way of being, in particular an emotional one: sometimes I hate my brain or my brain hates me—but that seems to mean that the brain hates itself; when my brain is said to feel "all sluggish and blocked" (Matzk 2008), it's really *I* who feel that way. Of course, the brain is also the agent of more cognitive experiences, such as when it is not "working right" or makes "weird associations."

Neuroscience serves to justify and naturalize differences. One self-advocate writes, "I know they are all individuals, and that we shouldn't blame every NT for the action of every other NT . . . but there is a common thread that ties them together and it is at the core of their being. It is more than cultural; it is how they are hardwired from the factory" (quoted in Brownlow and O'Dell 2006, 319). Similarly, Meyerding wonders, "If I could understand my life for the first time only by understanding how my brain was different from the majority of brains, how much did I really have in common with all those neurotypicals out there, compared to whom I'd been judged inadequate so many times? . . . Most of the ways I'm different from the neural norm can be disguised as eccentricities" (1998).

Brain metaphors and differences are frequently mobilized to construct autism in a positive light, whereas neurotypicals are largely depicted in negative terms. Both groups, however, believe in the "neurological origins of [their] exclusiveness" (Brownlow 2007, 138; Brownlow and O'Dell 2006, 319). At the same time that differences are naturalized, some autistic people believe that people with autism are less constrained by their biology than NTs are. Neurotypicals' genetic makeup determines their identity and lifestyle (Brownlow and O'Dell, this volume). They want to have the benefits of a clear and objective identity (biologically grounded) without paying the toll of weak or strong essentialism. Autism cannot be both a "natural" difference and one that is not (or is less) biologically constrained. Biology (and neurology) constrains everybody in the same way, not some people more than others.

Neurology thus functions as an instrument with which to erect identity frontiers. By a largely rhetorical reversal of the normalcy discourse, autistics may stress neurotypicals' strange behavior and satirically pathologize neurotypicality. Once he realized "how bizarre and illogical the NTs really are," self-advocate Archie found "that their comments and insults" had a greatly reduced effect; he could not "blame the people that are afflicted with neurotypicality," but, he remarked, "that does not mean that I am obligated to change my views to see values in traits I dislike" (quoted in Brownlow 2007, 140–41). Neuroscientific claims are mobilized in the construction of NT and autistic experiences so as to highlight their natural difference, yet at the same time even extreme self-advocates know how inextricably they are linked to the NT world. It would not be feasible, for example, to keep the utopian island of Aspergia free from NTs, as somebody in the Internet forum of Aspies for Freedom suggested: "If an aspergian man and woman get married and have an NT child would we have to kick it out of the country?" (Anonymous 2006).

The counterpart of the construction of identity differences based on neurological divergence is the belief in a certain ontological homogeneity. Although autism is considered a spectrum, some neurodiversity activists reject the distinction between its low- and high-functioning forms and consider differences across autistic populations as variations of degree not due to fundamental "underlying neurological differences" (Nadesan 2005, 208–9). In 2002, Meyerding explained that, since publishing her well-known 1998 essay "Thoughts on Finding Myself Differently Brained," she had "come to believe that the categorization of people into separate boxes labeled 'Asperger Syndrome' and 'autism' (or 'high-functioning autism') is seriously misleading"; she now prefers to identify herself "as autistic, period." Based on ethnographic research with online discussion groups, Brownlow and O'Dell (this volume) have identified two complementary strategies to counter the rhetoric of the ontological homogeneity of the neurotypical/Asperger binary. One relies on the "autistic cousins" group identity, which encompasses people with

different diagnoses as well as friends of autistics. The other advances the
notion of a neurodiverse spectrum, which includes everybody—autistic
and nonautistic people—within the continuum of human functioning,
thereby defying assumed notions of normalcy and pathology. The latter
fits discourses around biological citizenship, enabling a more heterogeneous view of autism and autism-related politics than the neurotypical/
Asperger binary. I deeply sympathize with Brownlow and O'Dell's pluralistic view of autistic identity formation and political organization.
I fully agree that autistic people navigate between different identity
positions, choosing which one is more appropriate for their particular
situations. Furthermore, I believe that assessing autism as a neurodiverse spectrum rather than a neurological difference can help to avoid
some pitfalls of identity politics to which I refer in the next section.
Yet, as Brownlow and O'Dell acknowledge, not only is the homogeneous
view dominant but also autistic activists are frequently confronted with
claims of not being "autistic enough." This is particularly important in a
context where parent and professional groups accuse activists of speaking in the name of all autistics, negating thereby cognitive and emotional differences along the autism spectrum. Against this framework,
ontological and neurological homogeneity has a deep political meaning.

Ontological homogeneity, however, is, to a large extent, a linguistic
effect, an impression that results from what we can read and hear both
online and off-line. The world of autistic self-advocacy shows the same
phenomenon Emily Martin observed during her fieldwork on bipolar disorder: remarks about the brain seemed to her "like clones: endlessly rep-
licating but not generating new connections" (2009, 7). The brain works
like a "confining metaphor" (Martin 2009, 2010) that cuts off links among
domains and groups of people. Yet the brain-centered vocabulary—a
"folk neurology" (Vrecko 2006) or a "folk neuropsychology" (Rodriguez
2006)—has not replaced psychological descriptions of subjective experiences. No amount of neuroscientific progress can make the mind go
away (Martin 2000).

It is perhaps this uniformity and redundancy that facilitates what I
characterize as a cohabitation of everyday ontologies. People shift registers, and, as we have seen, "my brain" may serve to designate "my mind"
or, perhaps more precisely, just "I" or "me." Presumably, this doesn't
mean that people are sloppy and say "brain" when they mean "mind."
Rather, the metaphors and metonymies express a more or less harmo-

nious coexistence of views and practices of the self, while at the same time contributing to give a bodily organ—the brain—the kind of depth usually, or formerly, attributed to the psyche.

Identity Politics and the "Neuroscience Revolution": A Challenge for Critical Autism Studies

Disability-studies scholars have noted that the celebration of disability has sometimes come together with an emphasis on differentiating comparisons and even hostility toward nondisabled people (Swain and Cameron 1999). Tom Shakespeare has highlighted the dangers of building an identity on victimhood and oppression resulting from the politics of disability identity. The victim position implied in both the medical and the social models of disability—people are victims of either their flawed bodies and brains or an oppressive society—denies the agency of disabled people as well as a positive engagement with their impairment and society. An identity politics fueled by the ideology of victimhood leads to "exaggerating the differences and the polarity between the minority group and the mainstream," resulting in a politics that is "more extreme, separatist, vanguardist and aggressive" (2006, 80).

For autistic self-advocates, the homogenization within the spectrum of autism constitutes an important political move that would counter the critiques of several parent and professional groups, who accuse them of speaking in the name of all autistics (Harmon 2004; Orsini 2009; Silverman 2008b). In this context, identity politics embodies the typologizing of brain difference at the expense of autistics' own individual differences and the emphasis on neurological uniqueness. Hence, neurological explanations are mobilized to erect identity frontiers and naturalize differences between autistic and NT populations, while differences across autistic populations are downplayed and neurotypical forms of life and experience criticized. It would be disingenuous to subsume all forms of the autistic spectrum under the "high-functioning" label or to claim that "if [autism] is mild, moderate or severe, it is still autism" (O'Neill 1999, 83) and then argue that autism is a lifestyle.[6] Autistic identity politics seems to ignore the common adage that states, "If you know about one autistic person, you know about one autistic person" (Hacking 2009b, 46; 2010b, 265), and paradoxically reinforces biomedical discourses, which treat autism as a kind of mind and/or brain and speak about "the" autistic child or "the" autistic mind. Thus, autistic identity politics constitutes the opposite trend to Hacking's reflections on autism. The former draws on neurology to justify and naturalize differences between autistics and neurotypicals, precluding intragroup differences. On the contrary, Hacking's "narrative" approach draws on self-testimonies and autobiographies to establish a bridge between autistic and neurotypical populations (and to dismantle the "alien" trope used by both autistics and NTs to refer to each other) and to stress the radical heterogeneity within the autistic population (2009a, 1472; 2009b, 56; 2010b, 275–76).

"Alien" metaphors used to describe the cultural gulf between autistics and NTs (Hacking 2009b) emphasize their mutual "otherness." However, as Susan Wendell stresses, to be the "other" or the "alien" has more implications—from emotional and institutional to clinical and political—for disabled than for nondisabled people (1996). Attempts to satirize NT behavior can easily be ignored by the majority of the NT population, whereas predominant degrading and pathologizing constructions of autism as the "other" of neurotypicality or the "alien" have further consequences for autistic people. Like other individuals regarded as "other," disabled people—including autistic people—frequently suffer different forms of sexual, verbal, and/or physical abuse. Otherness tends to make those people invisible. Their struggles, feelings, and aspirations are excluded from the mainstream understanding of human experience. Moreover, otherness not only is maintained by culture but also limits culture in a profound way. The cultural gulf "deprives the non-disabled of the knowledge and perspectives that people with disabilities could contribute to culture, including knowledge of how to live well with physical and mental limitations and suffering" (Wendell 1996, 65).

The neurodiversity movement is beginning to question itself, however. For instance, Jim Sinclair has condemned anti-NT prejudice (2005), and some commentators with Asperger Syndrome consider Aspergia an "Aspie 'Warsaw ghetto'" (Anonymous 2007). Judy Singer herself has recently warned that the movement is walking on the "dark side" of identity politics through "its eternal victimhood, its infantilism, its demand for unconditional love and acceptance without concomitant adult self-reflection, self-criticism, a measure of stoicism, and a willingness to see light and dark in oneself as well as in 'the Other'" (2007).

Singer thus suggests that self-advocates' use of brain-related terms has contributed to concealing important individual and institutional dimensions. The brain is a "confining metaphor" not open to other domains. Brain identity tends to hide conflicts, denial, repressions, and other uncomfortable processes going on consciously or unconsciously. In her description of a research participant, Ben, and his "construction of a positive autistic identity," Nancy Bagatell observed that the task of orchestrating the different discourses around him produced "a lot of discomfort—depression, anxiety and sensory overload—and he desperately wanted relief" (2007, 423). One of the persons diagnosed with bipolar disorder interviewed by Emily Martin remarked that his "brain contains both health and illness, strength and weakness, darkness and light" (2010, 371). These identitarian ambivalences are frequently ignored by radical activists within the disability movement and dismissed as internalized oppression or false consciousness (Shakespeare 2006). "Passing" is the expression used to describe those who hide their impairments or do not want to "come out" as disabled or autistic. This perspective ignores the complexities involved in identity constitution, the management of disclosure, and the complex process of coming out. Yet several scholars acknowledge that although coming out can be an important political and strategic process, it can also be a source of anxiety and discomfort (Bagatell 2007; Davidson and Henderson 2010). As Simi Linton writes, "Both passing and overcoming take their toll" (2010, 230).

By cerebralizing their condition, autistic self-advocates neglect the fact that "not all is for the best in this brave new world that the 'neuroscience revolution' delineates" (Singer 2007). Also, some people in the antipsychiatry movement "fear that the neurodiversity movement too readily embraces a neurological and medical model for all human behavior" (Zifendorf 2005). If, on the one hand, seeing oneself as neurodiverse bolsters one's self-esteem and helps erase the social stigma often associated with mental pathology, it may, on the other hand, somewhat solipsistically narrow the notion of what it is to be a person. To focus narrowly on relations with people sharing the same condition (autism or other disability) excludes or limits other important domains of human sociality that constitute our daily lives. Human identity is being constantly created and re-created through interaction with other individuals. It is formed by an enormous variety of beliefs, traits, and positions, the "shifting articulation of all these disparate elements or 'subject positions' which combine in various ways, occasionally and transiently under the direction of one particular dominant element, but other times without any particular hierarchy" (Douzinas and Gearey 2005, 194–95). It is important to listen to those who disagree with generalizations made by members of one particular category about the experiences of all members of that category (Wendell 1996). Thus, even if for some people autism or another disability defines who they are, for others that condition might be just a part (and not an important part) of their lives. As Susan Whyte reminds us, "It is, after all, a life and not an identity that people are usually seeking" (2009, 13).

Identity politics promotes identification with one condition or life aspect, "a single, drastically simplified group-identity which denies the complexity of people's lives, the multiplicity of their identifications and the cross-pulls of their various affiliations." It also hides intragroup struggles, reinforces intragroup domination, and "lends itself all too easily to repressive forms of communitarianism, promoting conformism, intolerance and patriarchalism" (Fraser 2000, 112).

Yet how can autistic people struggle against an oppression based on the category of autism without using the very same category and organizing themselves around it? "Is it possible to use a collective identity, preserve the differences we value, and undermine our 'Otherness' too?" (Wendell 1996, 76). Would the preservation of each member's singularity weaken the collective struggle? Such a "community of singularities" (Agamben 1993) would avoid the pitfalls associated with identitarian struggles. Yet would it help to pursue collective goals of improving access, accommodations, and social acceptance for autistic individuals, as well as to challenge predominant, degrading narratives of autism, which currently influence public opinion, policy, and popular culture? Anti-identity-politics approaches to autism such as Hacking's narrative approach can be more useful to this end than an identity politics that mobilizes brain metaphors to erect and naturalize identity frontiers, stressing the radical heterogeneity of autistic and nonautistic people and contributing to their mutual otherness and alien feelings.

In this chapter, I have tried to contribute to the burgeoning field of critical autism studies by analyzing the relationship between autistic people and their brains. I explored how a brain-related vocabulary has been mobilized by autistic self-advocates to deconstruct prevailing narratives of autism that are deficit-focused. I challenged the idea shared by several neuroethicists that neuroscience is radically transforming our notions of personhood and community. On the one hand, there is a cohabitation of everyday ontologies among autistic self-advocates. Individuals shift ontological registers, expressing a coexistence of views and practices of the self. Sometimes they draw on a more psychological, sometimes on a more neurological vocabulary to talk about themselves and their relation to others. The use of a brain-centered vocabulary does not make the mind go away, and people do not really believe they *are* their brains, or not *just* their brains. On the other hand, as ongoing ethnographic research on the neurodiversity movement shows (Brownlow 2007; Brownlow and O'Dell 2006; Brownlow and O'Dell, this volume; Ortega 2009), solipsistic and reductionist ways of being and sociality do not necessarily result from cerebral descriptions of personhood and community.

These seem to be the central dilemmas and debates of the neurodiversity movement and an important challenge for the exciting new field of "critical autism studies." Criticism must deconstruct degrading narratives of autism, but it must also examine the emancipatory discourses and practices sustained by autistic people themselves. Autistic self-advocates' search for community is in tension with its own reductionist identity politics, in which selves result from the mechanics of the brain. It seems that neurodiversity can be sustained as a value only when it becomes embodied in a community; but the community works in ways that obviously go beyond the functioning of isolated individual brains and exceeds the limits set by the concept of neurodiversity itself. Being "critical" in the framework of critical autism studies implies being aware of this paradox, its strengths and shortcomings, and being attentive to the fact that metaphors are never innocent and brain metaphors even less so.

NOTES

1. The use of the phrase "anthropological figure," when related to the "cerebral subject," does not intend to rehabilitate some form of anthropological philosophy and draw on a notion of essence, or universal and ahistorical human nature. Rather, it designates the processes of individuation and subjectivization in certain sociohistorical contexts, and does not exclude the cohabitation of different anthropological figures: cerebral selves, psychological selves, neurochemical selves, and others. In this sense, the cerebral subject as an anthropological figure of

our contemporary biomedicalized societies constitutes a radicalization of modern Western forms of constitution of naturalized and singularized individuals, as have been analyzed by Louis Dumont (1986), Michel Foucault (1978, 1985, 1986, 1988), Charles Taylor (1989), Norbert Elias (1969, 1982), and Alan McFarlane (1992), among others.

2. See, among others, Brownlow and O'Dell (2006); Chamak (2008); Davidson (2008); Davidson and Henderson (2010); Orsini (2009); Orsini and Smith (2010); Silverman (2008b); Sinclair (1993, 1999, 2005); and Solomon (2008).

3. Data pertaining to autistic people were gathered from published qualitative research dealing with autism in cyberspace, writings by autistic people, personal blogs of people diagnosed, and several discussion lists on the Internet, mainly in the United States, Canada, the United Kingdom, and Australia. I drew, as well, on personal blogs and Web pages of vocal autistic self-advocates, such as Jane Meyerding. Because they have higher media and public visibility and the potential of influencing other autistic persons, I wanted to see to what degree well-known autistic activists favored brain discourse to describe themselves and their relation with other autistic and nonautistic individuals and to claim rights and other forms of compensation. I also quoted from discussion lists of Aspies for Freedom and other Web sites related to the neurodiversity movement. Statements in which the topic of autistic identity was linked to the use of brain-related vocabulary were favored, drawing directly on the topics of autistic identity and neurodiversity (see Ortega 2009). A very different empirical research would be necessary to consider to what degree less-politicized autistic individuals also favor brain discourses. Given the visibility of the vocal self-advocates as well as the prestige of neuroscience in our societies, one can assume that brain discourses are widely incorporated in the self-understanding of autistic people with no political agenda. One example is the present currency of the term *neurotypical*.

4. The literature about patient groups and the health movement is enormous and increasing. For a recent overview, see Epstein (2008). See also Orsini (2008, 2009); and Orsini and Smith (2010).

5. Paul Rabinow coined the term *biosociality* to analyze the sociocultural and political implications of genetics and particularly of the Human Genome Project (1996). The term has been widely used in recent years to describe different forms of identity constitution and social practices that have genetics as a reference (Gibbon and Novas 2008). I agree with Scott Vrecko, who has argued that the concept of biosociality is generally used to refer to patient advocacy, identity, and activism, neglecting other social transformations arising from the new biosciences (2010, 220). I use the term to stress different processes of biological and somatic subjectivization and forms of sociality that are present in our contemporary biomedical societies, including neurological identities and socialities.

6. Here one should not confound two different issues. It is one thing to state that autistic categories and diagnostic labels are changing, problematic, or degrading for autistic people. Hence, Amanda Baggs rightly observes, "I don't fit the stereotype of autism. But who does? . . . The definition of autism is so fluid and changing every few years" (quoted in Davidson and Henderson 2010). It is another thing to infer from the first issue that differences across autistic populations do

not exist, and to declare autism as an alternative form of life, thereby negating the reality and suffering imposed by the impairment on individuals diagnosed and their families (Hodge 2005).

REFERENCES

Agamben, G. 1993. *The Coming Community*. Minneapolis: University of Minnesota Press.

Anonymous. 2006. "What I Think of the Aspergia Ideas," December 15. Aspies for Freedom. Accessed April 30, 2013, http://www.aspiesforfreedom.com/showthread.php?tid=5698.

———. 2007. "RE: Neuro City," November 17. Aspies for Freedom. Accessed July 12, 2013, http://www.aspiesforfreedom.com/showthread.php?tid 11062.

Antonetta, S. 2005. *A Mind Apart: Travels in a Neurodiverse World*. London: Penguin.

Bagatell, N. 2007. "Orchestrating Voices: Autism, Identity, and the Power of Discourse." *Disability and Society* 22 (4): 413–26.

Baron Cohen, S. 1995. *Mindblindness: An Essay on Autism and Theory of Mind*. Boston: MIT Press / Bradford Books.

Brownlow, C. 2007. "The Construction of the Autistic Individual: Investigations in Online Discussion Groups." PhD diss., University of Brighton.

Brownlow, C., and L. O'Dell. 2006. "Constructing an Autistic Identity: AS Voices Online." *Mental Retardation: A Journal of Practices, Policy, and Perspectives* 44 (5): 315–21.

Bülow, P. H. 2008. "Tracing Contours of Contestation in Narratives about Chronic Fatigue Syndrome." In Moss and Teghtsoonian, *Contesting Illness*, 123–41.

Bush, George H. W. 1990. Proclamation No. 6158, July 17. *Project on the Decade of the Brain*. Library of Congress. Accessed March 26, 2013, http://www.loc.gov/loc/brain/proclaim.html.

Chamak, B. 2008. "Autism and Social Movements: French Parents' Associations and International Autistic Individuals' Organizations." *Sociology of Health and Illness* 30 (1): 76–96.

Clarke, J., and G. van Amerom. 2007. "'Surplus Suffering': Differences between Organizational Understandings of Asperger's Syndrome and Those People Who Claim the 'Disorder.'" *Disability and Society* 22 (7): 761–76.

Corker, M., and S. French, eds. 1999. *Disability Discourse*. Buckingham, U.K.: Open University Press.

Davidson, J. 2008. "Autistic Culture Online: Virtual Communication and Cultural Expression on the Spectrum." *Social and Cultural Geography* 9 (7): 791–806.

Davidson, J., and V. L. Henderson. 2010. "'Coming Out' on the Spectrum: Autism, Identity, and Disclosure." *Social and Cultural Geography* 11 (2): 155–70.

Douzinas, C., and A. Gearey. 2005. *Critical Jurisprudence: The Political Philosophy of Justice*. Oxford: Hart.

Dowling, J. E. 2007. *The Great Brain Debate: Nature or Nurture?* Princeton, N.J.: Princeton University Press.

Dumit, J. 2003. "Is It Me or My Brain? Depression and Neuroscientific Facts." *Journal of Medical Humanities* 24 (1–2): 35–48.

———. 2004. *Picturing Personhood: Brain Scans and Biomedical Identity.* Princeton, N.J.: Princeton University Press.

———. 2006. "Illnesses You Have to Fight to Get: Facts as Forces in Uncertain, Emergent Illnesses." *Social Science and Medicine* 62 (3): 577–90.

Dumont, L. 1986. *Essays on Individualism: Modern Ideology in Anthropological Perspective.* Chicago: University of Chicago Press.

Ehrenberg, A. 2004. "Le Sujet Cerebral." *Esprit,* November 2004.

Elias, N. 1969. *The Civilizing Process.* Vol. 1, *The History of Manners.* Oxford: Blackwell.

———. 1982. *The Civilizing Process.* Vol. 2, *State Formation and Civilization.* Oxford: Blackwell.

Epstein, S. 2008. "Patient Groups and Health Movements." In *The Handbook of Science and Technology Studies,* edited by E. J. Hackett et al., 3rd ed., 499–539. Cambridge, Mass.: MIT Press.

Foucault, M. 1978. *The History of Sexuality: An Introduction.* Translated by Robert Hurley. Harmondsworth, U.K.: Penguin.

———. 1985. *The Use of Pleasure.* Translated by Robert Hurley. Harmondsworth, U.K.: Penguin.

———. 1986. *The Care of the Self.* Translated by Robert Hurley. Harmondsworth, U.K.: Penguin.

———. 1988. "Technologies of the Self." In *Technologies of the Self,* edited by L. H. Martin, H. Gutman, and P. H. Hutton, 16–49. Amherst: University of Massachusetts Press.

Fraser, N. 2000. "Rethinking Recognition." *New Left Review* 3 (May–June): 107–20.

Gibbon, S., and C. Novas, eds. 2008. *Biosocialities, Genetics, and the Social Sciences.* London: Routledge.

Goggin, G., and C. Newell. 2003. *Digital Disability: The Social Construction of Disability in New Media.* Lanham, Md.: Rowman & Littlefield.

Goggin, G., and T. Noonan. 2006. "Blogging Disability: The Interface between New Cultural Movements and Internet Technology." In *Uses of Blogs,* edited by A. Bruns and J. Jacobs, 161–72. New York: Lang.

Hacking, I. 1995. "The Looping Effects of Human Kinds." In *Causal Cognition: A Multidisciplinary Approach,* edited by D. Sperber, D. Premack, and A. James-Premack, 351–83. Oxford: Clarendon.

———. 2002. "Making Up People." In *Historical Ontology,* 99–114. Cambridge, Mass.: Harvard University Press.

———. 2006. "What Is Tom Saying to Maureen?" *London Review of Books,* May 11. Accessed May 2007, http://www.lrb.co.uk/v28/n09/hack01_.html.

———. 2007. "Kinds of People: Moving Targets." *Proceedings of the British Academy* 151: 285–318.

———. 2009a. "Autistic Autobiography." *Philosophical Transactions of the Royal Society B.* 364 (1522): 1467–73.

———. 2009b. "Humans, Aliens, and Autism." *Daedalus* 138 (3): 44–59.

———. 2010a. "Autism Fiction: A Mirror of an Internet Decade?" *University of Toronto Quarterly* 79 (2): 632–55.

———. 2010b. "How We Have Been Learning to Talk about Autism." In *Cognitive Disability and Its Challenge to Moral Philosophy,* edited by E. F. Kittay and L. Carson, 261–78. Chichester, U.K.: Wiley-Blackwell.

Harmon, A. 2004. "How about Not 'Curing' Us, Some Autistics Are Pleading." *New York Times*, December 20.

Hill, E. L. 2004. "Executive Dysfunction in Autism." *Trends in Cognitive Science* 8 (1): 26–32.

Hodge, N. 2005. "Reflections on Diagnosing Autism Spectrum Disorders." *Disability and Society* 20 (3): 345–49.

Hyman, S. E. 2007. "Can Neuroscience Be Integrated into the DSM-V?" *Nature Reviews Neuroscience* 8 (9): 725–32.

Illes, J., ed. 2005. *Neuroethics: Defining the Issues in Theory, Practice, and Policy.* Oxford: Oxford University Press.

Illes, J., et al. 2010. "Neurotalk: Improving the Communication of Neuroscience Research." *Nature Reviews Neuroscience* 11 (2): 61–69.

Kirmayer, L. 1988. "Mind and Body as Metaphors: Hidden Values in Biomedicine." In *Biomedicine Examined*, edited by M. Lock and D. Gordon, 57–93. London: Kluwer Academic.

Linton, S. 2010. "Reassigning Meaning." In *The Disability Studies Reader*, edited by L. J. Davis, 3rd ed., 223–36. New York: Routledge.

Luhrmann, T. 2000. *Of Two Minds: The Growing Disorder in American Psychiatry.* New York: Knopf.

Martin, E. 2000. "Mind–Body Problems." *American Ethnologist* 27 (3): 569–90.

———. 2007. *Bipolar Expeditions: Mania and Depression in American Culture.* Princeton, N.J.: Princeton University Press.

———. 2009. "Identity, Identification, and the Brain." Paper presented at the workshop "Neurocultures," Max Planck Institute for the History of Science, Berlin.

———. 2010. "Self Making and the Brain." *Subjectivity* 3 (4): 366–81.

Matzk, D. 2008. *Danni's Blog*, December 12. Accessed April 30, 2013, http://dannimatzk.co.uk/.

McCabe, D. P., and A. D. Castel. 2008. "Seeing Is Believing: The Effect of Brain Images on Judgments of Scientific Reasoning." *Cognition* 107 (1): 343–52.

McFarlane, A. 1992. "On Individualism." *Proceedings of the British Academy* 82: 171–99.

Meyerding, J. 1998. "Thoughts on Finding Myself Differently Brained." Personal blog. Accessed March 26, 2013, http://www.planetautism.com/jane/diff.html. Prefatory note added in 2002.

———. 2003. "The Great 'Why Label?' Debate." Personal blog. Accessed March 26, 2013, http://www.planetautism.com/jane/label.html.

Miller, D., and D. Slater. 2000. *The Internet: An Ethnographic Approach.* Oxford: Berg.

Morein-Zamir, S., and B. J. Sahakian. 2010. "Neuroethics and Public Engagement Training Needed for Neuroscientists." *Trends in Cognitive Sciences* 14 (2): 49–51.

Moss, P., and Teghtsoonian, K., eds. 2008. *Contesting Illness: Processes and Practices.* Toronto, Ont.: University of Toronto Press.

Murray, S. 2008. *Representing Autism: Culture, Narrative, Fascination.* Liverpool, U.K.: University of Liverpool Press.

Muskie. 2002. "About This Site," March 18. Institute for the Study of the Neurologically Typical. Accessed July 12, 2013, http://isnt.autistics.org/.

Nadesan, M. 2005. *Constructing Autism: Unravelling the "Truth" and Understanding the Social.* London: Routledge.

O'Neill, J. L. 1999. *Through the Eyes of Aliens: A Book about Autistic People.* London: Kingsley.

Orsini, M. 2008. "Hepatitis C and the Dawn of Biological Citizenship: Unravelling the Policy Implications." In Moss and Teghtsoonian, *Contesting Illness,* 107–22.

———. 2009. "Contesting the Autistic Subject: Biological Citizenship and the Autism/Autistic Movement." In *Critical Interventions in the Ethics of Health Care,* edited by S. Murray and D. Holmes, 115–30. London: Ashgate.

Orsini, M., and M. Smith. 2010. "Social Movements, Knowledge, and Public Policy: The Case of Autism Activism in Canada and the US." *Critical Policy Studies* 4 (1): 38–57.

Ortega, F. 2009. "The Cerebral Subject and the Challenge of Neurodiversity." *BioSocieties* 4 (4): 425–45.

Ortega, F., and F. Vidal. 2007. "Mapping the Cerebral Subject in Contemporary Culture." *RECIIS—Electronic Journal of Communication Information and Innovation in Health* 2 (1): 255–59.

———, eds. 2011. *Neurocultures: Glimpses into an Expanding Universe.* Frankfurt, Ger.: Lang.

Osteen, M., ed. 2008. *Autism and Representation.* London: Routledge.

Pellicano, E., et al. 2006. "Multiple Cognitive Capabilities/Deficits in Children with an Autism Spectrum Disorder: 'Weak' Central Coherence and Its Relationship to Theory of Mind and Executive Control." *Development and Psychopathology* 18 (1): 77–98.

Rabinow, P. 1996. "Artificiality and Enlightenment: From Sociobiology to Biosociality." In *Essays on the Anthropology of Reason,* 91–111. Princeton, N.J.: Princeton University Press.

Racine, E. 2010. *Pragmatic Neuroethics: Improving Treatment and Understanding of the Mind-Brain.* Cambridge, Mass.: MIT Press.

Rees, D., and S. Rose, eds. 2004. *The New Brain Sciences: Perils and Prospects.* Cambridge: Cambridge University Press.

Rodriguez, P. 2006. "Talking Brains: A Cognitive Semantic Analysis of an Emerging Folk Neuropsychology." *Public Understanding of Science* 15 (3): 301–30.

Rose, N. 2007. *The Politics of Life Itself: Biomedicine, Power, and Subjectivity in the Twenty-First Century.* Princeton, N.J.: Princeton University Press.

Rosenberg, C. E. 2002. "The Tyranny of Diagnosis: Specific Entities and Individual Experience." *Milbank Quarterly* 80 (2): 237–60.

———. 2006. "Contested Boundaries: Psychiatry, Disease, and Diagnosis." *Perspectives in Biology and Medicine* 49 (3): 407–24.

Shakespeare, T. 2006. *Disability Rights and Wrongs.* London: Routledge.

Shapiro, J. 2006. "Autism Movement Seeks Acceptance, Not Cures." National Public Radio. Accessed January 2010, http://www.npr.org/templates/story/story .php?storyId=5488463.

Silverman, C. 2008a. "Brains, Pedigrees, and Promises: Lessons from the Politics of Autism Genetics." In Gibbon and C. Novas, *Biosocialities, Genetics, and the Social Sciences,* 38–55.

———. 2008b. "Fieldwork on Another Planet: Social Science Perspectives on the Autism Spectrum." *BioSocieties* 3 (3): 325–41.

CEREBRALIZING AUTISM 95

Sinclair, J. 1993. "Don't Mourn for Us." *Our Voice* 1 (3). Autism Network International. Accessed December 2007, http://ani.autistics.org/dont_mourn.html.

———. 1999. "Why I Dislike 'Person First' Language." Internet Archive: Wayback Machine. Accessed April 30, 2013, http://web.archive.org/web/20090210190652/, http://web.syr.edu/~jisincla/person_first.htm.

———. 2005. "Autism Network International: The Development of a Community and Its Culture." Autism Network International. Accessed March 26, 2013, http://www.autreat.com/History_of_ANI.html.

Singer, J. 1999. "Why Can't You Be Normal for Once in Your Life? From a 'Problem with No Name' to the Emergence of a New Category of Difference." In Corker and French, *Disability Discourse*, 59–67.

———. 2007. "Light and Dark: Correcting the Balance." Neurodiversity.com. Accessed January 2010, http://www.neurodiversity.com.au/.

Solomon, A. 2008. "The Autism Rights Movement." *New York Magazine*, May 25. Accessed August 2009, http://nymag.com/news/features/47225.

Swain, J., and C. Cameron. 1999. "Unless Otherwise Stated: Discourses of Labeling and Identity in Coming Out." In Corker and French, *Disability Discourse*, 68–78.

Taylor, C. 1989. *Sources of the Self: The Making of Modern Identity*. Cambridge, Mass.: Harvard University Press.

Vidal, F. 2009. "Brainhood, Anthropological Figure of Modernity." *History of the Human Sciences* 22 (1): 5–36.

Vrecko, S. 2006. "Folk Neurology and the Remaking of Identity." *Molecular Interventions* 6 (6): 300–303.

———. 2011. "On the Political Economy of the 'Gambling Brain.'" In Ortega and Vidal, *Neurocultures*, 217–34.

Weisberg, D. S., et al. 2008. "The Seductive Allure of Neuroscience Explanations." *Journal of Cognitive Neuroscience* 20 (3): 470–77.

Welkowitz, L. 2009. "Got It: Obama's Diversity and the New Frontier." *Asperger's Conversations*, January 22. Accessed July 12, 2013, http://welkowitz.typepad.com/.

Wendell, S. 1996. *The Rejected Body. Feminist Philosophical Reflections on Disability*. New York: Routledge.

Whyte, S. R. 2009. "Health Identities and Subjectivities: The Ethnographic Challenge." *Medical Anthropology Quarterly* 23 (1): 6–15.

Wilson, S., and L. Peterson. 2002. "The Anthropology of Online Communities." *Annual Review of Anthropology* 31 (1): 449–67.

Zifendorf. 2005. "Neurodiversity (Idea)." Everything2. Accessed April 2011, http://everything2.com/user/Zifendorf/writeups/neurodiversity.

Autism as a Form of Biological Citizenship

Charlotte Brownlow and Lindsay O'Dell

In this chapter, we discuss the ways in which a biological explanation of autism has been refashioned into a neurological account of neurodiversity. The neurodiversity discourse functions as a critical tool with which people with autism may engage with negative and disabling mainstream models of autism. We outline the development of the neurodiversity movement, which claims autism as a difference from (and often as a superior identity to) "neurologically typicals" (NTs). The chapter draws on the concept of "biological citizens" alongside a construction of neurodiversity. The concept of biological citizenship has become part of a new critical engagement with various "disorders," such as bipolar affective disorder (Rose and Novas 2003) and autism (Orsini 2009) (although the validity of the label "autism" as a singular diagnostic category is contested; see, for example, Happé, Ronald, and Plomin 2006). We are not suggesting a biological determinant to autism; neither is our intention to add weight to the dominance of a biologized view of autism. Rather, we aim to explore how a renewed interest in biological explanations can be supportive and helpful for those claiming a positive autistic identity. Through the chapter, we consider our position in relation to the arguments made by Francisco Ortega, in this volume, and share his concerns about the dominance of a biological discourse of autism.

The concept of biological citizenship was first introduced by Adriana Petryna (2002) and can be considered a tool by which individuals can link with others through their shared claims to classification and therefore their claims to a shared identity with others based on such classification. Although Paul Rabinow is reported to have proposed the term *biosocial* partly as a joke to counter the dominance of sociobiological discourse in the early 1990s (see Hacking 2006), it is evident that biological explanations have become a discursive project, a convincing and powerful way to articulate an identity. Biological citizens can therefore organize themselves politically around particular diagnostic labels and form a potential force for collective action (Hughes 2009; Orsini 2009). Ian Hacking talks about "making up people," writing that "new kinds of people come into being, people characterized by a certain risk factor, who band together to create a social group" (2006, 94). Rabinow and Nikolas Rose draw on Foucault's notion of biopower and the ways in which the body is drawn into discourse as a way of regulating subjectivities. The notion of biological citizenship stems from this idea to consider the "forms of knowledge, regimes of authority and practices of intervention that are desirable, legitimate and efficacious" (Rabinow and Rose 2006, 197). Groups of biological citizens may therefore offer the potential to form powerful collectives and challenge the view of autism as a neurological impairment. Drawing on a discourse of neurodiversity, we seek to explore whether the identification of "neurobiological citizens" can offer the potential for autistic individuals to construct alternative understandings of autism, ones that are not dominated by a deficit-model focus.

Although there would seem to be a potential power in the formation of neurobiological collectives, Rose and Carlos Novas (2005) argue that as well as being a tool of collectivization, biological citizenship can also operate as a tool of individualization, through which individuals come to understand themselves and interpret their actions in terms of their own biology. They identify, for example, the Internet as being a powerful tool in enabling those motivated to gain information about their own diagnosis and thereby engage in a very individual process of "biomedical self-shaping" in their quest for information. Indeed, Rose and Novas postulate that there are many layers of complexity that may form our understanding of biological citizenship, including "informational bio-citizenship," whereby collectives incorporate and utilize quite specialist scientific and professional knowledge; "rights bio-citizenship," where collectives advocate for the rights of their groups; and "digital bio-citizenship," where new ways of forming collectives are invoked, such as Internet technologies. The potential roles that the Internet may play in public understandings of autism have been well documented (see, for example, Dekker 2000; Blume n.d.; Brownlow and O'Dell 2006); however, the role that the Internet may play in the experiential understandings of autism remains unclear. In this chapter, we briefly discuss the role of the Internet in the production of online autistic communities and of positive autistic identities (see also Davidson and Orsini, this volume).

In this chapter, we further seek to explore the concept of biological citizenship and extend considerations of it to challenge dominant (deficit) models of autism. We therefore seek to extend the concept of biopower to examine the ways in which people with autism can draw on a claim to neurobiological citizenship to construct identity and to (re)claim a position as different from neurologically typical individuals but with equal citizenship rights. Following Rose and Novas (2005), we therefore need to consider these questions: Who controls the definition of autism and the protocols for treating it? How are the lives of autistic people defined and controlled through biomedical means or diagnostic tools? Who are the experts, and whose concepts and assumptions will guide and define the world of autism?

In reflecting on these questions, we will draw on some of our previous research with four online discussion forums: two for people with autism, one for parents with an autistic child, and one for professionals who support families with an autistic family member. The research was conducted in the United Kingdom but included contributors from across the world. These were primarily based in the United Kingdom, North America, and Australia, although there were also key contributions from individuals based in Singapore and Indonesia. All of the discussion-list exchanges were in English, and in total 994 contributions were made to the four discussion forums. The research complied with university-research ethics and the British Psychological Society's guidance for researching online (2007). We present material for which contributors have given permission for its use, and we present their voices verbatim using pseudonyms.

A Critical Interest in Biology and Impairment

In considering our first question informed by Rose and Novas, we need to examine who controls the definition of autism and the protocols for treating it. The dominant view of autism in academic and clinical literature remains one of identifying the various "impairments" evident in autistic individuals: a strong focus on how such individuals can be considered "deficient" in their abilities and in need of some form of intervention (see, for example, American Psychiatric Association 2000; Frith 2003). For many years, the social model of disability has offered a series of critiques to deficit models of disability (see, for example, Barnes and Mercer 1996; Lawthom and Goodley 2005). It enables an examination of the social and cultural implications of disability and a disabling society, rejecting the view that disability is an illness, and in doing so maintains the need to separate the concepts of disability and impairment in order to potentially understand disability as a basis for identity politics (see, for example, Chappell, Goodley, and Lawthom 2001). This position is not without its tensions, however. Critical disability theorists such as Lennard Davis have questioned the foundational basis of "disability" as a fixed category (1995).

There have also been questions raised in the literature concerning the application of the social model of disability to learning difficulties (see, for example, Chappell, Goodley, and Lawthom 2001). Anne Louise Chappell argued that much of the disability literature has a tendency to define the concept of impairment in terms of the physical body; however, she asserts that there is nothing intrinsic about the word *impairment* to suggest a physical rather than an intellectual difficulty, providing a firm place for learning difficulties within such a model (1998). Chappell, Dan Goodley, and Rebecca Lawthom further these discussions of the neglect by the social model of disability of people with learning difficulties and argue that, because of this exclusion, an individualized model of disability is frequently applied to people with learning difficulties (2001).

In considering the application of the social model of disability to autism specifically, the separation of the concepts of disability and impairment has mixed implications for the understanding of autism. The concept of disability as defined by the Union of the Physically Impaired against Segregation (UPIAS 1976) raises important questions concerning whether being autistic should necessarily be a disability; however, the social model did provide an important theoretical platform on which to draw attention to politicized rights-based debates surrounding disability.

An issue for the theorization of autism drawing on the social model of disability is an emphasis on impairment as separate from disability and the biological from the social. Previous researchers have called for an examination of the construction of impairment rather than understanding impairment purely through biological means (see, for example, Abberley 1987; Hughes and Paterson 1997). "Second-wave" disability theorists such as Mark Rapley have called for recognition of the socially constructed nature of "impairments" (2004). Ortega (this volume) argues that neuroscience has become part of the dominant way in which people understand themselves. We and others argue that "impairments" are constructed through a biological discourse that accords the impairment an ontological status. In this chapter, we argue that using biologized discourse can be a powerful way for autistic people and their advocates to challenge mainstream understandings of autism. Rather than framing biology and neurology as a reductionist tool (as a way of closing off discussions of autism and constructing it as a singular biologically based deficit), we propose that the biological and neurological elements need to be foregrounded in discussions of the positioning of autism. We are not arguing that neuroscience can provide the facts through which to understand autism; rather, we are interrogating how (and why) a neurobiological explanation and a framing of autism in terms of neurobiological citizenship have become a key issue in critical autism studies and increasingly in popular accounts drawn on, for example, by parents of children with autism. We build on the work of Michel Foucault, Hacking, and others to argue that constructing autism in particular ways produces a set of material effects. We share Ortega's concerns about the dominance of neuroscience in contemporary culture and science but see a potential for examining the production of the autistic citizen through an engagement in neurobiological claims to identity, difference, and ontological homogeneity.

NT/AS Binaries and Neurodiversity

The concept of neurological difference has been a long-standing issue for autistic advocates in their discussions and within critical disability studies (see, for example, Dosch Brown 2011; Dekker 2000; Robertson 2010). Discussions center on a neurological explanation as a way of distinguishing people with autism (AS) from "neurotypicals" (NT). A key implication of the newly developing interest in a critical biological understanding of autism is that AS and NT people are distinctly different. The neurodiversity movement has become a significant critical voice in the past five to ten years of disability studies and disability advocacy. The neurodiversity movement, which is often playful in its approach, draws on a biologized discourse to position NTs as, at best, different from and often as inferior to autistic people. The discourse reifies neurological differences between autistic and neurotypical individuals, constructing the two groups as fundamentally different. For example, in an online discussion forum, Archie wrote, "I know they [NTs] are all individuals and that we shouldn't blame every NT for the action of every other NT . . . but there is a common thread that ties them together and it is at the core of their being. It is *more than cultural; it is how they are hardwired* from the factory" (our emphasis). In this quotation, Archie explains the difference between AS and NT as reducible to the "hardwiring" of neurological functioning. The notions of neurological difference are therefore being used to position NTs as "other" than people with autism through a discourse of biological essentialism. Constructing NTs as "strange" and problematic by implication can enable people with autism and their advocates to understand autism in a positive, enabling way. There has been much written by autistic people, and others, to promote the binary of NT/AS based on what is positioned as an irreducible neurological fact: it is "natural" that autistic people are seen as equal to but just different from NTs. Indeed, much discussion focuses on the "strangeness" of NTs. For example, a quotation from Ernie illustrates the "otherness" of NTs in his posting to an online discussion group run for and by people with autism. Ernie also makes a distinction between autistic people, NTs, and ACs (autistic cousins), which we discuss later in this chapter.

> As one of those struggling with the problems of human relationships, I had realized that NTs have amazingly peculiar lifestyles. I shall provide some of you here with a beginner's guide of their strangeness. . . . They often prize relational achievements more than intellectual achievements. . . . Their games often unfold in intricate ways, so vast in scope and powerful in calculated effect that if they catch you unprepared you will suffer heavily without even knowing who set you on fire. Some of their games would seem incomprehensible, but from what I do understand, they often consider solutions that ACs would rule out because of "unfairness," that these goes against one's morals or that it violates some rule systems such as the law. . . . They can insist on the principle that everyone has equally valid opinions worthy of respect and yet they often insist you comply with their opinions. . . . In conclusion, one would find it good curiosity to study the NT society, but not to live

in it. The NT lifestyle appears either totally inconherent or rather primitive, and NTs in general, remain slaves to their own genetic codes than master of them.

Ernie illustrates a view of an autistic community in which people with autism are seen to be neurologically different from NTs, their strangeness, and their genetics. Genetic makeup is presented here as being a "fixed" entity that determines the NTs' identity and lifestyle. The implication of Ernie's comments is that whereas NTs are determined by their neurology, autistic people are less constrained.

This returns to our consideration of the second question posed at the start of this chapter: How are the lives of autistic people defined and controlled through biomedical means? Biomedical understandings of autism may be twofold in their shaping of understandings and experiences of autism. From one perspective, biomedical understandings enable the positioning of difference in a positive way, through the potential validation of an autistic identity in a positive manner; however, the counterposition is that of individuals being determined by a reductionist, biologized discourse (see Ortega [this volume], who specifically addresses the difficulties inherent within this perspective).

There are implications of these two very different understandings of the role of biology in our understandings of autism, but what is clear is that, through drawing on a biologized discourse, a dichotomy is created between "autistic" and "nonautistic." The dichotomy of AS/NT constructs two distinct worlds. The view that there are two worlds of NT and AS is strongly felt by many autistic people and their families. For example, in a post to an online discussion group, Annie, the mother of an autistic child, wrote, "I feel that I live in two worlds. The 'NT' but I don't especially care for that term, and the AS b/c of my son."

The dualisms of AS/NT present autistic and nonautistic people as mutually exclusive groups, with a strong focus on the neurobiological foundation of such differences. However, contributors to the online discussion lists also reflect the complex issues involved when attributing a particular group membership to an individual and reflect competing and divergent voices in a multifaceted debate. The challenge presented to the binaries created takes the form of an AC group identity, which may bring into question the "fixed" boundaries between neurobiological collectives.

The group referred to as autistic cousins is particularly complex to define. On some occasions, "AC" is used to refer to a whole range of similar terms, encapsulating several diagnoses, including high-functioning autism and Asperger Syndrome; on other occasions, it refers to a distinct group of people without a specific diagnosis of autism but who have a close relationship with someone who is autistic. However, despite the seemingly flexible use of terminology, there remains a strong distinction between the group who might collectively be referred to as AC and the NTs, that is, neurologically typical people who are not autistic.

One way of defining AC interprets the category as comprising autistics and "cousins" who are friends of autistics. This implies that the boundaries between NT and AS are more fluid than would first appear; therefore, in terms of the defining of autism through biomedical means, this may be more of a fuzzy boundary. This is particularly evident in Archie's words: "Some NTs have experience with one of us and they suppress their innate rule enforcement protocols. We call these people Acs [autistic cousins] and we elevate them to a higher status than the run-of-the-mill narrow-minded NT. The fact is, though, that NTs don't become Acs easily. Like I said earlier, we Ass [autistics] do not go out and force our ways on others . . . it is not part of who we are. NTs, with the exception of Acs, do, and it takes special knowledge to make an NT into an AC." Here what confers the AC identity is not a label, "impairment," a diagnosis, or a particular style of biological functioning; rather, it is the "special knowledge" that this group of people is seen to possess. Although neurological understandings are invoked as a means of a political positioning of identity, it is clear that within such discourses remains an element of flexibility and an opportunity to maintain a heterogeneous thread running through what could be positioned as a homogeneous neurological discourse. However, such a definition of ACs does create a hierarchical structure to category membership, with NT being the least valued, AS the most valued, and a few "deserving" NTs promoted to a point midway between the two. This forms an inversion of the implicit, dominant view that "normal," and therefore NT, is best. As Archie says, "With any luck, she will soon be eligible for promotion to AS cousin, or whatever term you would rather use to describe an 'enlightened' NT."

Following Ortega (this volume), it could be argued that adopting a polarized position through the invoking of neurological differences works to minimize the differences between the group of NTs and the group of individuals with autism. However, consideration of the group identified as ACs may introduce an element of discursive flexibility in the boundaries between the two groups. "AC" offers a potential identity for contributors that lies somewhere in between autistic and nonautistic, thereby calling into question the "inevitable" reductionism of a neurobiological discourse.

A variation on the NT/AS dichotomy is also evident in the proposition of a neurodiverse spectrum. Rather than the focus on an oppositional identity politics inherent in the construction of distinct NT and AS worlds, a focus on neurodiversity makes the assumption that everyone is on a spectrum of functioning. Although the view of autism as a spectrum is evident in much traditional academic literature (see, for example, Frith 2003; Wing 1981), the proposition of a *neurodiverse* spectrum includes not only those with a label of autism but also NTs (and ACs) in order to account for the neurological functioning of everyone. The proposition of a neurodiverse spectrum challenges the assumed normalcy of NTs set against the assumed impairment of ASs by positioning everyone along a singular spectrum of functioning. This is evident in discussions by autistic people, advocates, and some in critical disability work (see, for example, Brownlow 2007; Yergeau 2010). Such representations may focus on the various distinctions not only between, for example, high-functioning autism and Asperger Syndrome but also between "social" and "nonsocial" people. Framing autism as a form of neurodiversity would seem to fit well with the positioning of autism as a form of biological citizenship; however, we must remain mindful that the deficit model of autism dominates much autism research, and the historical construction of "normality" and "abnormality" typically privileges the voices of professionals in constructing the seemingly homogeneous grouping of people with autism and the impairments associated with it. Indeed Ortega (this volume) argues that such neuroscientific theories have become more widely available, one consequence being that such representations of neurological patterns have been taken up in "commonsense" ways of understanding individuals. Such common representations may therefore construct a singular, biologized view of autism, with clear implications concerning the deficient nature of some neurological patterns. While the work of writers such as Hacking (2009b) highlights the plural nature of autistic communities, the homogeneous view enabled by a singular, biologized construction of autism still remains a dominant theme.

Communication and Neurobiological Citizenship

Communication between autistic people is key in developing and maintaining a discourse of neurobiological citizenship. Some off- and online communities allow autistic people to engage with others who share their interests and abilities, which can relieve them of the burden of having to explain to others the "idiosyncrasies" typically associated with being autistic (Bertilsdotter Rosqvist, Brownlow, and O'Dell 2013). The traditional boundaries of "normality" and "abnormality" are therefore questioned and often inverted in light of this exchange. This can be seen in previous quotations in this chapter, specifically when considering the binaries of NT and AS and the hierarchical group membership constructed when considering the AC identity. Following Rose and Novas (2005), autistic people may therefore be invoking the digital and rights biocitizenship models in a complementary crafting of a challenging collective.

Mitzi Waltz has previously discussed the lack of voice given to people with autism in academic literature; a professional third-person voice is typically adopted in order to lend an authoritative, factual style to descriptions and explanations of people with autism: a clear indication of the powerful control that the medical model continues to have over the definitions of autism and the protocols for treating it (2005). However, there are numerous and increasing numbers of texts written by people with autism (see, for example, Grandin 2011; Lawson 2008; Williams 1998) and examples of academic work analyzing such texts (see, for example, Davidson and Smith 2009; Hacking 2009a). The increase in writings by autistic individuals may serve to bring into the mainstream alternative representations of autism and therefore alternative understandings of the (constructed) competencies of people with autism. These texts often have a broad popular appeal in society; there is a strong need for many to be able to account for the diverse ranges of skills and attributes of autistic people that are not fully (and not positively) accounted for in mainstream research.

One area where there has been a great deal of engagement by people with autism is in new technologies and online communication (see Davidson and Orsini, this volume). The Internet provides unique possibilities for facilitating the sharing of biomedical knowledge and experiential understandings of autism among diverse populations, including autistic advocates, parents, and practitioners, and further enabling such sharing in a global community (Braun 2007). For Rose and Novas (2003), the Internet therefore provides opportunities for the "making up" of the biological citizen from individuals who identify with specific labels, providing a challenge to the shaping of individuals through the power of the state and the dominant power and knowledge of "psy professionals" who produce knowledge and "interventions" for autistic people. Transnational collections of autistic individuals, their advocates, and other ACs can be formed online in contexts where AS people make up the dominant majority, which is in contrast to the predominantly NT social world of face-to-face encounters off-line.

Indeed, the Internet has been shown to play a significant role in the crafting of more empowering autistic identities in some of our previous work (Brownlow 2010), where autistic people drew on alternative discourses of autism. These new ways of thinking about autism focus on a biological understanding of neurological difference, or neurodiversity. The new discourses have a broad appeal and have been taken up by autistic individuals, as well as some parents, indicating the potential for the movement of the collectives of such individuals online into a wider social arena.

The Internet is also being used in quite different ways by some parents of autistic individuals, in the development and refinement of their technical knowledge and language surrounding autism, enacting what Rose and Novas (2005) term "informational bio-citizenship." It can be argued that part of the position of power maintained by professionals is evident in the specialist discourse adopted by members of the profession, for example, by referring to psychometric terminology when presenting assessments of people with autism. The discourse utilizes terminology that is not commonly found in lay or nonscientific language. The use of such discourse maintains specialist knowledge and confirms that professionals working within the field are best suited to govern individual behavior through the identification of "problem" behavior and subsequent interventions. By drawing on other participants in online communities with relevant expertise, parents are able to draw on informational biocitizenship to enable them to challenge the previously exclusive "expert talk" of the psy professionals. Referring back to questions of who are the experts and whose concepts and assumptions will guide and define the world of autism, we argue that professional discourse of the psy professionals is increasingly taken up by individuals who are not in a position of traditional expert power. Here we offer an illustration from an online discussion forum set up for parents of autistic children. In this extract, Jennie, the mother of a child undergoing diagnosis, is using the group to gain information about the diagnostic processes:

> I was just wondering if anyone can tell me why the doctor needed to know my sons head circumference (he's currently being assessed for autism). (Jennie)
>
> Good question. I didn't think that there was any significance to head circumference. If there is, it is in a narrow range of disabilities that are probably rare. (Tim)
>
> Maybe the doctor is ruling out other disabilities before labelling him autistic. There are other disabilities that have autistic-like characteristics, but are actually another disability. I had a child in my internship that was being assessed for autism and the doctor checked his head circumference as part of a way to rule out Neurofibromatosis (some have enlarged heads); however, in this child's case he was diagnosed autistic, but it was good that the doctor assessed for other disabilities before labelling him. (Helen)

This discussion demonstrates that parents are not passively accepting received views of autism but are working up their accounts of what should be done to help themselves (or their children). They may either agree or disagree with professionals but use the discussion forum to gain knowledge with which to challenge professional intervention that is not seen to be helpful or supportive.

Informational biocitizenship was not confined to parents of people with autism. Several examples can be cited of adults not recognizing their autistic identity until they came across discussions on the Internet or in other media, such as newspapers or first-person accounts, which led them ultimately to pursue a diagnosis and/or to self-identify with an autistic label. For example, Richard writes, "I have Asperger's Syndrome, the highest-functioning form of autism and only found it out in the spring of 1995, as a result of reading an article in *The New Yorker* by Oliver Sacks." Examples such as this provide evidence supporting the existence of "self-help" culture that has developed around technologies and their potential uses in forming collectives of like-minded neurobiological citizens. Online communities may therefore provide opportunities for self-help and advocacy to challenge oppressive practices and disabling "interventions" as well as to provide friendship and support.

We have discussed earlier in this chapter the possibilities for constructing a positive autistic identity based on a view of the person as a neurobiological citizen with abilities equal, and possibly superior, to the "host" NT culture; however, Sujatha Raman and Richard Tutton remind us of the importance of not becoming distracted by the perceived power of biopolitics "from below" (2010). In addition to embracing the potentials of biological collectives as an empowering force, we must also be mindful of the continuing power of the role of the state in the management of citizens. Raman and Tutton cite the example of the Human Genome Project and its potential influence on societal choices and decisions. They argue that although individuals can be considered to make choices concerning issues of personal health and care, this is largely within the context of professional dominance and power. For example, in the United Kingdom, women are typically provided with the option of having a blood test at sixteen weeks of pregnancy to assess the likelihood that their babies have Down syndrome, and in Australia a national immunization register is kept on the immunization status of individual children. Both of these examples are positioned in public discourse as individual choice, but they are strongly governed in terms of the wider discourses of the medical model, which provides contexts for such choices.

The power of biological discourse may therefore remain a double-edged sword. Autistic activists draw parallels with biomedical research and cultural genocide, with the aim of research being to find a genetic marker for autism and ultimately remove autistic people from existence (Rose and Novas 2003). Indeed, several high-profile discussions about people with autism, such as the MMR debate, frame autistic children as "damaged goods" (O'Dell and Brownlow 2005). Some activists fear that, in a way similar to Down syndrome, if biological developments enabled the detection of an "autistic gene," many parents might opt to terminate pregnancies (Orsini 2009). We recognize that there are limitations and potential dangers in positioning autism as a biological fact. The scientific quest for a genetic marker for many stigmatized groups is ongoing and illustrates further the power of a biologized foundation for identity, as well as the need to construct an alternative biological discourse through which to counter these knowledge claims and scientific activities.

Neurobiological Citizens: Final Reflections

Returning to the questions posed at the start of this chapter, what might neurobiological citizenship mean for autistic individuals? There remain important questions to be considered concerning the challenge offered by a critical engagement in a biologized view of impairment. Ortega (this volume) argues that critical views of autism also homogenize autism by conceptualising it in terms of an NT/AS binary. Our view is that a framing of autistic people as citizens in a neurodiverse world may enable a more heterogeneous view of autism within critical discourses: citizens are diverse populations that may choose (in some circumstances) to engage, resist, or withdraw from the governing regime. We agree with Hacking that advances in biological, neurological, and genetic science have not provided us with answers to questions about identity and functioning: "Far from increasing determinism and limiting opportunity, the life sciences are creating more choices. On the one hand, in a sense, we have more biologies to choose from than we anticipated. On the other hand, new societies form along newly recognised (or at any rate, newly asserted) biological or genetic lines, forging new alliances and loyalties. Forging new identities" (2006, 82).

Equally, citizens are governed and surveyed and caught within regimes of power and knowledge that position them as particular kinds of person. Indeed, as Orsini and Smith highlight (2010), autistic activists are often confronted with claims that they are "not autistic enough" if they attain achievements that exceed expectations of what it means to be autistic. In the counter position, where autistic individuals celebrate their neurodiversity in a strategy to promote positive constructions of autistic difference, there remains a danger that they become essentialized as "ontologically different beings" (Orsini 2009).

To claim the status of a neurobiological citizen may therefore enable challenges and resistance to the positioning of autistic people in an NT-dominated world, but the true impact of this claim may not yet be realized.

Indeed, Hacking reflects on the complexities of and challenges posed to the established language that we have at our disposal to reflect on and construct autism (2009b). Alternative and new discourses of autism that draw upon "biological collectives" can reframe our understandings of what it means to be autistic. Ortega (this volume) argues that "neurodiversity can be sustained as a value only when it becomes embodied in a community." We argue that there are possibilities of establishing communities (both off- and online) that enable this sustaining. Working in such communities can enable autistic activists, their parents, friends, and ACs to gain knowledge and specialist language of the psy professions with which to represent and challenge dominant ideas. However, such individuals remain physically located within particular environments, which may be more or less AS friendly. Therefore, the possibilities are limited for some people.

There are also tensions concerning the understanding of autism in terms of a dichromatic difference from neurologically typical individuals and understanding autism as a spectrum. Biological citizenship can be claimed on the basis of two competing representations of autism: as a "neurodiverse spectrum" (drawing often on a medical, health discourse) or as "neurological difference" (drawing on a discourse of rights and political separatism). In the same way that other political activists (such as feminists and gay-rights and black activists) have claimed difference positively as an identity position, it may be politically expedient to conceptualize autism in terms of dualisms rather than as a spectrum on which everyone rests. Activists can position autism as a difference that has been stigmatized, oppressed, and devalued. Within this position, there are two separate worlds: the NT world and the AS world, through which AS people are required to travel and some interested NTs may choose to travel. Therefore, in positioning autism as a distinct grouping, individuals can align their self-identity with a clear set of values. This can become a clear political statement valuing and prioritizing autistic traits and challenging the dominance of neurotypicality in clinical and academic psychological literature. However, at times the construction of a single, neurodiverse world in which everyone falls on a spectrum of neurological functioning can also have leverage within public debates and understandings of autism. It is evident that autistic individuals draw upon the two discourses interchangeably, presenting the most appropriate argument for a given situation in which they find themselves.

In this chapter, we have argued that positioning people with autism (and, equally importantly, those without a diagnosis who consider themselves to be NT) as neurobiological citizens, who may adopt one of a range of identity positions, enables new understandings of autism and provides ways of challenging the NT dominance of the majority face-to-face world. In our commentary, we have drawn on "biology" and "neurological functioning" as discursive products rather than inescapable facts. The recourse to a biological discourse with which to challenge mainstream disabling concepts of autism has a currency at this time; however, we recognize that this discourse is a contingent and strategic alliance between critical disability studies, people with autism, and advocates, involving a biologized understanding of autism. It remains one of many ways in which critical autism studies could move forward.

REFERENCES

Abberley, P. 1987. "The Concept of Oppression and the Development of a Social Theory of Disability." *Disability, Handicap, and Society* 2 (5): 5–19.

American Psychiatric Association. 2000. *Diagnostic and Statistical Manual of Mental Disorders.* 4th ed. Washington, D.C.: American Psychiatric Association.

Barnes, C., and G. Mercer, eds. 1996. *Exploring the Divide: Illness and Disability.* Leeds, U.K.: Disability Press.

Bertilsdotter Rosqvist, H., C. Brownlow, and L. O'Dell. 2013. "Mapping the Social Geographies of Autism: On- and Off-Line Narratives of Neuro-Shared and Separate Spaces." *Disability and Society* 28 (3): 367–79. Accessed March 26, 2013, http://dx.doi.org/10.1080/09687599.2012.714257.

Blume, H. n.d. "Autism and the Internet; or, It's the Wiring, Stupid." MIT Communications Forum. Accessed July 13, 2011, http://web.mit.edu/comm-forum/papers/blume.html.

Braun, B. 2007. "Biopolitics and the Molecularization of Life." *Cultural Geographies* 14 (6): 6–28.

British Psychological Society. 2007. "Ethical Issues in Researching Online." British Psychological Society. Accessed September 22, 2011, http://www.bps.org.uk/publications/policy-guidelines/research-guidelines-policy-documents/research-guidelines-policy-documents.

Brownlow, C. 2007. "The Construction of the Autistic Individual: Investigations in Online Discussion Groups." PhD diss., University of Brighton, UK.

——. 2010. "Presenting the Self: Negotiating a Label of Autism." *Journal of Intellectual and Developmental Disability* 35 (14): 14–21.

Brownlow, C., and L. O'Dell. 2006. "Constructing an Autistic Identity: AS Voices Online." *Mental Retardation* 44 (315): 315–21.

Chappell, A. L. 1998. "Still Out in the Cold: People with Learning Difficulties and the Social Model of Disability." In *The Disability Reader: Social Science Perspectives,* edited by T. Shakespeare, 211–20. London: Cassell.

Chappell, A. L., D. Goodley, and R. Lawthom. 2001. "Making Connections: The Relevance of the Social Model of Disability for People with Learning Difficulties." *British Journal of Learning Disabilities* 29: 45–50.

Davidson, J., and M. Smith. 2009. "Autistic Autobiographies and More-Than-Human Emotional Geographies." *Environment and Planning D: Society and Space* 27 (5): 898–916.

Davis, L. 1995. *Enforcing Normalcy: Disability, Deafness, and the Body*. London: Verso.

Dekker, M. 2000. "On Our Own Terms: Emerging Autistic Culture." Beyond Autism. Accessed July 6, 2000, http://trainland.tripod.com/martijn.htm.

Dosch Brown, R. 2011. "'Screw Normal': Resisting the Myth of Normal by Questioning Media's Depiction of People with Autism and Their Families." Paper presented at the Minnesota Disability Studies Symposium, University of Minnesota, July 29–31. Accessed January 29, 2012, http://blog.lib.umn.edu/gara0030/iggds/Screw%20Normal FINAL_Dosch%20Brown.pdf.

Frith, U. 2003. *Autism: Explaining the Enigma*. 2nd ed. London: Blackwell.

Grandin, T. 2011. *The Way I See It: A Personal Look at Autism and Asperger's*. Arlington, Tex.: Future Horizons.

Hacking, I. 2006. "Genetics, Biosocial Groups, and the Future of Identity." *Daedelus*, Fall, 81–95.

——. 2009a. "Autistic Autobiography." *Philosophical Transactions of the Royal Society B: Biological Sciences* 364 (1522): 1467–73.

——. 2009b. "How We Have Been Learning to Talk about Autism: A Role for Stories." *Metaphilosophy* 40 (3–4): 499–516.

Happé, F., A. Ronald, and R. Plomin. 2006. "Time to Give Up on a Single Explanation for Autism." *Nature Neuroscience* 9: 1218–20. doi: 10.1038/nn1770.

Hughes, B. 2009. "Disability Activisms: Social Model Stalwarts and Biological Citizens." *Disability and Society* 24 (6): 677–88.

Hughes, B., and K. Paterson. 1997. "The Social Model of Disability and the Disappearing Body: Towards a Sociology of Impairment." *Disability and Society* 12 (3): 325–40.

Lawson, W. 2008. *Concepts of Normality: The Autistic and Typical Spectrum*. London: Kingsley.

Lawthom, R., and D. Goodley. 2005. "Community Psychology: Towards an Empowering Vision of Disability." *Psychologist* 18 (7): 423–25.

O'Dell, L., and C. Brownlow. 2005. "Media Reports of Links between MMR and Autism: A Discourse Analysis." *British Journal of Learning Disabilities* 33 (4): 194–99.

Orsini, M. 2009. "Contesting the Autistic Subject: Biological Citizenship and the Autism/Autistic Movement." In *Critical Interventions in the Ethics of Healthcare*, edited by S. J. Murray and D. Holmes, 115–30. Abingdon, U.K.: Ashgate.

Orsini, M., and M. Smith. 2010. "Social Movements, Knowledge, and Public Policy: The Case of Autism Activism in Canada and the US." *Critical Policy Studies* 4 (1): 38–57.

Petryna, A. 2002. *Life Exposed: Biological Citizens after Chernobyl*. Princeton, N.J.: Princeton University Press.

Rabinow, P., and N. Rose. 2006. "Biopower Today." *BioSocieties* 1: 195–217.

Raman, S., and R. Tutton. 2010. "Life, Science, and Biopower." *Science, Technology, and Human Values* 35 (5): 711–34.

Rapley, M. 2004. *The Social Construction of Intellectual Disability.* Cambridge: Cambridge University Press.

Robertson, S. M. 2010. "Neurodiversity, Quality of Life, and Autistic Adults: Shifting Research and Professional Focuses onto Real-Life Challenges." *Disability Studies Quarterly* 30 (1).

Rose, N., and C. Novas. 2005. "Biological Citizenship." In *Global Anthropology,* edited by A. Ong and S. Collier. London: Blackwell. Accessed June 30, 2011, http://www2.lse.ac.uk/sociology/pdf/RoseandNovasBiologicalCitizenship2002.pdf.

UPIAS. 1976. *Fundamental Principles of Disability.* London: Union of the Physically Impaired against Segregation.

Waltz, M. 2005. "Reading Case Studies of People with Autistic Spectrum Disorders: A Cultural Studies Approach to Issues of Disability Representation." *Disability and Society* 20 (5): 421–35.

Williams, D. 1998. *Nobody Nowhere: The Remarkable Autobiography of an Autistic Girl.* London: Kingsley.

Wing, L. 1981. "Asperger's Syndrome: A Clinical Account." *Psychological Medicine* 11: 115–30.

Yergeau, M. 2010. "Circle Wars: Reshaping the Typical Autism Essay." *Disability Studies Quarterly* 30 (1).

PART II. Researching the Politics and Practice of Care

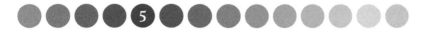

Autism and Genetics
Profit, Risk, and Bare Life

Majia Holmer Nadesan

In 2007, the U.S. Centers for Disease Control reported that autism-spectrum disorders affect 1 in 150 children. Parents, educators, medical professionals, and social-service providers demand that autism's causes be identified and its social and economic risks be addressed and managed, despite considerable controversy over what autism actually is (see Nadesan 2005). Some autism advocates see autism as an inborn or environmentally caused medical condition that requires treatment and cure, whereas others see autism as a difference that requires accommodation.

This chapter considers competing causal explanations and discusses the politics inherent within and informing these competing frameworks for interpreting and treating autism. The chapter critiques the politics of the inborn and genetic-based dominant frame governing autism research and public funding for autism in the United States by focusing on the allocation of funding for autism, the prioritization of pharmaceuticals, and expanding efforts to create autism-susceptibility tests. The chapter addresses the marginalization of environmental explanations for genetic changes that arguably derives from the research emphasis on finding susceptibility genes. The emphasis on inborn susceptibility has implications for people with autism and their families, as the search for genes may be prioritized over research and spending related to support, therapy, and accommodation in an economic context of public-spending cuts. People with autism and their families should consider carefully this formulation of autism as a heritable, genetic deficiency, because they will shoulder a growing share of the economic costs of accommodation and treatment as the austerity state cuts services.

Some autism advocates reject altogether the idea of "deficiency"; thus, the construct of autism as a heritable, genetic-based disorder may be troubling as autism-susceptibility testing expands. The heritable model of genetic deficiency could legitimize a new prenatal eugenics as families seek to limit the economic and social impacts of having a child with autism. Autism becomes in this dystopic vision a marker of a devalued life form, or bare life.

Autism Research Priorities: Genes, Dollars, and Susceptibility Tests

Expert discourses have carved out a definition of autism operationalized through behavioral criteria. The *DSM-IV* stipulates that a diagnosis of autism (299.00 Autistic Disorder) requires that the patient exhibit symptoms (a total of six or more items) from a triad of behavioral or communication impairments, including: (1) impairments in social interaction, including impairments in nonverbal behaviors ("eye contact," "facial expressions," "body postures," and "gestures to regulate social interaction"), impairments in the ability to develop appropriate peer relationships, and impairments in emotional reciprocity (such as pleasure in other people's happiness); (2) impairments in communication, including delays in expressive language, impairments in conversational competence, use of stereotypic or repetitive language, and lack of spontaneous make-believe play; and (3) "restricted repetitive and stereotyped patterns of behavior, interests, and activities." Onset of delays and/or impairments must occur before the age of three for a diagnosis of autistic disorder (American Psychiatric Association 1994, 70–71). With few substantive differences, the diagnostic criteria stipulated in the *ICD-10* by the World Health Organization (2009) basically mirror these criteria. Neither system specifies that mental retardation be an essential diagnostic feature of autism. Because of the heterogeneity of autistic expressions, both the *ICD-10* and the *DSM-IV* include a diagnostic category for atypical expression: "Atypical Autism" in the *ICD-10* requires that the patient meet fewer of the diagnostic criteria stipulated for autism, as does "Pervasive Developmental Disorder: Not Otherwise Specified" (299.80 PDD-NOS) in the *DSM-IV*. In the *DSM-IV*, late age of onset requires a diagnosis of PDD-NOS in the absence of other diagnostic possibilities (such as schizophrenia).

Most medical and popular accounts of autism represent the disorder as involving brain damage, usually perceived as caused by genetic mutations or alleles (see Herbert 2005). The brain damage is believed to manifest in the triad of impairments that constitute the disorder's diagnostic criteria. Today, functional magnetic resonance imaging (fMRI) and other brain-scanning technologies can identify precise areas of the brain believed to be affected. Brain-imaging technologies can be employed to create "neural phenotypes" (Ramus 2006, 247), which are seen as necessary for establishing clear relationships between (1) brain and mind and (2) brain and gene, as researchers seek to map cognitive symptoms of autism (mind) onto specific brain areas. After this first step, researchers strive to link targeted brain areas with gene alleles that may contribute to the disorder by affecting the brain's development in those areas.

Finding autism genes might be regarded as the Holy Grail of autism research. Autism is typically understood in the medical and scientific literature as *primarily* a genetic disorder, although the literature occasionally acknowledges the mediating role of exogenous factors (for example, see Lauritsen and Ewald 2001; Ozand et al. 2003). Findings of areas linked to autism include regions on chromosomes 7q21-35, 17q, and 11. However, this research has revealed no consistently replicable genetic markers despite more than two decades of research (Geschwind 2008; Losh et al. 2008). The phenotypic and etiological complexity of the disorder may complicate discovery of replicable genetic or other bio-based markers. Autism may be caused by multiple risk alleles of small effects, making it difficult to identify using genetic-linkage analysis. New DNA-imaging technologies have revealed de novo structural variations (those not seen in parents), such as microdeletions and duplications in DNA segments linked to autism, particularly on chromosome 16. However, most of the copy-number variations detected in microarray research appear to be "rare, essentially private, mutations in simplex (one affected child) autism families" (Geschwind 2008, 394). Viruses, environmental contaminants, and ionizing radiation all emerge as potential exogenous factors figuring into susceptibilities for mutations. However, very little research actually addresses the role of environmental factors in producing the de novo genetic mutations that have been recently linked to autism. Hence, genetic explanations remain severed conceptually from environmental contaminants.

Despite the ambiguity about the role of genes in causing autism, the public has been educated to regard autism as a hereditary disorder. Popular Web sites such as WebMD typically prioritize genetics in their introductory accounts of autism, as illustrated here in "Autism: Topic Overview": "Autism tends to run in families, so experts think it may be something that you inherit. Scientists are trying to find out exactly which genes may be responsible for passing down autism in families. Other studies are looking at whether autism can be caused by other medical problems or by something in your child's surroundings" (2010). Likewise, *Parenting Magazine* notes in a 2012 article titled "New Autism Facts and Figures" that "we're getting closer to understanding the possible causes [of autism]. Groundbreaking research last year pinpointed what scientists are calling autism 'susceptibility' genes, which regulate how the brain develops and how connections between cells are made." The article acknowledges, however, that individuals who have the susceptibility genes do not necessarily have autism.

This framing of autism as a heritable genetic disorder has dominated public-research priorities, expert discourse about autism in the media, and commercial product developments pertaining to autism. For instance, the same WebMD topic explains, under the heading of "What Autism Research Is Being Done?" that "the National Institute of Neurological Disorders and Stroke, part of the National Institutes of Health (NIH), is studying brain abnormalities that may cause autism and is looking for genes that may increase the risk of autism" (2010). Funding agencies such as the NIH have prioritized the research goal of finding autism-susceptibility genes. For instance, in 2004, the NIH issued a "Request for Proposal for Identifying Autism Susceptibility Genes," which would make $4,295,000 available in fiscal year 2005. The focus on autism-susceptibility genes in the absence of discussion of environmental mediations implies that autism is simply inherited through the convergence of susceptibility genes.

Furthermore, in 2007, three of the six Autism Centers of Excellence (ACE)[1] research awards focused on brain-imaging studies, two focused on genetic-based causes (one of which also used neuroscience), and one focused on behavioral interventions (National Institute of Mental Health 2007). In 2008, the ACE Center award was for a study seeking to identify rare genetic variations believed to play a role in autism (National Institutes of Health 2008). In 2008, ACE Network award recipients included three grants, studying genetics; pharmaceutical treatment with Buspar; and, atypically, environmental risk. A study of NIH funding priorities for autism from 1980 to 2007 by Mark Blaxill, Sallie Bernard, and Theresa Wrangham (2008) found that genetic and imaging grants were strongly favored. Treatment using pharmaceuticals and screening were also prioritized, whereas environment-only studies were strongly de-emphasized when funding was allocated. In 2009, Johns Hopkins University Bloomberg School of Public Health announced receipt of an ACE award to study the intersection of genetics and autism. This list of funded research priorities illustrates the strong emphasis placed on genetic research and neuroscience and, to a lesser extent, research on biomarkers, screening, and drug treatment. It also illustrates the de-emphasis on environmental factors, which, when investigated at all, are cast in relation to genetic susceptibilities. Funding prioritizes research that simply aims to identify genes linked to the disorder and/ or brain anomalies that deviate from the neural profiles of "normal" populations. Research assessing the appropriateness and effectiveness of actual therapeutic practices is almost nonexistent. Federal and private funding for autism privileges research that studies autism as a genetic and brain-based disorder. In contrast to research funding, public funding for *services* for people with autism does not exist to any significant degree at the national level in the United States. Furthermore, national funding for research developing and assessing nonpharmaceutical treatment protocols is extremely limited, as I will discuss presently. States within the United States are therefore responsible for providing the limited funding that does exist for actually treating people diagnosed with autism. These treatment protocols are primarily nonmedicinal and emphasize instead sensory-integration therapy, speech therapy, and cognitive and behavioral-skills training. Some autism advocates argue that the transmission of the majority of private and public autism dollars to large, institutional, and often commercially driven research programs may result in relatively fewer social or medical benefits for people diagnosed with the disorder. The prioritization of genetic and, increasingly, neuroscientific research frameworks that presume biological deficiency and damage raises concern among some autism advocates (for example, Blaxill, Bernard, and Wrangham 2008; Rimland 1997; "U.K. Autism Research" 2004). Advocates worry that public funding for practical therapies for people with autism may be rejected in favor of investing those public dollars in commercially viable or commercially "sexy" research projects conducted at high-profile public and private research labs. Genetics and neuroscience are "in," whereas cognitive therapy is not.

This attitude toward prioritizing high-profile, commercially viable research in genetics and neuroscience was illustrated by the 2009 appointment of Francis S. Collins to head the National Institutes of Health (NIH) after he stepped down from his position as director of the National Human Genome Research Institute at the NIH, which he held from 1993 to 2008. Although Collins publicly eschews genetic determinism, his research has prioritized it; after his appointment to the NIH, Collins's first research priority for mental health was "applying genomics and other high throughput technologies" (Collins 2010; see also Blumberg 2006). Collins's 2010 "Director's Report to the 224th National Advisory Mental Health Council Meeting" emphasized genetic approaches to autism and schizophrenia. In his role as director at the NIH, Collins encouraged the National Institutes of Mental Health, which is subordinate to the NIH, to embrace genetic explanations and pharmacological treatment of mental illness. Collins's stance reinforced the trend to approach autism as a brain-based disorder caused by genetic mutations or alleles.

Despite its popularity and institutional support, the genetic brain-based approach has failed to deliver on its promises to explicate the "causes" of autism and has failed to lead to new autism treatments. Genes believed to increase susceptibility in one population are difficult to find in other populations. Penetration is typically uneven, as identical twins with autism do not uniformly share the disorder (Bruder et al. 2008). Unknown environmental factors and other independent variables, such as father's age, may contribute to genetic mutations linked to the disorder as susceptibilities. The relationship between phenotypic autistic traits (such as behavioral and cognitive traits) and specific genes remains very unclear, although researchers suspect that genotype–phenotype relationships may exist (Thompson, Cannon, and Toga 2002).

It is difficult to deny the monetary significance of genetic research. Many gene alleles and processes believed to play a role in the disorder have been patented. Genes can be patented after their sequence is decoded. The World Intellectual Property Organization recognizes patents on at least two autism-susceptibility genes. (Patents also exist for ADHD-susceptibility genes.) The U.S. Patent Office has also patented a method for screening genetic markers associated with autism (Nadesan 2010). Genes have been transformed into commodities, shaping research trajectories and problem/solution frames (Nelkin 2001, 558; Rose 2008).

Patenting of autism genes and other genes linked to illness or undesirable states raises a variety of ethical issues and concerns. Patents can dictate and restrict research trajectories and may be used to generate revenue streams. Thus, disorders such as autism can become business opportunities for bioengineering and pharmaceutical companies. Autism circulates in a growing bioeconomy that is viewed as vital to reestablishing national economic competitiveness (Gottweis 1998; Rajan 2006). Although geneticists studying autism formally acknowledge the role of environmental mediations, it is their ability to target susceptibility genes (over environmental contributions) that produces commercial revenue streams. By shifting our focus from environment to genes, the marketization of autism genes absolves the state of regulatory responsibility for monitoring and governing those diverse contaminants known to confer risk and susceptibility to developmental disorders, such as lead, mercury, ionizing radiation, and industrial chemicals (such as phthalates) and pesticides (including organophosphate pesticides). Genes, as opposed to environments, are viewed as risk-laden. The shift in risk from environments to persons implied in the formulation of gene-based autism susceptibility can usher in a dangerous politics of life and death.

Not all genetic research is driven by the profit motive, however. Moreover, not all biological research is genetic. Nonetheless, the seductive combination of genes and dollars has the potential to crowd out other research trajectories and autism-funding priorities. The concern here is that knowledge and products developed by the pharmaceutical-research complex will likely promote autism detection (tests) and pharmaceutical "management" over the more costly (in terms of initial investments) therapeutic approaches that are labor- and resource-intensive (such as sensory-integration therapy and special education services) and over alternative research approaches that might curtail industry profits by foregrounding environmental explanations for autism and other syndromes and diseases.

Environmental research on autism receives limited federal funding, and nonpharmaceutical research on autism prevention emphasizing environmental remediation is almost nonexistent. Environmental-health research addresses environmentally mediated causes of autism and other syndromes, including cancer. This research seeks to identify toxic or carcinogenic environmental contaminants or processes that give rise to diseases. Sometimes, this research examines genetic susceptibility in conjunction with environmental harms. At other times, this research emphasizes the role of chemicals and ionizing radiation in destroying subcellular processes, for instance, in breaking the chemical bonds of DNA. This biological research assumes that there are causes to disorders such as autism and that these causes can be identified and acted upon (for example, see Landrigan 2010). However, this biological research does not typically lead to profitable pharmaceuticals and may be unpopular with industries that are responsible for producing environmental hazards. As I shall examine in greater detail, this research is underfunded and underreported in the popular media, because financial incentives and domestic austerity are together crowding out alternative approaches and basic treatments for people with autism.

Risk Management and Autism-Susceptibility Testing

Autism-susceptibility tests are seen as a strategy for detecting childhood autism early in development, before behavioral-based testing outlined by the *DSM-IV* can be employed. As Patrick Walsh and colleagues remark: "there is an intensive search for biological markers for autism. Such biomarkers could not only reveal causes of the condition but could also be clinically useful in complementing or improving the behavioral diagnosis of autism and in enabling earlier detection of the condition" (2011, 603).

Autism-susceptibility tests presume that people with autism are born biologically different and that their differences from "normal" populations are significant enough to enable detection by focusing on biological markers. Susceptibility testing could involve prenatal testing for the presence of autism-susceptibility genes. This approach would be problematic for the reasons discussed in the previous section but may in fact be developed if costs for sequencing are reduced. Commercial efforts to develop susceptibility tests are also pursuing other biomarkers that might be linked to the disorder. Biomarkers are the "surface" manifestations of the underlying biological differences that constitute the disorder.

The possibility that gene-based susceptibility tests might be developed has raised considerable concern within particular subsets of the autism-advocacy movement. For example, for a time there existed online an "autism genocide clock" that purported to count down years, days, and minutes to the seemingly inevitable development of an autism prenatal test that would result in an autism holocaust. This clock was uploaded in 2001 in response to concerns that genetic knowledge about autism would lead to the patenting of susceptibility genes, which in turn could be used to develop commercial prenatal tests. Private fertility clinics have been scanning embryos for gene-linked diseases for years, so these concerns were not unwarranted. A recent survey of 999 U.S. residents seeking genetic counseling found that 75 percent supported genetic tests for the elimination of mental retardation (Naik 2009).

The online research Web site Autism Research and Prenatal Testing observed in July 2011 that, today, concerns about a gene-based autism-susceptibility test have been largely put to rest, because the genetic research has failed to identify consistent markets and because of opposition from autism advocates who fear an impending autism holocaust ("Ventura Fanfiction Universe" 2011). Still, each new announcement of the identification of autism-susceptibility alleles affords clinical-testing services a new opportunity to capitalize on autism. For instance, in 2010, identification of yet another autism-susceptibility allele was broadcast through the media (see Sousa et al. 2010). Furthermore, Walsh and colleagues report that chromosomal microarray testing can be used to identify submicroscopic deletions and duplications that have been linked with autism (2011). These findings could stimulate further efforts to develop commercial autism-susceptibility tests.

Indeed, patents have been granted for screening techniques aimed at detecting genetic errors linked to birth defects. A new method called comparative genomic hybridization obtained two patents in the 1990s to detect sequence deletions, duplications, and translocations in targeted areas of an individual's genome. The abstract for patent 5,965,362 explains:

> Disclosed are new methods comprising the use of in situ hybridization to detect abnormal nucleic acid sequence copy numbers in one or more genomes wherein repetitive sequences that bind to multiple loci in a reference chromosome spread are either substantially removed and/or their hybridization signals suppressed. The invention termed Comparative Genomic Hybridization (CGH) provides for methods of determining the relative number of copies of nucleic acid sequences in one or more subject genomes or portions thereof (for example, a tumor cell) as a function of the location of those

sequences in a reference genome (for example, a normal human genome). . . . Amplifications, duplications and/or deletions in the subject genome(s) can be detected. (Pinkel et al. 1999)

Comparative genomic hybridization is currently being used for prenatal diagnostics to identify fetuses potentially susceptible to particular syndromes caused by, or linked to, deletions or additions of genetic material (Stein 2008). Concern already exists that this type of genetic screening could be used to identify susceptibilities for a wide range of disorders linked, but not caused, by genetic factors. Comparative genomic hybridization transforms a child's risk into suspect absences or duplications of alleles prior to his or her birth. Risk becomes the punctuation of one's genome.

Researchers recently announced that they were able to sequence the entire genome of a fetus using a sample of the mother's blood (Marcus 2012). A news article heralding this accomplishment stated that the development would make it easier to predict fetal genetic defects with little risk. The researchers demonstrated their technique on a mother with DiGeorge syndrome, a genetic condition that can cause cardiac problems. They successfully determined that the fetus inherited the condition. The article notes that making sense of the information poses the most significant challenge because of limited information available about the relationships between genes and diseases. This innovation reinforces the emphasis on the punctuation of one's genome as the precursor for adult health and cognition, thereby marginalizing important environmental factors, including the conditions of the prenatal environment.

Autism-susceptibility tests need not rely on genes. In 2010, researchers declared that they could use MRI scans to measure and detect deviations in brain circuitry representative of autism (Lange et al. 2010). The research was promoted as offering an alternative route for detecting autism in very young children, although the researchers acknowledged that their system was not ready for clinical practice (McClean Hospital 2010). Other strategies suggested for early detection of autism include using serum samples for proteomic profiling and urine samples for metabolic profiling (see Walsh et al. 2011). Saliva-based susceptibility tests have also been proposed (see Castagnola et al. 2008).

The article by Walsh and colleagues on the ethical implications of autism-susceptibility testing (2011) raises ethical quandaries stemming from the contingency and uncertainty of autism diagnoses and outcomes. The authors recognize the potential for eugenic applications of autism testing, a concern that I raised in previous work (Nadesan 2005). Given the risk of eugenic applications, the authors recommend that autism advocates be involved with the development and assessment of autism-susceptibility tests. Their recommendations are worthy, but the commercial enterprises that develop autism-susceptibility tests—to be marketed with other tests for home and clinical use—are not likely to be swayed by these recommendations, which could impinge on profitable products. Indeed, in a 2010 article published in the Canadian *Globe and Mail,* the director of Canada's Centre for Applied Genomics, Stephen Scherer, observed that he believes people will be able to purchase mail-order genetic tests that scan for autism-related genes in the "near future," even if the information is "dubious at best" (see Abraham 2010).

Moreover, it is possible that even the most sensitively developed and marketed autism-susceptibility tests could have adverse effects for public support and medical insurance for people diagnosed with the disorder. Parents who "choose" to carry a susceptible embryo to term could be held responsible for their child's care by insurance companies and society alike if the child develops autistic symptoms. Likewise, it is possible that susceptibility tests marketed directly to prospective or new parents (see Castagnola et al. 2008) might be implemented in the absence of social and therapeutic supports, leaving parents terrified, but ill-equipped, to evaluate the long-term prospects for their "risky" fetus or infant.

In 2006, the *New York Times* published a troubling essay by Elizabeth Weil titled "A Wrongful Birth." In her essay, Weil describes a legal suit of wrongful birth brought by a woman whose baby was born with a gene duplication and a gene deletion on his fourth chromosome. The baby was diagnosed with Wolf-Hirschhorn syndrome, which often involves physical and mental disabilities. The mother sued her medical providers for failing to detect problems with the fetus, whose weight and size were abnormally low. The multimillion-dollar lawsuit charged that the obstetrician's neglect disallowed her the right to abort the fetus. Weil observes that this case and others like it reveal new beliefs about reproduction:

> And what those cases are exposing is the relatively new belief
> that we should have a right to choose which babies come into the
> world. This belief is built upon two assumptions, both of which

have emerged in the past 40 years. The first is the assumption that if we choose to take advantage of contemporary technology, major flaws in our fetus's health will be detected before birth. The second assumption, more controversial, is that we will be able to do something—namely, end the pregnancy—if those flaws suggest a parenting project we would rather not undertake.

A third assumption not identified by Weil is that *the* measure of a child's perfection exists in a form of genetic normalization that may be read off genetic sequences. Development of ever more sophisticated and less invasive prenatal testing devices encourages the idea that the seeds of perfect normalization are located in our genes, that prenatal testing can measure a child's propensity for this form of perfection, and that we have an implicit responsibility to know and decide upon the birth of a child before she or he is born.

Prenatal testing is an ethically complex field. It is therefore not surprising that autism advocacy surrounding issues of autism detection and treatment is a heterogeneous terrain notable for its fragmentation. Some autism advocates push for finding autism's causes and cures and might welcome autism-susceptibility tests. The organization Defeat Autism Now illustrates this approach to advocacy. This approach toward cause and cure is itself fragmented between those who see autism as a gene-based order and those who stress environmental causes for the disorder, ranging from vaccinations to inorganic chemicals such as pesticides and endocrine-disrupting phthalates.

In contrast to the approach emphasizing cause and cure, other autism advocates argue that people with the disorder are simply different, not deficient.[2] Advocates within this group argue that the overarching emphasis on cause and cure can distract attention from the more important goal of helping people diagnosed with the disorder live meaningful and comfortable lives. Some advocates within this second group reject the disease model altogether and all approaches that aim to cure the disorder. Advocacy by this group, often by people diagnosed with autism, has grown in visibility as the Internet enables autism-spectrum individuals to communicate comfortably their concerns about how "neurotypical" persons view and attempt to normalize autistic differences (Nadesan 2005). Advocates in this group often share a sense of a unifying common biology that presents challenges but also offers special contributions to society. These advocates promote assistance that does not seek to eradicate difference but, rather, seeks to promote individual growth and development. For advocates who reject medicalization, autistic individuals are simply "wired differently" (Nadesan 2005). This idea has been promoted by the field of cognitive neuroscience. Autism has been a cash cow for neuroscience research and has garnered publicity for the discipline's efforts to map cognitive traits, aptitudes, and behaviors directly onto the brain (see Ortega and Vidal 2011; Nadesan 2005, 2008a). Neuroscience aims to create neural phenotypes of autistic brains that may be linked to physiological causes, such as gene alleles. Using technologies such as fMRI and PET (positron emission tomography), researchers claim to identify patterns of neural activity representing "normal" and "deviant" (for example, autistic) cognition and affect. Autistic phenotypes can be generalized from patterns of "autistic" cognition and affect created through the neural scans. Ultimately, such research hopes to identify gene alleles that correlate with specific neural phenotypes, bridging brain and gene (and behavior or trait). This research has a variety of ontological and methodological problems that will not be rehearsed here (see Ortega and Vidal 2011; Ortega, this volume; Uttal 2001). What is of interest for this chapter is that neuroscientific knowledge claims have been used by some autism advocates to affirm autistic differences.

Yet this strategy of affirming difference by seizing upon neuroscience's ontology of autistic brains can have dangerous implications, particularly for those who fear susceptibility testing will produce a veiled eugenics. The growing awareness of autism may actually increase parental fears about having and raising a child with autism, particularly in a contracting economy characterized by government austerity. Biological susceptibility tests may effectively reduce unborn autistic persons to a form of biological, but nonhuman, "bare life" that enables annihilation by reducing the entire person to a small set of biological markers regarded as deviant or abnormal. Tests that evaluate genetic and/or biomedical susceptibility to autism risk producing a "thanatopolitics"—a politics of death—for autism. Prenatal autism tests, for instance, have the potential to reduce life from *bios*, the life proper to an individual within a polity, to *zöe*, or bare life that can be killed with impunity (see Agamben 1998).

The decision to abort an autistic fetus stems from a perception of irreparable damage done to the fetal brain by deficient or damaged genes, or by other physiological events or processes. The potential becoming of the fetus is calibrated only in terms of autistic characteristics or deficiencies. The fetus becomes bare life, denied becoming and personhood (see, for example, Tremain 2005, 2006). To raise concern about this type of reduction of human life to disposability does not necessarily imply a strident "pro-life" bias, nor does it necessitate sentimentalizing autistic persons. Rather, the concerns being raised are twofold. First, the cultural adoption of prenatal testing signals ascendancy of a technocratic determinism that rejects uncertainty, the unpredictable processes of becoming, and the work of parenting. Second, the technologies of prenatal testing may make parents financially responsible for choosing children with special needs in the context of increasingly austere social supports. Finally, technologies of detection may usurp environmental policies and technologies of prevention, because the former provide opportunities for capitalization, whereas the latter imply greater monitoring and regulation of industry, processes which are costly to government and industry.

Austerity and Personal Responsibility in the Great Recession

Having explored the limitations and financial and ethical implications of genetic-based and deterministic models of autistic brains, this chapter now turns to examine autism within the contemporary socioeconomic context. In chapter 6 of this volume, "Caring for Autism: Toward a More Responsive State," Kristin Bumiller demonstrates that the life chances of people with autism are significantly impacted by the state policies that structure and enable opportunities and financial support. She argues that recent trends toward privatization of care shifts responsibility onto families. Bumiller's concerns about the "responsibilization" of families for the care of those with disabilities takes on heightened significance in the context of the massive cuts in social spending that have occurred in the United States and Europe over the last five years. The shift in governmental priorities away from the social welfare of dependent and vulnerable populations may impact their valuation in public attitudes and expert opinions. Formulations of disability that emphasize growth and development through intensive supports and accommodation may fade from public consciousness as more deterministic and less resource-intensive formulations emerge. Indeed, the formulation of "irrevocably brain-damaged" autistic persons might gain credence within this social context because of its economic expediency. Irrevocably damaged persons demand less therapeutic remediation than persons who have the capacity to grow and develop within intensive (and costly) therapeutic supports and accommodations. Early detection of people classified as autistic could be used for nefarious purposes as well as for optimizing ones. This section examines these arguments, focusing on the challenges of providing educational and therapeutic services for autistic people in the context of economic recession.

The global recession that began in 2007 has hit the United States particularly hard, exacerbating three decades of slow decline as U.S. jobs were automated and outsourced abroad. The American middle and working classes have been severely impacted. The Center for American Progress issued a report titled "Recession, Poverty, and the Recovery Act: Millions at Risk of Falling out of the Middle Class" in February 2009. The report documents rising unemployment, loss of health insurance, and growing poverty before concluding, "Our economy is in a perilous state. Millions of middle-class families are likely to fall into poverty if Congress does not take swift action" (Kvaal and Furnas 2009). In September 2011, 49.9 million Americans had no health insurance, and employer-sponsored private insurance covered only 55 percent of the population ("Bleak News" 2011). The U.S. stimulus, the National Recovery Act, fell short of delivering adequate relief and job growth to an increasingly fragile middle class and an increasingly desperate working class (Hilsenrath and Leo 2009; Kroll 2011).

Calls for fiscal austerity in the United States by "deficit hawks" and the decimated budgets of public entities such as states, school districts, and cities are eroding health, social-welfare, and educational support and spending in the United States. The reign of "disaster capitalism" (Klein 2007, 6) terrorizing all those citizens who are dependent upon public spending promises to significantly curtail supports for children and adults whose social vulnerability and/or biomedical differences require greater health, welfare, or educational spending than is allocated to wealthier, healthier, or more "optimized" populations.

Public services are stretched thin as demand is rising while public budgets are contracting. Public education has been particularly affected by the recession. Public schools in the United States derive most of their funds from local property taxes. Today's property taxes reflect the inflated housing values of the real-estate bubble, the collapse of which precipitated the recession. As property valuations are adjusted downward over the next several years, schools will face significant declines in revenue. The National Conference of State Legislatures predicts that schools' funding will metaphorically drop "off a cliff" when the American Recovery and Reinvestment Act (that is, the stimulus) funds expire (see Shreve 2009). Even the socially and economically conservative *Forbes* magazine observes, "Unless major changes are made, or taxes raised sky-high, spending on baby-boomer retirements (Social Security, health care, public employee pensions, etc.) will eat up almost every morsel of discretionary funding that could otherwise go to services like schools" (Finn and Petrilli 2009). Out of necessity, schools will raise class sizes and cut elective programs such as art, music, and physical education. For instance, the *Wall Street Journal* reported that 75 percent of California's elementary schools would increase class size in 2010 (Tuna 2010). Likewise, Georgia school districts are facing $700 million in cuts, leading state lawmakers to consider temporarily waiving state-mandated class-size limits.

Strapped schools will have difficulty providing aids and needed resources such as speech therapy, occupational therapy, and physical therapy to children with special needs. Federal funding for special education is limited. The 1975 Individuals with Disabilities Education Act (IDEA) specified that the federal government would compensate schools for 40 percent of excess special education costs by 1982. However, funding has never reached the 40 percent level and is believed to account for far less. The U.S. Department of Education's own data (2010) attribute only about $1,700 in federal dollars per student toward states' grants funding students qualifying under IDEA in 2009 and 2010.

The crisis in funding is also stressing state, county, and city budgets. These entities are cutting funding for programs for the poor, the elderly, and the disabled. The Center on Budget and Policy Priorities reported in May 2010 that at least thirty states had cut funding for low-income families eligible for health insurance or care, and at least twenty-five states were cutting programs for the elderly and disabled (Johnson, Oliff, and Williams 2011). Efforts to halt budget cuts to people with disabilities using injunctions have not been successful in states such as

Arizona (Arizona Center for Disability Law 2010). State budget short-falls anticipated for 2011 were expected to total approximately $121 billion and would exceed the 2010 and 2009 shortfalls (Center on Budget and Policy Priorities 2010). Further cuts for services and programs for disabled and vulnerable populations seem inevitable. Home health-care services for the elderly and disabled have been targeted for cuts, even though these programs are cost-efficient and are a vital lifeline for those who receive their services (Leland 2010).

States such as Arizona and California must run balanced budgets, but the federal government operates using a fiat currency model and therefore can run extensive deficits. The financial bailout of the insolvent U.S. banking system and unprecedented military spending have resulted in massive federal deficits. Given the ease with which the federal government runs up deficits, one must question why austerity is being enforced in social-welfare spending. The federal government could replace lost state funding necessary for operating social services. Instead, it is allowing extreme state-level austerity measures that cripple services to the old, disabled, and ill.

Disasters allow neoliberal authorities and various other "reformers" to downsize social-welfare programs and services (Klein 2007). Austerity measures typically target vulnerable populations lacking the resources to lobby against them, as is evidenced in the disaster capitalism that occurred in the wake of Hurricane Katrina (Nadesan 2008b). Austerity measures are often accompanied by the circulation of neoliberal cultural discourses that render individuals responsible while delegitimizing the logic of social welfare (Nadesan 2008a, 2010). Poor populations, those with disabilities or chronic illnesses, the long-term unemployed, the elderly, children, and every other conceivable group that fails to achieve the neoliberal idealization of entrepreneurial autonomy become second-class citizens.

Neoliberalism dovetails smoothly with the amorality of Randian narcissism. Indeed, Ayn Rand's philosophy, marked by intolerance for anything less than perfect human autonomy, captured the imagination and loyalty of the long-term Federal Reserve chairman Alan Greenspan (Taibbi 2010). The fusion of neoliberal market valorization and Randian intolerance and arrogance enabled and legitimized the plundering of the wider population and the systematic dismantling of Keynesian social-welfare equalization and redistribution systems. The ruthless, predatory capitalist ethos held in check by Keynesian-era reforms and values has now been fully unleashed. The vast majority of the American population is vulnerable to wage repression and austerity measures, and no population is more vulnerable than those with autism.

Cuts in state- and community-level public funding for autism research are likely to exacerbate the already-existing public-policy bias that frames autism as a biological, gene-based disorder in search of a pharmaceutical cure. Future autism research priorities and commercial product developments are likely to reflect the interests of the pharmaceutical and biotech companies still able and willing to "invest" in autism.

Family members of people with autism will be "responsibilized" for their care without the benefits of supports as states, counties, cities, and school districts shed services. The potential expansion of autism-susceptibility testing may have the potential of refiguring risk so that parents of autistic children are made financially responsible for the "choice" to keep (that is, not abort) their autistic children. The brain-based model of irreparable autistic harm will circulate more widely as medical and public authorities alike struggle to rationalize elimination of funding for therapeutic programming for people with autism. This dystopic scenario is not the fruit of wild extrapolation but the logical consequence of current trajectories.

Another important effect of neoliberal approaches toward health research and management is the disinvestment in and symbolic marginalization of environmental research on autism and related disorders. A recent research study publicized by Reuters found that children exposed to organophosphate pesticides have higher risks of ADHD (2010). If these pesticides can be directly and positively correlated with ADHD, it seems probable that they could just as likely be correlated with autism, given that many researchers see ADHD as part of the autism spectrum because of commonalities in executive-function deficits (see, for example, Corbett et al. 2009). Indeed, Philip Landrigan's research suggests that a wide array of common environmental toxins could play a role in producing autism (2010). Martha Herbert, a prominent researcher in the area of autism and environmental health, agrees, although she is more optimistic about physiological interventions for children who have suffered environmentally induced injuries.[3] Yet the U.S. approach to regulating chemicals remains lax despite growing evidence of chemical harms to human and animal life.

The Children's Environmental Health Center at Mount Sinai Hospital reports that only 20 percent of the more than 80,000 new chemicals produced since World War II have been tested for toxicity in children (Kristof 2009). In August 2007, the U.S. Government Accounting Office (GAO) published a report comparing the lax U.S. regulatory framework for chemicals with a recently enacted European framework called REACH. The GAO report explains that under the current regulatory system in the United States, companies do not have to develop information on the health or environmental impact of chemicals unless specifically required by ruling of the Environmental Protection Agency (EPA). Consequently, the EPA relies on voluntary programs for gathering information from chemical companies to evaluate and regulate new chemicals under the provisions of the 1976 Toxic Substances Control Act (TSCA).[1] The GAO report's recommendation that the burden of risk be shifted to the chemical companies was not adopted by the administration of George W. Bush, even after the President's Cancer Panel found a strong link between environmental toxins and cancer (see Layton 2010b; President's Cancer Panel 2008–2009). In 2010, a new regulation to overhaul the now-outdated 1976 TSCA was introduced, but so far nothing has been passed (see Layton 2010a; "Momentum Builds" 2010, Safer Chemicals, Healthy Families 2011).

Chemicals are not the only environmental factor that may be implicated in autism. Ionizing radiation has received almost no attention in the environmental research on autism, yet in my opinion it is considerably likely that it may play a role in the disorder. Research has demonstrated that even low doses of ionizing radiation can cause childhood leukemia (Little, Wakeford, and Kendall 2009). Environmental researchers have pointed out that radiation risk-exposure standards are oriented toward adults, and children are a sensitive subpopulation whose biological vulnerabilities have not been properly assessed for risk-management standards (see Fucic et al. 2008; Preston 2004). Furthermore, natural killer (NK) cells that have been implicated as being deficient in children with autism (Enstrom et al. 2008) are particularly susceptible to damage from ionizing radiation (Vokurková et al. 2010). The nuclear power and weapons industry has been very successful in deflecting attention away from radiation as an environmental risk.

Two research centers study environmental factors and autism: the University of Medicine and Dentistry of New Jersey / Robert Wood

Johnson Medical School in Piscataway, and the University of California at Davis ("New Centers" 2002). However, efforts to regulate environmental factors implicated in human disease and disorders face formidable challenges from industry, ranging from industry science to corporate lobbyists (see McGarity and Wagner 2008). Epidemiological evidence that chemicals cause harm is often riddled with contingencies that offer fuel to the corporate science aimed at debunking environmental-health research. Most important, contingency complicates efforts to calculate definite harms using financial logics and methodologies. Contingency calculates poorly within neoliberal economic calculi used for assessing risk when costs are involved. Neoliberalism is inherently biased toward protecting industry when regulation is at issue. Even when harms are established, opposition to environmental legislation typically overwhelms support. Business claims that environmental regulation will raise costs, or force industry to export production abroad, are powerful persuaders.

The compelling body of research documenting environmental factors in producing autism is likely to be marginalized for the foreseeable future. The fiscal significance of autism may very well wane as public expenditures on health care and services for people with autism are cut. As risk shifts to individuals, government has fewer financial incentives for battling industry and enforcing commercially costly enhanced environmental regulations. In contrast, public dollars for university and commercial research on the genetic causes of autism will continue, since this type of funding is represented as promoting biotech innovation and professional job creation. The same can be said for pharmaceutical development. Pharmaceuticals that manage autistic symptoms simultaneously provide cost-effective strategies for managing people with autism and fulfill the mantra of fostering innovation while promoting economic growth.

Conclusion

This chapter has considered some of the competing causal explanations for autism and has discussed the politics inherent within and informing these competing frameworks for interpreting and treating the disorder. The chapter critiqued the politics of the inborn and genetic-based dominant frame governing autism research and public funding for autism in the United States, by focusing on the allocation of funding for autism, the prioritization of pharmaceuticals, and expanding efforts to create autism-susceptibility tests. The chapter emphasized the latent dangers lurking in a geneticization of autism devoid of environmental mediation. Concerns were raised also about the potential for the dominant framework to produce prenatal testing, potentially ushering in a new eugenics cloaked in the guise of personalized "technologies of the self"; that is, autism advocates see prenatal testing as shifting eugenic decision making to prospective parents who then are made financially responsible for their children's conditions. Finally, the chapter raised the possibility that the economic and social stressors of the ongoing financial-economic crisis could amplify the prioritization of inborn-genetic frameworks and that this prioritization could undermine support for costly educational and therapeutic supports, thereby having the potential to reduce autistic persons to a form of bare life denied social equality and political representation.

NOTES

1. The passage of The Children's Health Act of 2000 (P.L. 106-310) mandated that the NIH assist a new platform of at least five centers of excellence focusing on autism and related disorders. The Autism Centers of Excellence (ACE) program consolidates two previously existing programs, the Studies to Advance Autism Research and Treatment (STAART) and Collaborative Programs of Excellence in Autism (CPEA), into a single research effort. The CPEA program began in 1997 and emphasized genetic, immunological, and environmental factors. The STAART program emphasized causes, diagnosis, early detection, prevention, and treatment (National Institutes of Health 2006). It appears the two programs were combined in 2007.

2. Autism advocates in this second group are a diverse group. Some notable advocates include Stephen Shore, Phil Schwartz, Frank Klein, and Jim Sinclair, all of whom have published writings and other material on the Internet.

3. Martha Herbert, correspondence with author, May 4, 2011.

4. Passed in 1969, the National Environmental Policy Act (NEPA) initiated policy actions addressing biological and ecological impacts of synthetic environmental chemicals (Frickel 2006). NEPA mandated the creation of the Environmental Protection Agency (EPA) and the Council for Environmental Quality. NEPA requires an annual report on the state of the environment and environmental-impact assessments using data collected from the EPA. The EPA was afforded additional regulatory authority with the passage of the 1976 Toxic Substances Control Act (TSCA), which enabled the EPA to control chemicals known to pose unreasonable risks to human or environmental health.

REFERENCES

Abraham, C. 2010. "Genetic Finding Paves Way for Controversial Autism Testing." *Globe and Mail*, June 9. http://www.theglobeandmail.com/news/national/genetic-finding-paves-way-for-controversial-autism-testing/article1597861/.

Agamben, G. 1998. *Homo sacer: Sovereign Power and Bare Life*, translated by D. Heller-Roazen. Stanford, Calif.: Stanford University Press.

American Psychiatric Association. 1994. *Diagnostic and Statistical Manual of Mental Disorders*. 4th ed. Washington, D.C.: American Psychiatric Association.

Arizona Center for Disability Law. 2010. "Legal and Policy News." Accessed November 17, 2012, http://www.acdl.com/legalpolicynews.html.

"Autism: Topic Overview." 2010. WebMD, April 12. Accessed December 20, 2011, http://www.webmd.com/brain/autism/autism-topic-overview.

Blaxill, M., S. Bernard, and T. Wrangham. 2008. "NIH and Autism: A Case Study in Barriers to Progress in Environmental Medicine." SafeMinds. Accessed November 11, 2012, http://www.safeminds.org/research/case-study-barriers-progress-environmental-medicine.pdf.

"Bleak News on Health Insurance." 2011. *New York Times*, September 14.

Blumberg, M. S. 2006. *Basic Instinct: The Genesis of Behavior*. New York: Basic Books.

Bruder, C., et al. 2008. "Phenotypically Concordant and Discordant Monozygotic Twins Display Different DNA Copy-Number-Variation Profiles." *American Journal of Human Genetics* 82 (3): 763–71.

Castagnola, M., et al. 2008. "Hypo-phosphorylation of Salivary Peptidome as a Clue to the Molecular Pathogenesis of Autism Spectrum Disorders." *Journal of Proteome Research* 7 (12): 5327.

Center on Budget and Policy Priorities. 2010. "Recession Continues to Batter States." Center on Budget and Policy Priorities. Accessed July 7, 2010, http://www.cbpp.org/cms/?fa=view&id=711.

Collins, F. S. 2010. "Director's Report to the 224th National Advisory Mental Health Council Meeting." National Institutes of Mental Health. Accessed February 11, 2011, http://www.nimh.nih.gov/about/advisory-boards-and-groups/namhc/reports/directors-report-to-the-224th-national-advisory-mental-health-council-meeting-february-11-2010.shtml.

Corbett, B. A., et al. 2009. "Examining Executive Functioning in Children with Autism Spectrum Disorder, Attention Deficit Hyperactivity Disorder, and Typical Development." *Psychiatry Research* 166 (2–3): 210–22.

Enstrom, A. M., et al. 2008. "Altered Gene Expression and Function of Peripheral Blood Natural Killer Cells in Children with Autism." *Brain, Behavior, Immunology* 23 (1): 124–33.

Finn, C. E., and M. J. Petrilli. 2009. "Will the Recession Kill School Reform?" *Forbes*, January 29. http://www.forbes.com/2009/01/29/school-reform-education-funding-opinions-contributors_0129_chester_finn_michael_petrilli.html.

Frickels, S. 2006. "When Convention Becomes Contentious: Organizing Science Activism in Genetic Toxicology." *New Political Sociology of Science: Institutions, Networks, and Power*, 185–210. Madison: University of Wisconsin Press.

Fucic, A., et al. 2008. "Genomic Damage in Children Accidentally Exposed to Ionizing Radiation: A Review of the Literature." *Mutation Research / Reviews in Mutation Research* 658 (1–2): 111–23.

Geschwind, D. H. 2008. "Autism: Many Genes, Common Pathways?" *Cell* 135 (3): 391–95.

Gottweis, H. 1998. *Governing Molecules: The Discursive Politics of Genetic Engineering in Europe and the United States.* Cambridge: MIT Press.

Herbert, M. R. 2005. "Autism: A Brain Disorder, or Disorder That Affects the Brain?" *Clinical Neuropsychiatry* 2 (6): 354–79.

Hilsenrath, J., and L. D. Leo. 2009. "Economic Revival Shown Less Robust." *Wall Street Journal,* November 25.

Johns Hopkins Bloomberg School of Public Health. 2009. "NIH Autism Center of Excellence Network Announces Launch of Most Comprehensive Study of Earliest Possible Causes of Autism." News release, June 9. Accessed July 7, 2010, http://www.jhsph.edu/news/news-releases/2009/earli.html.

Johnson, N., P. Oliff, and E. Williams. 2011. "An Update on State Budget Cuts: At Least 45 States Have Imposed Cuts That Hurt Vulnerable Residents and the Economy." Center on Budget and Policy Priorities. Accessed February 9, 2011, http://www.cbpp.org/cms/?fa=view&id=1214.

Klein, N. 2007. *The Shock Doctrine: The Rise of Disaster Capitalism.* New York: Metropolitan.

Kristof, N. D. 2009. "Cancer from the Kitchen." *New York Times,* December 5. http://www.nytimes.com/2009/12/06/opinion/06kristof.html?_r=1&th=&a dxnnl=1&emc=th&adxnnlx=1260118877-5+EHIHVAw+7zDpAR7b+Kmw.

Kroll, A. 2011. "McEconomy: Is America's Middle Class Doomed to Low-Wage Jobs and a Poor Standard of Living?" *AlterNet,* May 8. Accessed May 10, 2011, http://www.alternet.org/economy/150872/mceconomy%3A_is_america%27s_middle_class_doomed_to_lowwage_jobs_and_a_poor_standard_of_living/?page=entire.

Kvaal, J., and B. Furnas. 2009. "Recession, Poverty, and the Recovery Act: Millions at Risk of Falling out of the Middle-class." Center for American Progress. Accessed September 7, 2009, http://www.americanprogress.org/issues/2009/02/pdf/recession_poverty.pdf.

Landrigan, P. 2010. "What Causes Autism? Exploring the Environmental Contribution." *Current Opinion in Pediatrics* 22 (2): 219–25.

Lange, N., et al. 2010. "Atypical Diffusion Tensor Hemispheric Asymmetry in Autism." *Autism Research* 3 (2): 350–58.

Lauritsen, M. B., and H. Ewald. 2001. "The Genetics of Autism." *Acta Psychiatrica Scandinavica* 103: 411–27.

Layton, L. 2010a. "Lautenberg Bill Seeks to Overhaul U.S. Chemical Laws." *Washington Post,* April 15.

———. 2010b. "US Facing 'Grievous Harm' from Chemicals in Air, Food, Water, Panel Says." *Washington Post,* May 7.

Leland, J. 2010. "Cuts in Home Care Put Elderly and Disabled at Risk." *New York Times,* July 16. http://www.nytimes.com/2010/07/21/us/21aging.html?th&emc=th.

Little, M. P., R. Wakeford, and G. M. Kendall. 2009. "Updated Estimates of the Proportion of Childhood Leukaemia Incidence in Great Britain That May Be Caused by Natural Background Ionising Radiation." *Journal of Radiological Protection* 29 (4): 467–87.

Losh, M., et al. 2008. "Current Developments in the Genetics of Autism." *Journal of Neuropathology and Experimental Neurology* 67 (9): 829–37.

Marcus, A. D. 2012. "Mother's Blood Shows Birth Defects in Fetal DNA." *Wall Street Journal*, July 5.

McGarity, T. O., and W. E. Wagner. 2008. *Bending Science: How Special Interests Corrupt Public Health Research*. Cambridge, Mass.: Harvard University Press.

McLean Hospital. 2010. "Major Step toward First Biological Test for Autism." *ScienceDaily*, December 2. Accessed December 12, 2010, http://www.science daily.com/releases/2010/12/101202124335.htm.

"Momentum Builds in Congress to Overhaul U.S. Chemicals Policy." 2010. Earthjustice. Press release, July 23. Accessed August 7, 2010, http://www .earthjustice.org/news/press/2010/momentum-builds-in-congress-to-overhaul-u-s-chemicals-policy.

Nadesan, M. 2005. *Constructing Autism: Unravelling the "Truth" and Understanding the Social*. London: Routledge.

———. 2008a. *Governmentality, Biopower, and Everyday Life*. Routledge Studies in Social and Political Thought. New York: Routledge.

———. 2008b. "Hurricane Katrina: Governmentality, Risk, and Responsibility." *Controversia* 5 (2): 67–90.

———. 2010. *Governing Childhood into the Twenty-First Century: Biopolitical Technologies of Childhood Management and Education*. New York: Palgrave.

Naik, G. 2009. "A Baby, Please. Blond, Freckles—Hold the Colic." *Wall Street Journal*, February 12.

National Institute of Mental Health. 2007. "NIH Funds New Program to Investigate Causes and Treatment of Autism." Science update, October 30. National Institute of Mental Health. Accessed September 8, 2010, http://www.nimh .nih.gov/science-news/2007/nih-funds-new-program-to-investigate-causes-and-treatment-of-autism.shtml.

National Institutes of Health. 2004. "Request for Proposal for Identifying Autism Susceptibility Genes." RFA-MH-05-007. National Institutes of Health. Accessed July 30, 2010, http://grants.nih.gov/grants/guide/rfa-files/RFA-MH-05-007.html.

———. 2006. "Request for Proposal for Autism Centers of Excellence." RFA-HD-06-016. National Institutes of Health. Accessed July 30, 2010, http://grants .nih.gov/grants/guide/rfa-files/RFA-HD-06-016.html.

———. 2008. "Newly Awarded Autism Centers of Excellence to Further Autism Research." *NIH News*, April 1. Accessed July 30, 2010, http://www.nih.gov/news/ health/apr2008/nimh-01.htm.

Nelkin, D. 2001. "Molecular Metaphors: The Gene in Popular Discourse." *Nature*, July, 556–59.

"New Autism Facts and Figures." 2012. *Parenting Magazine*, July 5. http://www .parenting.com/article/new-autism-facts-and-figures.

"New Centers to Focus on Autism and Other Developmental Disorders." 2002. *Environmental Health Perspectives* 110 (1): 20–21. http://www.ncbi.nlm.nih.gov/ pmc/articles/PMC1240703/pdf/ehp0110-a00020.pdf.

Ortega, F., and F. Vidal. 2011. *Neurocultures: Glimpses into an Expanding Universe*. Frankfurt: Lang.

Ozand, P., et al. 2003. "Autism: A Review." *Journal of Pediatric Neurology* 1 (2): 55–67.

Pinkel, D., et al. 1999. "Comparative Genomic Hybridization." Patent 5,965,362, October 12. http://patft.uspto.gov/netacgi/nph-.

President's Cancer Panel. 2008–2009. *Reducing Environmental Cancer Risk: What We Can Do Now.* Annual report. Accessed July 15, 2010, http://deainfo.nci.nih.govADVISORY/pcp/pcp08-09rpt/PCP_Report_08-09_508.pdf.

Preston, J. R. 2004. "Children as a Sensitive Subpopulation for the Risk Assessment Process." *Toxicology and Applied Pharmacology* 199 (2): 132–41.

Rajan, K. S. 2006. *Biocapital: The Constitution of Postgenomic Life.* Durham, N.C.: Duke University Press.

Ramus, F. 2006. "Genes, Brain, and Cognition: A Roadmap for the Cognitive Scientist." *Cognition* 101 (2): 247–69.

Reuters. 2010. "Pesticides Tied to ADHD in Children in U.S. Study." May 17. Accessed August 1, 2010, http://www.reuters.com/article/idUSTRE64G41R20100517.

Rimland, B. 1997. "Genetics, Autism, and Priorities." *Autism Research Review International* 11 (2): 3.

Rose, N. 2008. *The Politics of Life Itself.* Princeton, N.J.: Princeton University Press.

Safer Chemicals, Healthy Families. 2011. "The Safe Chemicals Act." Legislative update. Accessed September 7, 2010, http://www.saferchemicals.org/safechemicals-act/index.html.

Shreve, D. 2009. "Cliff Jumping Pirates in Aqua-Cars: Making Sense of Federal Education Programs in 2009." National Conference of State Legislatures. Accessed February 14, 2010, http://www.ncsl.org/?tabid=19343.

Sousa, I., et al. 2010. "Polymorphisms in Leucine-Rich Repeat Genes Are Associated with Autism Spectrum Disorder Susceptibility in Populations of European Ancestry." *Molecular Autism* 1 (7). Accessed October 7, 2010, http://www.ncbi.nlm.nih.gov/pmc/articles/PMC2913944/.

Stein, R. 2008. "Fetal Gene Testing Spurs Hope, Alarm." *Arizona Republic,* October 26.

Taibbi, M. 2010. "Will Goldman Sachs Prove Greed Is God?" *Common Dreams,* April 24. Accessed April 30, 2010, http://www.commondreams.org/view/2010/04/24.

Thompson, P., T. D. Cannon, and A. W. Toga. 2002. "Mapping Genetic Influences on Human Brain Structure." *Annals of Medicine* 34 (7–8): 523–36.

Tremain, S. 2005. *Foucault and the Government of Disability.* Ann Arbor: University of Michigan Press.

———. 2006. "Reproductive Freedom, Self-Regulation, and the Government of Impairment in Utero." *Hypatia* 21 (1): 35–53.

Tuna, C. 2010. "Fiscal Woes Push Up Class Size." *Wall Street Journal,* February 19. http://online.wsj.com/article/NA_WSJ_PUB:SB100014240527487043370045750600300026160638.html.

"U.K. Autism Research 'Is Lacking.'" 2004. BBC News, March 2. Accessed June 9, 2010, http://news.bbc.co.uk/go/pr/fr/-/2/hi/health/3522935.stm.

U.S. Centers for Disease Control. 2007. "1 in 150 Children Has Autism Spectrum Disorder." *Autism Research Review* 21 (1): 1.

U.S. Department of Education. 2010. "Fiscal Year 2011 Budget Summary." Section III.B, "Special Education and Rehabilitative Services," under "Special Education State Grants: Grants to States." ED.gov. Accessed September 30, 2010, http://www2.ed.gov/about/overview/budget/budget11/summary/edlite-section3b.html#spedstate.

U.S. Government Accounting Office. 2007. *Chemical Regulation: Comparison of U.S. and Recently Enacted European Union Approaches to Protect against the Risks of Toxic Chemicals.* GAO-07-825, August 17. Accessed May 5, 2009, http://www.gao.gov/docdblite/details.php?rptno=GAO-07-825.

Uttal, W. R. 2001. *The New Phrenology: The Limits of Localizing Cognitive Processes in the Brain.* Cambridge, Mass.: MIT Press.

"The Ventura Fanfiction Universe." 2011. Autism Research and Prenatal Testing. Accessed August 2, 2011, http://www.ventura33.com.

Vokurková, D., et al. 2010. "Radiosensitivity of CD3_CD8þCD56þ NK Cells." *Radiation Measurements* 45 (9): 1020–23.

Walsh, P., et al. 2011. "In Search of Biomarkers for Autism: Scientific, Social, and Ethical Challenges." *Nature Reviews Neuroscience* 12 (10): 603–12.

Weil, E. 2006. "A Wrongful Birth." *New York Times Magazine,* March 12. http://www.nytimes.com/2006/03/12/magazine/312wrongful.1.html?pagewanted=all.

"What Autism Research Is Being Done?" 2010. WebMD, October 15. Accessed October 22, 2010, http://answers.webmd.com/answers/1193900/What-autism-research-is-being-done.

World Health Organization. 2009. *ICD-10: International Statistical Classification of Diseases and Related Health Problems.* 10th rev., vol. 1. Geneva: World Health Organization.

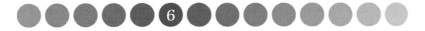

Caring for Autism
Toward a More Responsive State

Kristin Bumiller

Fewer than thirty years ago, the biomedical definition of autism gained acceptance over psychological explanations that often placed blame on the family (Bumiller 2009). This change in the understanding of autism ushered in new possibilities for treatment and forms of parent advocacy (Silverman 2011). This transformation was coterminous with a major shift in responsibility for the care of disabled children that began in the late 1970s. Children with disabilities were no longer fated to become wards of the state; the movement for family-based care revolutionized the disability world. The deinstitutionalization of care transformed expectations about the potential for a normal life for disabled individuals and made parents responsible for meeting their children's needs at home while claiming their share of public resources through rights-based entitlements. But it is also important to recognize that as the system of institutionalized care diminished, so did assumptions about protecting the home from the burdens of caretaking for the disabled. The state was no longer invested in protecting the middle-class family from the extraordinary demands of caring for a disabled child in order to preserve the normalcy of family life (Eyal et al. 2010).

These transformations are dramatic and recent; the first generation of children raised outside of institutions achieved an unprecedented level of independence. Disability advocates, many of whom worked in or had children who resided in the state homes for the "feeble-minded," ardently romanticize this change for good reasons—it brought an end to public institutions that warehoused the disabled and allowed for abominable treatment "behind closed doors." The move to community-based care also came with the promise of empowering parents to make decisions about their children, support for independent living, opportunities for social inclusion, and social justice for people with disabilities ("Community Imperative" 1979; Gleeson 1997; Lakin and Bruininks 1985).

Despite its intent to bring people into the community, this chapter argues that the advent of the biomedical model (with its shift to parental responsibility), in conjunction with the growth of neoliberal social policies, has created a system of privatized care for children with autism.[1] Drawing primarily on the context of the United States (in ways that may apply broadly to other Western democratic societies), the consequences of this shift to community-based care for families are explored, as well as the implicit model of state responsibility it furthers. This shift brought "community" integration in name only, for the location of care has moved from public institutions to the isolation of the household. Under this new system, the state plays a limited role in supporting the work that takes place inside private homes and in most cases will not allow for cash benefits to families. The state's narrowed responsibility for children with disabilities primarily resides with public schools, and the viability of this option is almost entirely dependent upon an adequate individualized education plan. Although community-based care for children with disabilities held the promise of granting greater autonomy and decision-making power to parents, this chapter demonstrates that the exercise of this power is highly variable. As a consequence, the idealization of normal life in the public sphere is threatened when inclusion policies appear unsuccessful and parents and children face intolerance in their community. The focus on the family often deflects attention from the failure of public institutions (including schools, Social Security disability, employment services, housing programs, and medical care) to cope with all the immediate challenges presented by the growing number of autistic children.

These issues are profoundly important for critical autism studies. Much of critical scholarship has been driven by efforts to construct an autism identity that recognizes the positive uniqueness of characteristics of people on the autism spectrum while also acknowledging that personhood is not defined in totality by one's disability. The focus on identity has fueled high expectations for the lives of people with autism, yet it has also drawn attention away from the centrality of material resources in creating more opportunities. Concerns are raised, most frequently by neurodiversity advocates, that popular culture and some advocacy groups place too great an emphasis on how autism is a burden to both the individual and society (Bagatell 2010). It is therefore crucial to break down the seeming contradiction between focusing on either identity or resource issues. Moreover, it is important to take into account the growing number of adults with autism and the resulting changes in the social and political landscape. These changes include the broadening of the definition of the condition, the increasing number of people identifying as autistic who have not received a medical diagnosis, the shift from the understanding of autism as a rare disease to a common condition, and the growing number of individuals desiring to advocate for themselves (Grinker 2010).

This analysis will show how the life chances of people with disabilities, in particular those with autism, are highly determined by the state policies that structure opportunities and provide financial support. Moreover, this chapter offers a critical perspective on how the recent history of the treatment of children with disabilities and proscriptions for future policies are directly connected to the changing nature of state responsibility. It presents the argument that an expansion in the role of the state in providing opportunities for people with disabilities is essential for persons with autism to satisfy their high expectations for involvement in the community. It also examines how the recent trend toward privatization of care is shifting responsibility onto families and how it is more generally affecting people with autism. In response to this worsening situation, it is necessary to reimagine the responsibilities of the state in the hope of creating a more socially inclusive future for people with autism.

The Complexities of Parent Advocacy

How we envisage responsibility for caring for people with autism depends greatly on how the disability is framed as a public problem. Increasingly, cultural narratives focus on genetic explanations for autism and their potential value in finding a cure. This has a profound impact on how affected families perceive their role as advocates, particularly their role in promoting autism awareness and championing biomedical research. In the contemporary context of disability activism, parents and other family members play an important role in the leadership of the major autism-advocacy organizations. In the United States, the most prominent of these organizations is Autism Speaks, an umbrella organization that primarily supports medical research. Undoubtedly, the rise of parent advocacy has had a significant impact on the changing understanding of and treatment for autism and has brought legitimacy to the agenda promoted by highly skilled parents. Chloe Silverman's research has documented this successful and complicated alliance between parents and professionals (2011).

However, this alliance has led to disputes between the more established advocacy organizations and parents and autistic individuals who have other agendas. Most notably, the more established advocacy groups have clashed with the "Mercury Moms," who claim that there is a link between vaccines and autism, as well as with the neurodiversity movement, which criticizes advocacy organizations' negative depiction of autistic people (Bagatell 2010; Bumiller 2008, 2009). Importantly, an active adult autism community that resists efforts to normalize autism has challenged the whole idea of parent advocacy. This is most acutely seen in the controversies regarding ABA (applied behavior analysis) therapies, which have produced a direct conflict between parents who struggle to obtain state funding and spokespersons for Asperger organizations who see such therapies as actually harmful (Bagatell 2010).

Moreover, a recent study of parental response to medicalization in Australia found that the expectation of "choice" was problematic when parents with autistic children were placed in a complex system of service provision. For parents who were overwhelmed by the information offered by experts, choice was a disempowering experience, and more active parents didn't exercise real choice under current conditions of resource constraint and service rationing. Regardless of apparent passivity or assertiveness, parents sorted through a "maelstrom of information" and made decisions based upon contested evidence, complex ethical considerations, and their own capacity to purchase services (Valentine 2010, 956). This reality is at odds with advocacy organizations' idealization of good parent advocates for their capacity to function alongside professionals.

Although the new biological understanding of autism has empowered some parents and increased their status vis-à-vis professionals, it is important to consider whether it has actually improved families' day-to-day circumstances. This question cannot be fully addressed without more empirical data about the relationship between parents and professionals and detailed information about the impact on families' lives. The question also raises issues at the heart of critical autism studies, such as whether the desired social outcome is reducing the incidence of autism, providing accommodations, or creating societal acceptance of autistic traits. In addition, it is vital to consider the socioeconomic factors that may enable families with more resources to take fuller advantage of their role as advocates and to gain the respect of professionals. Also at issue, as Majia Holmer Nadesan discusses in this volume, is whether monetary support of genetically focused autism research comes at the cost of providing direct services for families and people with autism. Finally, the success of these new forms of activism also should be measured in terms of the interest and desires of people with autism (who are independent from and potentially different from their families).

Shifting Responsibility

As parents have taken a larger role in advocacy focused on medical intervention, the family-empowerment philosophy that fueled the movement for community-based care is no longer at the forefront of disability advocacy. The movement, as originally conceived, was about respecting parents as experts about their own children and relying upon their leadership to further their children's integration into the community. The nature of the disabling condition was less important than the need of children, both in the present and as future adults, to enjoy the same opportunities as other citizens. The objective of the movement was not only to end institutionalization but also to eradicate the social stigma that justified hiding away children with disabilities. The philosophical commitment of the movement rested on the idea that a better life emerged from exercising one's right to become a fully participating member of the community.

Achieving the full ambitions of the movement for community-based living is profoundly compromised by the difficulties parents face in navigating a highly compartmentalized system of disability services for children with autism, including public-school-based special education, in-home care, family-empowerment programs, rehabilitation programs, adult independent-living communities, and Social Security. In their efforts to navigate these systems, successful parents must create a master narrative about their children's disability and needs that offsets the lack of direction and planning among multiple service providers

(Keenan et al. 2010). The art of parent advocacy is about coordinating children's services within systems and through mandatory transitions. As children age, parents are frequently at risk of losing support systems that have been put in place. At each stage, parents often confront new challenges to eligibility that require them to strategically reinforce definitions of disability to assure the continuation of services. Programs have limited formal or informal mechanisms that allow them to work together, creating more reliance on parental coordination. The separation of programs by age group and sphere of life activity, as well as the growth of "professionalized" approaches, makes it rare for any one program to address the child as a whole. This problem is accentuated by the fact that the specialized nature of disability services allows for little consideration of race, ethnicity, and unique family arrangements. If a good parent advocate fails in her efforts to put a functioning program in place, such as a specialized school program, the results can be catastrophic given the amount of support some autistic children need to function in any environment. Parents with insufficient advocacy skills often repeatedly fail to maintain the most basic services and are left with little more than day-to-day crisis management. Moreover, the work of caring for disabled children and adults, usually undertaken by mothers, is unpaid and socially invisible. Much of this work involves the physical care of children and is often extraordinary in comparison to typical child-care responsibilities (Baker and Drapela 2010).

The end result is that parents essentially function as quasi-governmental organizations by assuming a case-manager position. Coordinating public services is especially taxing because of the overall inadequacy of those services. Given the unique challenges of managing the life of a person with special needs, conflicts between professionals and parents are almost inevitable (Hodge and Runswick-Cole 2008; Dillenburger et al. 2010). Professionals tend to evaluate the competence of their parenting in a fashion similar to parents of typical children; parents need to show that they can discipline their children, prepare them for schooling, be responsive to teachers' criticisms, and provide a stable home life. Often, professionals treat failure as a problem with parents (related to depression, stress management, poor parenting skills, and the like) rather than a result of the unique requirements of the child or the extraordinary requirements of case management (Weiss and Lunsky 2011).

This creates a situation where the greatest challenge in parenting a child with autism may be related not to the condition itself but to managing the child's life in the public domain (Neely-Barnes et al. 2011). Although care needs in the home may be considerable, these responsibilities are made even more significant by the demands outside of the home. This shift to in-home care, incongruously, comes with more exposure to and with greater demands for functioning in the public domain. This can be particularly overwhelming in relation to autistic children, where the unpredictability of a public setting is often more difficult than living comfortably at home. Acting appropriately in public is often a major undertaking and involves support to understand social cues as well as functioning under conditions where the environment is difficult to control. Even more pressure is created in situations where a child's success or failure in the public domain leads to a judgment about the quality of parenting. This places an enormous burden on parents of autistic children that is separate and distinct from the day-to-day issues of living with the disability. Sociologist David Farrugia, in an empirical study of the experiences of parents of children with autism, finds that these parents describe an unusually high degree of stigma compared to parents of children with other disabilities. He found that "regular breaches of social norms in social situations can lead to feelings of shame and humiliation, as well as exclusion from normal social activities" (2009, 1013). This situation was compounded by the fact that the "normal" appearance of children with autism made it more likely that parents were compelled to provide an explanation for their children's unruly behavior. This was necessary to avoid stigmatizing "views of their children, and, by association, their families and themselves" (1013). He also found that the management of stigma was particularly difficult in anonymous public situations, and parents often resorted to the difficult process of trying to use medical definitions to explain their child's behavior (1024). Even in school settings, parents had to struggle to counteract accusations that parenting was the cause of deviant behavior by employing medical explanations or the assistance of experts.

There are other ways that the caretaking function disrupts parents' participation in the public sphere; families report that friends and acquaintances are unwilling to spend time in their home because of the modifications that are associated with an "autism household" (Farrugia 2009, 1017). Whole households are structured around the needs of a child with autism, such that all activities are governed by strict routines.

This restructuring of family life creates a household environment distinct from the larger community (1019). Another study found that parents of children with high-functioning autism "restricted their social lives to accommodate the potentially disturbing encounters that could arise from their child's inappropriate public behavior" (Gray 2002, 741). Parents often experience hostile staring and rude comments in public situations (Gray 2002). Bystanders assuming that public incidents are manifestations of bad behavior rather than neurological difference accentuate these reactions.

In evaluating the shift of responsibility onto the family, it is critical to acknowledge that the consequences are not gender-neutral. Single mothers are heads of household in a significant percentage of families of children with autism (Graetz 2010). In two-parent (bi-gender) families, more responsibility is often placed on mothers in a manner that extends the preexisting unfairness inherent in the gendered division of labor within American households. The isolation of the autistic household, as well as the need to negotiate stigmatized identities in public settings, places additional burdens above and beyond the usual physical and emotional costs of mothering children. Feminist theorist Marjorie Devault elaborates how the high stress of meeting the needs of children with disabilities is often related to accommodating social and institutional demands. She also notes that deinstitutionalization has operated on the assumption that families provide "infinitely flexible emotional safety nets" (Devault 1999, 61). Moreover, in a study by David E. Gray, mothers frequently experienced stigmatizing encounters in public (2002, 743–45). Persistent stereotypes about the inadequacy of women's care of male children (including failure to discipline, lack of male role models, failure to prevent criminal involvement, and other stereotypes associated with motherhood) are often applied to mothers who must publicly deal with their children's challenging behaviors. The additional burden placed on mothers is often discounted in a social and market economy that devalues the efforts of women.

Hence, the move to deinstitutionalize is a complex and unfinished process with untold effects on family life. The shift to community care leaves families in the situation of providing and coordinating complex systems of care with minimal respite, and free-market forces end up replacing the public good in the home health-care business (Peter et al. 2007). In most cases, moreover, parents must continue both to provide the care at home and to coordinate services when their children become adults (Graetz 2010). The excessive personal and financial investment in managing children with disabilities is warranted, because the success of adults in the labor market and the achievement of other milestones of independent living are highly related to the benefit of exceptional parenting (Pascall and Hendey 2004).

Privatizing Cost

At the same time that parents have assumed a delineated role as advocates and have taken responsibility for coordinated service provision for their children, the state has also redefined its role and responsibilities in regard to citizens who need care. A fuller picture of the historical transformation in disability policy requires examining the connections between the shift of responsibility onto the family and the devolution of the welfare system in the United States and other Western democracies. In the United States, the "end of welfare" is justified by a new moral consensus based upon an "ethic of personal responsibility" (Mink and Solinger 2003). The Personal Responsibility and Work Opportunity Reconciliation Act of 1996 (PRWORA) activated the discourse of responsibility in regard to welfare recipients and has had a broad influence in a wide range of policy debates fueled by the crumbling of redistributive welfare and the fiscal crisis of the state (Albelda and Withorn 2002). The policy debates regarding provisions for people with disabilities are influenced by the same logic and rhetoric, in particular, the belief that poverty is alleviated through independence and employment. In a social-welfare state, disability creates a welfare entitlement on grounds similar to childhood and old age, based upon the notion of inherent dependency. Subsumed under this category, welfare policy casts the disabled as worthy of government assistance because of their need to be "cared for" throughout the life span (Priestly 2000). As a policy justification, this is particularly incongruent with the notion of independence and the diverse manifestation of autism within a lifetime and among people on the spectrum.

Specifically, welfare reform, as we know it in the United States and in other countries experiencing a retrenchment in the social-welfare state, is about replacing financial support with work incentives. On its face, this shift to the new welfare seems to be consistent with the efforts of disability activists who push for financial independence through paid work and the removal of barriers to full inclusion in the workplace. However, there is a clear difference between disability activists who see workplace participation as a "right" and welfare policies in which "workfare" is a punitive measure to prevent overreliance on public assistance (Galvin 2004, 346). Similarly, the problem of access to work, as defined by disability activists, is linked to failure to provide accommodations in the employment environment; and in welfare policy the problem is deemed to be the lack of individual initiative (Galvin 2004).

The advent of neoliberal social policy also has far-reaching consequences for the deinstitutionalization process. In the United States (and many other countries), deinstitutionalization is incomplete and has failed to result in desirable independent-living situations (Mansell 2006). This has been primarily due to the implementation of a market-based approach to the delivery of services. In community-delivered programs, people with disabilities are deemed "consumers," and the term "service user" has become widely used. Peter Beresford notes how such language is not neutral; it denotes "little more than an administrative category of welfare consumption" and "may create and perpetuate a different and inferior identity for those associated with it" (2005, 476). Moreover, the market model has encouraged the development of generic and cost-efficient services. This model is particularly ill suited for people with autism; rather than calling for skilled and preventative behavior management, the dominant model of care is unskilled minding (Mansell 2006). The continuing process of deinstitutionalization is moving toward the de-differentiating disability; this allows for the minimum standards across disabilities and eliminates the need for specialized expertise. The overarching concerns are twofold: that services are delivered to meet "good enough" standards rather than to support the full range of potential among people with disabilities; and, ultimately, that the poor results of community care will justify a return to institutionalized arrangements (Mansell 2006, 73).

The high costs associated with caring for autism has created a particular challenge to prevailing postwelfare consensus. There has been a dramatic growth in the potential costs to families and society, and in this market context, the primary pressure for meeting such costs are pushed into the private sphere. Nadesan further explores this issue in this volume, noting that both private and public funding is focused on biomedical research and large national institutions, whereas there is extremely limited funding at the state and local levels for treatment and family services. Although the notion of an autism epidemic is highly disputed, it is nonetheless the case that, starting in the late 1990s, there has been a rapid increase in the number of children diagnosed on the autistic spectrum (Wazana, Bresnahan, and Kline 2007). Whether or not the future brings a slowing or a reduction in incidence, there is currently a large cohort of children with autism who are reaching adulthood and who will require lifetime support.

The potential costs of lifetime support will be enormous, and parents of children with autism will not be well situated to assume those costs. In a recent study, Harvard Public Health School professor Michael Ganz claims that the "lifetime per capita incremental societal cost of autism is $3.2 million" (2007, 348). This figure is based upon an attempt to estimate both the direct and indirect costs of autism, where direct costs are a measure of goods and services, and indirect costs are a measure of lost productivity.[2] However, the increase in medical expenses is insubstantial compared to the lost productivity of both people with autism and their parents. The most significant costs, according to Ganz's economic model, are constituted by the unemployment of individuals with autism and their parents. In the long run, unemployment reduces the capacity of parents to cope with lifetime care needs. As parents and children age, the combined effect of the adult child's limited income and the decreased income and savings of parents who have financially supported their child will create an even greater financial burden on these families (348).

Adopting the prevailing "ethic of personal responsibility," Ganz suggests that parents might be able to seek "financial counseling" to plan for these lifetime costs. Yet Ganz's own model suggests that this is an unrealistic expectation to place on parents. Even with the best financial planning, it is unlikely that families can compensate for the economic disadvantages created by caring for a child with autism. In fact, studies show that parents of children with disabilities have a distinctively lower sense of well-being and professional attainment in midlife (Selzer et al. 2001). Moreover, privatizing the economic burden has disproportionate consequences for women. Ganz fails to take into account how gender inequalities place disproportional time demands on women in the home and result in less earning capacity in the workplace.[3] His model is also based upon a household definition that fails to take into consideration different family configurations; a family is constituted by a mother, a father, and one child with autism. Consequently, the economic model fails to account for a common family arrangement for children with autism: families headed by single mothers. Dana Lee Baker and Laurie Drapela show that there are adverse employment effects for parents of children with autism, and the most severe impacts are experienced by mothers (2010).

The privatization of all categories of costs—medical, nonmedical, and in-home care and adult supports—potentially puts families at increased risk for poverty and accentuates preexisting gender differences in labor-market participation. As I emphasized earlier, these consequences are rapidly emerging as the incidence of autism increases and as a large cohort of people with autism is reaching adulthood. The effect on families is also highly related to how other institutions, such as schools and social-services agencies, respond to the growing incidence of autism. In particular, it is important to consider how even more pressure is placed on families when they are faced with inflexibility or retrenchment of services. The next sections examine how increased stress on institutional structures results in further shifting of the costs of disability onto the private sphere.

Educational Policy

In the context of a declining role of the state in providing social supports for families, the primary forum for treatment of children with autism has been the public schools. This creates a situation where successful social inclusion is almost entirely dependent upon obtaining services from school districts. The Individuals with Disabilities Education Act (IDEA), enacted by Congress in 1990, was conceived as an instrument of deinstitutionalization and the primary means to move children from state homes and other restrictive placements to "free and appropriate" educational settings. The act invests rights in the child, but its enforcement is dependent upon the parent aggressively pursuing those rights. Parents, until recently (as modified in court decisions), had no independent rights or interests in their children's educational opportunities. IDEA has narrower eligibility requirements than earlier special education provisions under section 504 and is more specifically aimed at improving educational results for students with disabilities (Weber 2009). The explicit purpose of a free and appropriate education is to prepare children for productive roles in society, especially employment.

Under IDEA, special education methodologies tend to be normalizing. That is, the goals focus on improving a child's ability to function in mainstream educational settings rather than transforming the educational environment to suit the needs of children with disabilities. Despite the requirements of IDEA to address the after-school, home, and summer recreation needs of children, such programming is the most difficult to extract from districts. The result is that in-school programming is generally all that most children receive; this, in effect, puts a low priority on the child's recreation, social needs, and quality of family life. Moreover, neither school districts nor parents have incentives to provide services that meet the needs of more than one child. In fact, privacy regulations get in the way of groups of parents realizing they have common concerns and need similar educational modifications.

The number and cost of children with autism qualifying for services under IDEA have taxed the educational system and its funding mechanisms. From 1993 to 2002, the number of children (ages 6–21) receiving services under IDEA increased 805 percent. Moreover, the cost of educating children with autism under IDEA has risen to three times the amount of educating children without a disability ($18,760 versus $6,556; Marlett 2009, 62). As a result of this dramatic increase, courts have minimized the demands on local school districts by restricting eligibility (in ways inconsistent with the original intention of the act) and placed the burden of proof on parents by providing services only in response to the child's serious academic failure.

The most significant change in the policies came in 2004, when the Individuals with Disabilities Education Improvement Act (IDEIA) was passed in order to make IDEA consistent with the goals of the No Child Left Behind Act (NCLB). These changes led to greater imbalances regarding the burden of proof and more restrictions on the recovery of attorney and expert fees. The new regulations also included children with disabilities under district-wide performance rankings and defined performance goals as the same for all students. Commentators who were critical, more generally, of the use of standards in NCLB saw promise in the attempt to align IDEA with NCLB. It was hoped that these requirements brought into focus how the issue of providing resources and improving the quality of education for children with disabilities was linked to the education of all children. Although this alignment creates incentives for school districts to employ high standards in teaching children with disabilities, it may also narrow the performance goals to testable skills. This strengthens the tendency, already underpinning IDEA, that the purpose of special education is to help children develop employable skills rather than to meet the broader skills necessary for full inclusion.

At the same time, the alignment raises a larger issue related to the persistent failure of school districts to comply with special education regulations. The districts with the poorest records of compliance often serve urban areas and are not meeting the needs of students more generally. These school districts face a wide range of issues, including growing achievement gaps, low student and teacher retention, lack of parental involvement, budget constraints, deteriorating facilities, waning public confidence, and negative racial attitudes. In a recent survey of major urban public-school systems about the most pressing needs, administrators ranked special education "twenty-third out of forty-three listed" (MacArdy 2009, 879). The study demonstrates that administrators in urban school districts often see a trade-off between addressing the educational needs of children with disabilities and meeting other demands. Although the stresses on urban schools might be seen as a justification for reducing the expectations placed on school districts and relaxing compliance standards for failing schools, another strategy is to integrate the goals of IDEA into an overall approach of reforming education.

However, the enforcement mechanisms of IDEA work against this strategy. IDEA allows parents to advocate for programming that is specifically designed to remedy their children's disabling condition and is based on the assumption that special education techniques work best if tailored to a child's unique needs. This approach to special education fundamentally prevents school systems from addressing group issues across disabilities and coordinating efforts to help children with other needs. Special education funnels resources to children with documented disabilities and does little to improve the education of disadvantaged students more generally.

The enormous difficulties involved in enforcing IDEA, particularly for children with autism who require specialized programs and well-trained teachers, may have made less-inclusive options more attractive to parents who desire to obtain the best-quality services. Disability advocates are making the case for revising the requirement for the least restrictive environment that is a core component of IDEA. Law professor Ruth Colker suggests that mainstreaming is no longer necessary; instead, more emphasis should be placed on attaining high-quality approaches to mitigate the disabling condition (2006). She claims that mainstreaming is often inappropriate and that Congress should modify the standards for a less restrictive educational environment to allow for a subjective, case-by-case approach. Other special education scholars have joined Colker to support a "modern incarnation of the mainstreaming requirement" that relaxes restrictions on segregated education for "children with ASD [autism spectrum disorder] because of the inherent tensions between the underlying principles of mainstreaming and the clinical features of autism" (McDonough 2008, 1255–56). In the reincarnated model, inclusion in regular classrooms is no longer viewed as presumptive, for three reasons. The first is that the stigmatization that results from segregated settings does not apply in the education of autistic children. This conclusion is based upon evidence that finds that autistic children "do not tend to report accurately social acceptance nor do they appear to express loneliness despite lower social acceptance" (McDonough 2008, 1256). The second reason is that treatments for autism require extensive time spent one-on-one with a therapist. It is suggested that autistic children may benefit more from time working with a therapist than from being mainstreamed with nondisabled peers (McDonough 2008, 1257). Finally, the importance of mainstreaming is questioned because of the lack of efficacy of behavioral therapies in teaching social skills. If autistic children have no "intrinsic desire" to enact social skills, then it is assumed that they are better off being taught useful "communication skills" rather than being provided a mainstream environment to allow for normal social interaction (McDonough 2008, 1258). All three arguments are based upon debatable assumptions about autistic children's capacities for emotional connection, their deeper understanding of the social sphere, and their capacity for more complex learning. Critical autism studies has challenged such reductionist interpretations of the emotional life of people with autism and has provided a cautionary perspective on efforts to downplay the advantages of mainstreaming.

In the context of inadequately trained teachers, school administrators hostile to inclusion, and the need for frequent monitoring to assure the adequacy of mainstreaming programs, parents are given a strong incentive to abandon inclusive educational approaches. Courts have already shown a willingness to side with parents who feel that an appropriate education for their children involves therapies outside of regular classrooms (McDonough 2008, 1259). This inclination is furthered by biomedical knowledge that puts a strong emphasis on intensive early intervention as opposed to creating opportunities for children to interact with other, nonautistic children.

The diminishing demand for social inclusion is a distressing and consequential trend. It has the potential to erode the ideological foundations of the movement for deinstitutionalization. This push is often led by parents and advocates with the most resources and experience in combating institutional resistance. This is due in part to the fact that they see the best opportunities for their children in programs outside of the mainstream. This trend poses the risk of drawing limited resources to specialized settings and bringing an end to the most ambitious efforts to transform traditional classrooms according to the principles of special education. These programs also set a precedent for establishing less costly segregated programs for children who do not benefit from strong parental advocacy. As I have argued, the process of deinstitutionalization remains incomplete, and the failure to maintain cost-effective services in community settings may justify the return to education in institutionalized settings. Most importantly, the overriding philosophical arguments for inclusion are being eclipsed by seemingly practical and/or individualistic concerns. The impetus to reverse the mainstreaming priority weakens the vision of community participation and empowerment at the core of the movement for community-based living.

Social Security

In the United States, the Social Security disability system that is currently in place originated in 1960, when Congress eliminated the age limit (of 50) in programs that covered workers who became disabled prior to retirement. Changes in 1965 and 1972 opened eligibility to those without permanent disabilities and with no prior work experience, and this dramatically increased the numbers receiving disability benefits. Subsequently, Congress has enacted several measures in an attempt to reduce the rolls by excluding those who are able to participate in any kind of substantial gainful work (Colker 2007). Disability payments are approximately 16 percent of the Social Security budget.

Supplemental Security Income (SSI) is the only form of cash benefit available to people with disabilities and to low-income parents of children with disabilities. However, the program is not designed to provide income maintenance or long-term support. SSI only mitigates poverty; it does not lift recipients above the poverty line (Berry 2000). The system was created primarily to address temporary disabilities, and its policies are essentially incompatible with the notion of lifetime disabling conditions. Yet parents of children with disabilities often experience loss of income and unemployment, and new provisions such as the Family Leave Act are grossly insufficient to deal with such demands on these parents. No other comprehensive social programs recognize or compensate families for the unpaid caretaking and nonreimbursable resources required to provide for children with disabilities.

There is no "security" in Social Security for the disabled. When disability benefits are available, they function more like public assistance than social insurance, because provisions are deemed temporary and subject to frequent eligibility determinations. The system is administered in a highly bureaucratic and punitive fashion in which most reviews end up in automatic denial of benefits, a situation that is resolved only through a lengthy appeal process. Achieving earnings that barely exceed Social Security levels results in elimination of Medicare eligibility that is often essential to people with disabilities. Moreover, the program creates disincentives to employment and strict limitations on resource accumulation. The Social Security system, in effect, sets up poverty as the norm for the disabled population.

Policy makers have long recognized that SSI exists in synergistic relationship with public assistance and unemployment insurance. Specifically as a result of the PRWORA, all children receiving SSI need a re-eligibility determination at eighteen years of age, and the Social Security Administration recommends cessation for 56 percent of recipients entering adulthood (Berry 2000). In fact, PRWORA provided for a "marked effort to restrict access to the SSI program" (Auxter et al. 1999, 196). The intent of the legislative change was to redetermine the eligibility of all children on the rolls who qualified under the "individualized functional assessment due to maladaptive behavior" (Davies, Howard, and Rapp 2000, 9). Although Medicaid benefits were supposedly grandfathered, many parents lost Medicaid during the redetermination process. A study of the overall effects of these changes found that parents compensated for the loss of SSI benefits by entering the labor force and, if they were already working, by increasing their work hours. However, despite these actions, overall family income decreased. The effect was to further impoverish families with children with disabilities: "Others suffered greater reductions in total family income after SSI benefits were lost because work hours had to be reduced in order to meet child care demands. Finally, many families turned to other public assistance programs to replace SSI income" (7). Families subject to these eligibility determinations have reported that they were too frightened and intimidated by Social Security Administration personnel to challenge the cutoffs ("SSI Families" 1998). Yet, given the decrease in Temporary Assistance for Needy Families benefits since 1996, receiving SSI benefits may be the best means to increase the probability that families will receive the extra income necessary to be lifted out of extreme poverty levels (Duggan and Kearney 2007).

Despite the inadequacy of the SSI program, commentators pushing forward the neoliberal agenda of welfare reform have targeted Social Security disability as wasteful government spending and as an area in which there is a need to shift the public/private boundary by using "market-reform" strategies to divest the state of its obligations. Such calls for fiscal austerity adversely impact people with disabilities who already are a low priority for government funding (Nadesan, this volume). Henry Olsen and John Flugstad, for example, have claimed that Social Security disability is a prime example of one of the programs growing at an unsustainable rate, and they categorize it as one of the "forgotten entitlements." They lampoon the word *disabled* as it is applied by the Social Security Administration, claiming that it should evoke "quadriplegics and speechless stroke victims" but that actually people on disability insurance are those with "back pain, mental problems, and other hard to diagnose maladies" (2009, 43). Olsen and Flugstad argue that SSI and SSDI (Social Security Disability Insurance) should "clean up the eligibility criteria and appeals process to help establish an expectation of work" (51). Disability advocates are already taking up the solutions offered by market reformers. Their hope is to shift the burden of treatment costs to private insurers. In this regard, autism advocates, led by Autism Speaks, are lobbying for legislative reforms that make certain behaviorally based treatments medical expenditures.

Although Social Security disability was created as a temporary benefit provided for low-income families with disabled children and disabled adults, the program is not linked to comprehensive rehabilitation efforts. In line with "workfare" created by welfare reform, the Social Security Administration created the Ticket to Work Program; however, this program has received limited funding and has been applied only to recipients who have the greatest chance of moving to employment. Robert Wilton and Stephanie Schuer argue that in the contemporary context, disabled persons are put "in a precarious position between an increasingly hostile welfare state and a labour market in which the 'able-body/mind' remains a largely unquestioned norm" (2006, 186). They note how such programs, often portrayed as liberating disabled people from dependency, focus on using employment experts to train individuals rather than creating more accommodating and accessible contexts for employment. They also suggest that we need to understand disabled persons' work opportunities in the context of the rise of low-wage service employment. They raise concerns about exploitation, especially in situations where employers are eager to hire people with disabilities because they perceive them as more compliant. They found that employers in food service, custodial, and care work recruited people with disabilities because they saw these people as "grateful for work and willing to tolerate downgraded service jobs" (193). Although the incentive to hire compliant workers may have made more jobs available, it did not open up possibilities for better-quality work.

Under current policies, the predominant type of job offered to disabled persons is in the form of assisted employment. This model has largely involved placing clients in segregated workshops or providing job coaching rather than finding competitive employment in private markets (Hendricks 2010). People with autism are a rapidly growing group of individuals requiring vocational services, and there is evidence that they have less successful employment outcomes (Cimera and Cowan 2009). This failure is linked to the fact that vocational models designed for people with intellectual disabilities may not be appropriate for many adults with autism (Muller et al. 2003). Adults with autism may not fit well into assisted employment venues, and often such positions may allow for neither mainstreaming into the employment sector nor the possibility of meaningful work. One issue is that individuals with autism have significantly different vocational-counseling needs than people with developmental disabilities (Hendricks 2010). Assisted employment is also often provided in only limited venues and may not allow individuals to exercise their highest capacities.

The available evidence suggests that more than half of adults with autism are not receiving a working wage (Graetz 2010). Not surprisingly, studies have found that participation in vocational rehabilitation programs does not increase the likelihood of obtaining employment, possibly because most individuals need structured and long-term supports to remain employed (Berry 2000). Those who are employed are often underemployed (Hendricks 2010). Interviews with individuals with autism utilizing vocational services show that these individuals have diverse career interests (rather than fitting any stereotyped idea of autistic interests) but are highly likely to have had negative work experiences because of lack of specific supports and accommodations (Muller et al. 2003). People with autism are "challenged by the need to negotiate the complex sensory geographies of everyday life" (Davidson 2010, 311). Consequently, employment opportunities could be broadly expanded for people with autism simply by recognizing the differences in their sensory experiences and, in many cases, by making relatively minor adaptations of the work environment. Only when vocational efforts are attuned to the functional diversity of people with autism will supports lead to the highest level of success (Schall 2010).

Imagining a Responsible State

Overall, the privatization of care has highly regressive consequences: it potentially enables success for families of means but reinforces the disadvantages of the poor. Limited resources to assist families are also in direct competition with other social-welfare programs and funds for educating children with other disadvantages. In the case of people with autism, the situation is hiding an emerging crisis; the growing number of children and adults requiring services has not been matched by an adequate, or even realistic, commitment of public funds.

Some disability activists have given up on the full realization of the movement for social inclusion. Philosophers Adrianne Asch, Jeffrey Blustein, and David T. Wasserman articulate this view: "Neighbours have increasingly become strangers, and social life has increasingly become fragmented and compartmentalized. Even if there was the will and wherewithal to integrate people with severe disabilities into the community, the community itself has become an elusive target" (2008, 161). They also argue that the family itself has become less involved in the wider community and less able to rely upon an expansive network of relatives. In these terms, the failure of movement is linked to the demise of community more generally. This explanation, however, may rest upon an idealization of family and community as autonomous sources of support. Moreover, it fails to recognize the essential dynamic of deinstitutionalization: more expectations are being placed on the private sphere without regard for the costs imposed.

Although there are compelling reasons for parents to retreat from inadequately designed efforts for maintaining their children in public schools and the community, further retrenchment from an already diminished public sphere is not the answer. The difficulties families face in promoting social inclusion are a direct result of the evolving process of deinstitutionalization and its unprecedented shift of the costs of disability onto the private sphere.

The objectives of disability activism should be firmly grounded in achieving the broadest ambitions for the exercise of citizenship for people with disabilities and their families. From this perspective, it is important to imagine how people with autism will participate in *all aspects* of employment, social life, and intimate relationships. It is also vital to push for change in public institutions (whether it is structural, in regard to job environments, or about societal attitudes toward people who appear different) so that they are constituted in ways that are autism- and disability-friendly. Such efforts would begin from a broader definition of inclusion than was originally conceived by the movement for community-based living.

The foundation for continued disability advocacy, therefore, should not be a focus on individual rights but a call for a public sphere more densely laden with opportunities for participation, enjoyment, and productivity. In this respect, advocates need to go beyond considering the merits of an institutional setting versus those in community life. Asch, Blustein, and Wasserman take the position that some institutional-care arrangements will continue to exist and should be thought of as the best alternative by some people with disabilities and their families. They argue that, given this reality, it is crucial to develop ethical standards and open up the possibilities to innovation within institutionalized settings: "Many of the real advances in enabling disabled people to live in the world have come from outside the political and social mainstream, in particular, the disability rights movement. . . . This is clearly a prime area for innovation: for experiments, pilot projects, and partnerships between public and private organizations" (2008, 166). Asch, Blustein, and Wasserman are calling for an affirmation of the fundamental inspiration of the disability-rights movement: a redesigning of human possibilities within public space. The most powerful examples are found in situations where disability awareness leads to transformation of public spaces occupied by individuals with a full range of abilities. In this regard, the best expansion of IDEA is to apply its principles more generally to all school-age children (Seligmann 2008). This expansion would transform curriculum to accommodate for a wide variety of learning styles and would affirm the right of all persons with autism to demand the accountability of a public education.

The first step is moving from a system that encourages dependency to support structures that affirm broad participation in the public sphere. This begins by challenging the foundational premise of both the ADA and the Social Security system that participation in the workforce, even if employment is insufficient to raise individuals above the poverty level and does little to further personal development, is the ultimate goal for people with disabilities. Incorporation in the labor force should not be the only option for sustaining an independent life. New, various, and meaningful opportunities for contributing to the common welfare should be made available to persons with disabilities. This involves creating ways of "pluralizing the public": bringing activities associated with the private sphere into the public domain. In the case of autism, this would mean creating more space in public settings amenable to the unique characteristics of persons with autism rather than expecting that these differences should be hidden away in "autism households."

Finally, we need a concept of public life that is compatible with a variety of care arrangements. The movement for community living was based on a static and idealized notion of the family, and its aspirations were dependent on the readiness of all families to serve as centers of advocacy. A new model of community needs to recognize the challenges and costs of inclusion that families experience.

Moving forward to preserve the interests and meet the needs of people with disabilities in general, and with autism in particular, can begin only with a reimagining of the public responsibilities of the state. My argument comes at an inauspicious moment in the United States, as state-level budget cutting driven by the recession has disproportionately affected disability-related programs. These devastating cutbacks come close to eliminating the already-underfunded infrastructure of programs that support children and adults in the community. Moreover, if this era follows the pattern of previous historical periods of financial crisis, then it is likely to lead to new state strategies in dealing with vulnerable populations and more inequality in general. This is all the more reason for disability-rights activists to clearly articulate their ambitions for social inclusion and to think creatively about how to further meaningful participation in public life.

NOTES

1. This chapter considers these consequences for children with a wide range of disabilities, but it places particular emphasis on their impact on children with autism.

2. Ganz describes his measurement as follows: "Direct medical costs were obtained either from the literature or from an analysis of the Medical Expenditure Panel Survey (MEPS) and the National Health Interview Survey (NHIS). Special education, transportation, child care and babysitting, respite care, out-of-home placement, home and vehicle modifications, and supported employment services are typical components of direct nonmedical costs.

"Indirect costs are the value of lost or impaired work time (income), benefits, and household services of individuals with autism and their caregivers because of missed time at work, reduced work hours, switching to a lower-paying but more flexible job, or leaving the workforce. Indirect costs were computed using a human capital approach that combines average earnings, benefits, and household services with information on average work-life expectancies and labor force participation rates for men and women at different ages" (2007, 344).

3. In Ganz's analysis, the productivity lost by parents was measured by predicting that the unemployment levels of fathers would be 10–20 percent and that of mothers would be 55–60 percent (2007, 344).

REFERENCES

Albelda, R., and A. Withorn, eds. 2002. *Lost Ground: Welfare Reform, Poverty, and Beyond.* Boston: South End Press.

Asch, A., J. Blustein, and D. T. Wasserman. 2008. "Criticizing and Reforming Segregated Facilities for Persons with Disabilities." *Bioethical Inquiry* 5 (2–3): 157–67.

Auxter, D., et al. 1999. "The Precarious Safety Net: Supplemental Security Income and Age 18 Redeterminations." *Focus on Autism and Other Development Disabilities* 14 (4): 194–203.

Bagatell, N. 2010. "From Cure to Community: Transforming Notions of Autism." *Ethos* 38 (1): 33–55.

Baker, D. L., and L. Drapela. 2010. "Mostly the Mother: Concentration of Adverse Employment on Mothers of Children with Autism." *Social Science Journal* 47 (3): 578–92.

Beresford, P. 2005. "'Service User': Regressive or Liberatory Terminology?" *Disability and Society* 20 (4): 469–77.

Berry, H. G. 2000. "The Supplemental Security Income Program and Employment for Young Adults with Disabilities." *Focus on Autism and Other Developmental Disabilities* 15 (3): 176–81.

Bumiller, K. 2008. "Quirky Citizens: Autism and the Anti-normalization of Politics." *Signs: Journal of Women and Culture in Society* 33 (4): 967–91.

———. 2009. "The Geneticization of Autism: From New Reproductive Technologies to the Conception of Genetic Normalcy." *Signs: Journal of Women and Culture in Society* 34 (4): 875–98.

Cimera, R. E., and R. Cowan. 2009. "The Costs of Services and Employment Outcomes Achieved by Adults with Autism in the US." *Autism: The International Journal of Research and Practice* 13 (3): 285–302.

Colker, R. 2006. "The Disability Integration Presumption: Thirty Years Later." *University of Pennsylvania Law Review* 154: 789–862.

———. 2007. "The Mythic 43 Million Americans with Disabilities." *William and Mary Law Review* 49 (1): 1–64.

"The Community Imperative: A Refutation of All Arguments in Support of Institutionalizing Anyone because of Mental Retardation." 1979. Opinion paper. Center on Human Policy, Syracuse University.

Davidson, J. 2010. "'It Cuts Both Ways': A Relational Approach to Access and Accommodation for Autism." *Social Science and Medicine* 70 (2): 305–12.

Davies, P., I. Howard, and K. Rapp. 2000. "The Effect of Welfare Reform on SAA's Disability Programs: Design of Policy Evaluation and Early Evidence." *Social Security Bulletin* 63 (1): 3–11.

Devault, M. L. 1999. "Comfort and Struggle: Emotion Work in Family Life." *Annals of the American Academy of Political and Social Science* 561 (1): 52–63.

Dillenburger, K., et al. 2010. "Living with Children Diagnosed with Autistic Spectrum Disorder: Parental and Professional Views." *British Journal of Special Education* 37 (1): 13–23.

Duggan, M., and M. Kearney. 2007. "The Impact of Child SSI Enrollment." *Journal of Policy Analysis and Management* 26 (4): 861–86.

Eyal, G., et al. 2010. *The Autism Matrix: The Social Origins of the Autism Epidemic*. Cambridge: Polity.

Farrugia, D. 2009. "Exploring Stigma: Medical Knowledge and the Stigmatisation of Parents of Children Diagnosed with Autism Spectrum Disorder." *Sociology of Health & Illness* 31 (7): 1011–27.

Galvin, R. 2004. "Can Welfare Reform Make Disability Disappear?" *Australian Journal of Social Issues* 39 (3): 343–55.

Ganz, M. L. 2007. "The Lifetime Distribution of the Incremental Societal Costs of Autism." *Archives of Pediatrics and Adolescent Medicine* 161 (4): 343–49.

Gleeson, B. 1997. "Community Care and Disability: The Limits to Justice." *Progress in Human Geography* 21 (2): 199–224.

Graetz, J. E. 2010. "Autism Grows Up: Opportunities for Adults with Autism." *Disability and Society* 25 (1): 33–47.

Gray, D. E. 2002. "'Everybody Just Freezes Everybody Is Just Embarrassed': Felt and Enacted Stigma among Parents of Children with High Functioning Autism." *Sociology of Health and Illness* 24 (6): 734–49.

Grinker, R. R. 2010. "Commentary: On Being Autistic and Social." *Ethos* 38 (1): 172–78.

Hendricks, D. 2010. "Employment and Adults with Autism Spectrum Disorders: Challenges and Strategies for Success." *Journal of Vocational Rehabilitation* 32 (2): 125–34.

Hodge, N., and K. Runswick-Cole. 2008. "Problematising Parent-Professional Partnerships in Education." *Disability and Society* 23 (6): 637–47.

Keenan, M., et al. 2010. "The Experiences of Parents during Diagnosis and Forward Planning for Children with Autism Spectrum Disorder." *Journal of Applied Research in Intellectual Disabilities* 23 (4): 390–97.

Lakin, K. C., and R. H. Bruininks, eds. 1985. *Strategies for Achieving Community Integration of Developmentally Disabled Persons.* Baltimore, Md.: Brookes.

MacArdy, A. 2009. "Jamie S. v. Milwaukee Public Schools: Urban Challenges Cause Systematic Violations of the IDEA." *Marquette Law Review* 92 (4): 857–88.

Mansell, J. 2006. "Deinstitutionalization and Community Living: Progress, Problems, and Priorities." *Journal of Intellectual and Development Disability* 31 (2): 65–76.

Marlett, C. 2009. "The Effects of the IDEA Reauthorization of 2004 and the No Child Left Behind Act on Families with Autistic Children: Allocation of Burden of Proof, Recovery of Witness Fees, and Attainment of Proven Educational Methods for Autism." *Kansas Journal of Law and Policy* 18: 53–72.

McDonough, C. B. 2008. "The Mainstreaming Requirement of the Individuals with Disabilities Education Act in the Context of Autistic Spectrum Disorders." *Fordham Urban Law Journal* 35: 1225–61.

Mink, G., and R. Solinger, eds. 2003. *Welfare: A Documentary History of U.S. Policy and Politics.* New York: New York University Press.

Muller, E., et al. 2003. "Meeting the Vocational Support Needs of Individuals with Asperger Syndrome and Other Autism Spectrum Disabilities." *Journal of Vocational Rehabilitation* 18 (3): 163–75.

Neely-Barnes, S., et al. 2011. "Parenting a Child with an Autism Spectrum Disorder: Public Perceptions and Parental Conceptualizations." *Journal of Family Social Work* 14 (3): 208–25.

Olsen, H., and J. Flugstad. 2009. "The Forgotten Entitlements." *Policy Review* 153: 41–54.

Pascall, G., and N. Hendey. 2004. "Disability and Transition to Adulthood: The Politics of Parenting." *Critical Social Policy* 24 (2): 165–86.

Peter, E., et al. 2007. "Neither Seen nor Heard: Children and Homecare Policy in Canada." *Social Science and Medicine* 64 (12): 1624–35.

Priestly, M. 2000. "Adults Only: Disability, Social Policy, and the Life Course." *Journal of Social Policy* 29 (3): 421–39.

Schall, C. M. 2010. "Positive Behavior Support: Supporting Adults with Autism Spectrum Disorders in the Workplace." *Journal of Vocational Rehabilitation* 32 (2): 109–15.

Seligmann, T. J. 2008. "An Idea Schools Can Use: Lessons from Special Education Legislation." *Fordham Urban Law Journal* 35 (5): 1225.

Selzer, M. M., et al. 2001. "Life Course Impacts of Parenting a Child with a Disability." *American Journal on Mental Retardation* 106 (3): 265–86.

Silverman, C. 2011. *Understanding Autism: Parents, Doctors, and the History of a Disorder.* Princeton, N.J.: Princeton University Press.

"SSI Families Say They Are Too Frightened and Intimidated to Challenge Funding Cutoffs for Disabled Children." 1998. *Human Rights: Journal of the Section of Individual Rights and Responsibilities* 25 (1): 22–24.

Valentine, K. 2010. "A Consideration of Medicalisation: Choice, Engagement, and Other Responsibilities of Parents of Children with Autism Spectrum Disorder." *Social Science and Medicine* 71 (5): 950–57.

Wazana, A., M. Bresnahan, and J. Kline. 2007. "The Autism Epidemic: Fact or Artifact?" *Journal of the American Academy of Child and Adolescent Psychiatry* 46 (6): 721–30.

Weber, M. C. 2009. "The IDEA Eligibility Mess." *Buffalo Law Review* 57 (1): 83–160.

Weiss, J., and Y. Lunsky. 2011. "The Brief Family Distress Scale: A Measure of Crisis in Caregivers of Individuals with Autism Spectrum Disorders." *Journal of Child and Family Studies* 20 (4): 521–28.

Wilton, R., and S. Schuer. 2006. "Towards Socio-spatial Inclusion? Disabled People, Neoliberalism, and the Contemporary Labor Market." *Area* 38 (2): 186–95.

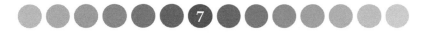

Participatory Research with Autistic Communities

Shifting the System

Dora Raymaker and Christina Nicolaidis

The relationship between scientists, minority communities, and mainstream society is complex and interconnected. Interactions between scientists and minorities can affect how society views, treats, and funds both community projects and academic research. Each year in the United States, hundreds of millions of dollars are poured into programs and research for people on the autism spectrum. But how many of these projects address the priorities of individuals on the spectrum?

Traditional approaches to science—which typically do not include members of the population being studied in the development of the research—have a history of failing minority communities. Minority communities, in turn, have a history of distrusting researchers. Studies that are conducted on minority "subjects" without understanding either the community's culture or the individuals who comprise the population may suffer from compromised sampling, weak study validity, and low intervention effectiveness. Minorities may feel angered by studies that are not helpful to them or that further marginalize them. Minorities' distrust of science and scientists' failure to include minorities in research development often create a feedback loop that further widens the divide between the two groups. In traditional approaches to autism research, the community of autistic individuals—like other minority communities defined by race, ethnicity, sexual preference, beliefs, or disability—also experiences this problematic dynamic.

Participatory approaches to research offer a way to change these dynamics. Instead of viewing a minority population as simply a source of raw data, researchers conduct participatory inquiries with representatives from the minority group as full members of the research team. Community-based participatory research (CBPR) works to make the scientist–minority relationship more beneficial for both parties. This chapter opens with an overview of some key issues in minority–scientist social dynamics and examines how they shape traditional autism research. It then explores how CBPR challenges traditional approaches to research, drawing examples from a CBPR project with autistic adults led by this paper's two coauthors: an autistic self-advocate and systems scientist; and a CBPR researcher, parent, and physician. Through the lens of these multiple perspectives, this chapter both examines and enacts a shift to participatory modes of knowledge production.

The Traditional Knowledge-Production System

Our critique of research dynamics is based on an understanding of traditional knowledge production as a complex system. Systems can be defined as collections of parts having relationships to each other and to an environment (Lendaris 1986). Highly complex systems, such as social systems, have properties that can make them difficult to understand and affect. Trends may emerge over long time spans, and thus may be difficult to perceive. Parts of a system influence one another simultaneously with feedback. The behavior of a system as a whole is often synergistic and emergent, with its overall behavior neither reflective of nor deducible based on its parts in isolation. Complex systems are decentralized, their behavior emerging from the dynamics of the system itself rather than from an identifiable master control or initial motivator, which can make connections between cause and effect elusive. Finally, the structure of complex systems is generative: how the parts relate to one another is what creates the overall system behavior. This means that one needs to understand the system's structure (the parts) and its dynamics (the relationships between the parts) in order to affect the system (Lendaris 1986; Senge 1990; Sterman 2000).

The "machine" of scientific research is a highly complex system. Science depends on funding, funding priorities shift with public pressures, and even the questions asked by science can be influenced or generated by complex social forces. Though there is at times a polite delusion that science can remain "pure" or "objective" in the face of social pressure, academia operates in conjunction both with the larger society and, in the case of human-subjects research, with the populations it studies. Complex systems such as science are difficult and slow to change. Feedback interactions exist both among the parts of the system and within each part individually (for example, scientists influencing other scientists). These feedback loops make it hard to tease out what, exactly, is responsible for a particular outcome, as subtle shifts often have surprising, unanticipated, or indirect effects. A simplified model of the system of traditional research with minority communities is shown in Figure 7.1.

In this model of traditional dynamics, the relationship between scientists and the members of mainstream (majority) society is very strong. Scientists disseminate theory and findings to the mainstream both directly and through the media. Majority society provides scientists with much of their research funding while setting the cultural environment, priorities for inquiry, and values within which scientists operate. It also strongly influences the minority community by shaping its values, molding public perceptions, and controlling the provision of services.

The interactions between the minority community and other parts of the system, however, are less significant. Members of the minority community are typically seen by scientists as simply sources of raw data. Although scientists may perform treatments or provide interventions in the minority community, most contact occurs within the context of a

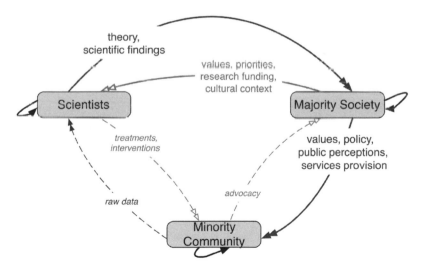

FIGURE 7.1. *A model of the traditional knowledge-production system with minority communities*

research study being conducted on the population. The minority community is able to influence the mainstream through advocacy, but often this connection is weak because of the stigmatization, social exclusion, and lack of resources typically faced by marginalized people. These dynamics suggest that although scientists and mainstream society strongly influence each other, and both directly affect minorities through existing power structures, minority communities can influence science only indirectly, by advocacy within the social mainstream—a path that may not always lie open.

In order to create significant social change through science or to push science to a new level, we must challenge and shift the traditional relationships within this system. Although this process is inescapably slow and difficult, understanding interactions within the system offers clues to help locate structural points of leverage where change might most readily be realized (Senge 1990).

Minorities and Research

The traditional system has frequently failed minorities, both ethically and pragmatically. In the 1956–1971 Willowbrook study, individuals with intellectual disabilities were injected with hepatitis and had treatment withheld so that scientists could track the development of the disease (Girod n.d.). More insidiously, research has been (and sometimes still is) used to support stigmatizing, stereotyping, or prejudicial points of view. For example, drawing causal links between race and health disparities without considering contextual factors such as culture and socioeconomic status can lead to an erroneous perception of ethnic minorities as inherently inferior or unhealthy (Bhopal 1997). Stigmatization can also be cloaked in the casual language of academic discourse; we have seen people on the autism spectrum compared to brain-dead monkeys (Cowen 2009), and girls with Rett disorder repeatedly described in a public, professional setting as "hav[ing] no souls." Even when it is not directly harmful, research sometimes misses its objectives by misunderstanding minority contexts, priorities, or needs (Institute of Medicine 1997; Minkler and Wallerstein 2003; Mittelmark et al. 1993; Steuart 1993; Susser 1995). Moreover, minorities are often underrepresented as research participants in general (Moorman et al. 2004; Murthy, Krumholz, and Gross 2004). We should, therefore, not be surprised that some minority communities distrust science and scientists so completely that they decline participation in studies, even when the studies might be beneficial to the community (Corbie-Smith, Thomas, and St. George 2002).

Laypeople who have not been given the skills to critically evaluate research are often told that science is about "facts" and that if a study "proved" something, it must be true. Likewise, there is a common misconception that "experts in the field" have a full grasp of all topics within a broader domain; for example, a researcher working with animal models of autism who has never interacted with a single person on the autism spectrum may still be given credibility when discussing what people need. Given the structure of the traditional system, both scientists and members of mainstream society are likely to accept an expert's assessment, even if that assessment is as extreme and inappropriate as a determination of soullessness.

Scientists working within the prevailing system may miss information that is key for successful research because they fail to directly engage the subjects of their studies on a level deeper than data points. Study materials may be inaccessible to the population being studied, the population may lack access to the researcher's recruitment methods, and/or the research methods may be inappropriate to the study's aims. For example, AIDS-education programs developed in the United States and Europe failed to have an impact in Brazil in the 1980s because researchers did not consider Brazil's radically different paradigm of homosexuality (Parker 1987). Scientists who do not understand their subjects' cultural contexts or abilities are more likely to design faulty research methods and draw questionable conclusions from their data. They are also more likely to produce studies that are harmful (Hatch 1993; Minkler and Wallerstein 2003; Thomas and Quinn 1991).

Because all parts of the knowledge-production system are connected through feedback loops, poor relations between researchers and the minorities they study can harm all parts of the system. A reinforcing feedback loop occurs when marginalization of minorities is continuously amplified, research systematically limits minority access to power (Fals-Borda and Rahman 1991; Hall 1992; Hatch 1993; Israel, Schulz, et al. 1998; Maguire 1996; Minkler and Wallerstein 2003; Wallerstein 1999), and science is unable to make the progress it needs to upset the status quo.

Minority Communities Defined by Disability

Community is a "readily available, mutually supportive network of relationships on which one [can] depend" (Sarason 1974). A community is characterized by shared symbols, history, identification, and perceived emotional safety (Dalton, Elias, and Wandersman 2007; McMillan and Chavis 1986; McMillan 1996). Minority communities are typically defined by geography, race, sexual orientation, or ethnicity. Although disability is at times considered an outcome for minority populations, disability itself also comprises a legitimate minority. And, like any minority, people with disabilities define their own communities.

The larger disability community in the United States has been leading a civil rights movement since the 1970s, inspired by the African American and women's rights movements. The disability community has achieved substantial social change in the past fifty years, including the enactment of influential national civil rights policies such as the Americans with Disabilities Act (ADA) and its resultant large-scale modifications in infrastructure and services, such as accessible transportation and buildings, captioning, and systems supporting students with disabilities at state universities (National Council on Disability 1997). Rather than a singular entity, the disability community consists of a loose (sometimes fractious) coalition of smaller communities defined by specific types of physical or mental diversity. Community boundaries may be shaped by various factors, including shared culture and language (as in the Deaf community), shared experiences (as in the community of psychiatric consumers/survivors), and shared use of a specific technology (as in the community of alternative- and augmentative-communication users).

Communities of individuals on the autism spectrum have also developed, particularly in recent decades, as the increasing availability of text-based communication technologies both accommodates the social-communication needs of many people on the spectrum and makes it easier for a sparse, geographically dispersed population to connect (Biever 2007; Murray and Aspinall 2006; Jordan 2010; Robertson 2007). For example, Autism Network International is an international community that meets online, informally in private homes, and at annual conferences, drawn by shared experiences of autism. The community has its own evolving set of customs, rules, distinctive terms, in-jokes, and expressions. It offers members belonging and the sense that it's okay to be autistic (Sinclair 2005).

Like other minority groups, Autistic communities experience troubled relationships with researchers and provide a shared space in which critiques can be developed and circulated. For example, in 2006, the mainstream media reported that autistics don't daydream (Pearson 2006), based on research conducted at the University of California examining brain-state differences between autistic and nonautistic individuals. Although the study—unlike the press—did not make any statements about daydreaming, it did conclude that autistic brains failed to go into a rest state and speculated that autistics' thoughts were, instead, fixated on concrete things such as "calendars, maps, or schedules" (Kennedy, Redcay, and Courchesne 2006). The media report raised concerns from the Autistic community, starting with the fact that it conflicted with first-person knowledge that daydreams can comprise a good portion of an autistic individual's daily experience. Further scrutiny of the research within the Autistic community revealed additional problems and questions. For example, the community questioned whether the research design was valid for the population, given that it required rapid mental task-switching and instructed participants in terms that could mislead the literal-minded (Raymaker 2006). The community also feared the study would perpetuate damaging and incorrect stereotypes. The idea that individuals on the autism spectrum lack imaginative capacity can easily be challenged by considering, for instance, the works of Vernon Smith in mathematics, Tito Mukhopadhyay in poetry, and Larry Bissonette in the visual arts.

The study also leads to larger questions of systemic marginalization and ethics. Although the daydreaming study was likely well-intentioned, it has potential to detrimentally affect the way society treats people on the autism spectrum and assesses their value and humanity. A study questioning the capacity of autistic people for introspection has potential to reduce the chance that scientists seek introspective first-person knowledge that would dispel the stereotype (for a refreshing example of researchers working with first-person knowledge, see Chamak et al. 2008). Ethically, there are questions about whether it's right to portray study participants in exclusively negative terms in publications without disclosing that intention to potential participants. Ultimately, there are also questions about how studies like the daydreaming study realistically improve the lives of individuals on the autism spectrum.

Building a Better System: Participatory Approaches to Research

As structure generates behavior for complex systems such as the knowledge-production system, one way to address these issues in traditional research is by changing the relationships between the parts of the system to generate a new overall behavior. Participatory research is based on collaboration between minority individuals or communities and scientists with the goal of an equitable exchange of power and expertise. The "subjects" of the research become members of the research team. Members of a minority community are valued not just as informants but as individuals with their own strengths and skills to actively contribute to the project.

There is no single, formalized way to conduct participatory research. The approach may consist of casual consultations with community representatives, close work with a single individual from a community, formal partnerships with many individuals, or other configurations. Participatory research has evolved in various fields of inquiry, with early examples emerging in organizational management and the social sciences in the mid-twentieth century (Argyris 1955; Lewin 1946). Although participatory studies are most commonly conducted with communities defined by race, ethnicity, location, or occupation, participatory approaches to research have been successfully used as well with communities defined by disability, such as the community of psychiatric consumers/survivors (Nelson et al. 1998). Participatory research has also been conducted with communities that are multiply marginalized, such as a project involving Latino youth with disabilities, which improved intervention efficacy while empowering advocates to break ties with an exploitative service organization and to develop their own bilingual sign-language programs (Balcazar et al. 1998). Another project with African Americans and Latinos with disabilities caused social change by both increasing community access for people with disabilities and improving participants' capacity to continue to advocate for civil rights (Oden, Hernandez, and Hidalgo 2010).

The community-based participatory research model was developed in health sciences with the express purpose of stimulating systems change and improving minority involvement. CBPR is a well-defined framework, formalized by individuals such as Barbara Israel, Eugenia Eng, and colleagues (2005). It acknowledges communities as core units of identity deeper than simply a population of individuals sharing a characteristic. CBPR builds on community strengths and resources, developing them as needed, and facilitates collaborative, egalitarian partnerships in all aspects of the research initiative. It engages researchers and community members in a reciprocal process of learning and capacity building, in order to generate knowledge and foster social change through cycles of action and critical reflection on both the process and outcomes of the project. It is driven by community-based perceptions of relevance, broad definitions of health and well-being, and an ecological approach that resists simple, reductive readings of individuals and social systems. Results and findings are disseminated in forms that are appropriate for both community and academic audiences. CBPR projects demand a great deal of time and effort but often evolve into long-term productive learning partnerships (Israel, Eng, et al. 2005).

Rather than indicating a specific set of methods or research topics, participatory research involves commitment to these guiding principles. These principles are intended to change the structure of the relationships between scientists and minority communities, strengthening their connection, reducing the likelihood of ethical trespass, and facilitating both the production of knowledge and shifts in the mainstream (Israel, Eng, et al. 2005).

The principles of community as a unit of identity and community relevance are particularly important with respect to autism research. A 2008 analysis of major funders by the Interagency Autism Coordinating Committee showed that of $22,459,793 in private and federal monies spent on autism research, 37 percent went to questions of causation and prevention, 24 percent to treatments for autism, and 18 percent to trying to understand what autism is or to explain its symptomatology. Only 5 percent was allocated to questions surrounding services (Office of Autism Research Coordination 2009). Clearly, the priorities in the United States for autism research are causes, cures, and remediation.

Anyone not steeped in the politics of autism may miss the vast divide that often separates families with autistic members, professionals, and self-advocates (Chamak 2008). These groups have historically held conflicting agendas, with the self-advocate community at times actively opposing the actions of parent or professional communities by staging protests (Wallis 2009) or lobbying for the cessation of stigmatizing public-service campaigns (Kaufman 2007; Ne'eman 2007). CBPR can certainly be conducted with parents, professionals, and other "people who have something to do with autism," but it recognizes that it is the individuals on the autism spectrum themselves who are in the position of the oppressed, excluded minority.

The current autism-funding priorities in the United States may be relevant to some parent or professional communities, but for the Autistic community, questions related to improving quality of life are more germane than causes, cures, and remediation. For an adult on the autism spectrum, particularly one who views his or her autism as a positive aspect of identity, research to decrease health-care disparities, improve service provisioning, or disprove harmful stereotypes holds more relevance than research to extinguish autistic existence. However, within the current system, it is very difficult for minority communities such as the Autistic community to have their perspectives about relevance heard, let alone heeded. Indeed, individuals on the autism spectrum are often either perceived as lacking the capacity for introspection and social communication that self-advocacy requires or dismissed by those who say that autistics who can speak for themselves are "not autistic enough" to represent the interests of "real" autistic people. At a summit of more than 150 autism policy makers sponsored by the Association of University Centers on Disability, held in Seattle, Washington, in 2010, only one autistic self-advocate was evidently in attendance. The structure of the traditional knowledge-production system limits the Autistic community's ability to advocate for its own needs in the autism-research agenda. CBPR provides a way for the Autistic community to directly engage with scientists about research topics it finds relevant.

Figure 7.2 shows a participatory knowledge-production model. The minority community still provides raw data to scientists, but it is now able to influence scientists directly. The community is able to communicate its own values and priorities, to share its cultural expertise, community resources, and insights, and to give scientists access to a larger population of study participants. The scientists may still provide the community with interventions and treatments, but because the minority community has been steering the research agenda, scientific find-

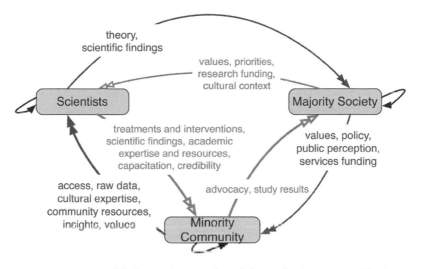

FIGURE 7.2. *A model of a participatory knowledge-production system with minority communities*

ings are more likely to be of actual use to the community. Scientists additionally offer the community academic expertise, resources, capacitation, and credibility, which the community can then use for more effective advocacy. Increased advocacy and community-relevant study results can then influence mainstream society. This could in turn change the nature of research funding, priorities, mainstream values, and overall cultural context as society feeds back to scientists (Wallerstein and Duran 2006). These claims may seem optimistic, yet the impact of CBPR has been well documented; for instance, one project in low-income communities of color in Southern California created large-scale environmental-policy change in their region (Israel, Eng, et al. 2005).

Participatory Autism Research: AASPIRE's Experience

Although the Autistic community experiences similar issues regarding research and majority society as do other minorities, to date the majority of community-based participatory research has been conducted with local communities defined by race or ethnicity. Because of its collaborative foundation, CBPR is an extremely social approach to conducting research. It requires continuous feedback between team members, keen group-facilitation skills, and a significant amount of communication and translation between scientists and laypersons across cultural boundaries and power relationships. Nonetheless, it has been successfully implemented with Autistic communities (Nicolaidis, Raymaker, McDonald, Dern, Ashkenazy, et al. 2011; Nicolaidis, Raymaker, McDonald, Dern, Boisclair, et al. 2013).

Like many CBPR partnerships, the Academic Autistic Spectrum Partnership in Research and Education (AASPIRE) emerged organically at an intersection between community need and available scientific expertise. The organization was formed when we, the authors, began critiquing autism research. We quickly became frustrated by issues of relevance, ethics, value, and validity, and by the great divide that seemed to exist between the types of research that the Autistic community was seeking and the work that traditional autism research was producing. AASPIRE's mission is to encourage the inclusion of adults on the autism spectrum in matters that directly affect them; to include adults on the autism spectrum as equal partners in research about the autism spectrum; to answer research questions that are considered relevant by the autistic community; and to use research findings to effect positive change for people on the spectrum (Nicolaidis, Raymaker, McDonald, Dern, Ashkenazy, et al. 2011).

Unlike minority communities in most CBPR partnerships, the Autistic community is not local, and its boundaries can be hard to define. It is also characterized by atypical interaction and communication, necessitating new ways of thinking about how to successfully conduct studies using CBPR. To include community members, AASPIRE has been operating online via text-based chat or e-mail, and has provided multiple modes for communicating input. This has sometimes set the nonautistic scientists at a disadvantage and has helped equalize power by displacing scientists' privilege during group communications (Nicolaidis, Raymaker, McDonald, Dern, Ashkenazy, et al. 2011).

Throughout the research process, both the community partners and the academic partners bring expertise that differs in content but not in value or significance. Figure 7.3 shows AASPIRE's model of CBPR (Nicolaidis, Raymaker, McDonald, Dern, Ashkenazy, et al. 2011). In the initial development stage of a CBPR project, when the focus of the inquiry evolves, the study is designed, and the funding is procured, community

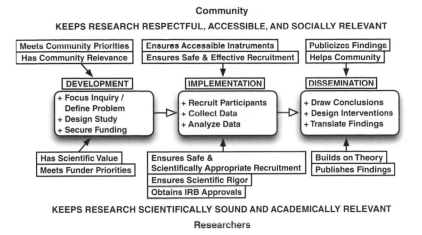

FIGURE 7.3. *A model of community-based participatory research. From Nicolaidis, Raymaker, McDonald, Dern, Ashkenazy, et al. (2011).*

members ensure that their priorities and values are met and that the inquiry is relevant to the community, while scientists safeguard the project's scientific value and adherence to funder priorities. In AASPIRE's case, due to the dearth of autism research meeting community priorities, many study topics were discussed, including employment, empathy, intimate relationships, special interests, services, and bullying. Given the partnering scientists' areas of expertise and the importance of the issues, ultimately the group decided to start with health, health care, and the relationship between Internet use, sense of community, and well-being. Studies were then designed with the dual purpose of advancing science and generating something of practical use for the community. For example, a health-care study was designed in part to generate statistical data about health-care disparities (Nicolaidis, Raymaker, McDonald, Dern, Boisclair, et al. 2013), which could be used to lobby for policy change, to produce qualitative data about health-care experiences to help explain the statistics and to improve the training of those providing care, and to support applications for funding to create practical tools to improve health-care access. From the project's inception, the Autistic community involved had control over what was researched, how it was researched, and how it was funded. Some large potential funders were rejected because of conflicts with community aims and values.

During the implementation phase of a CBPR project, again the community is involved in all stages of the research process. The community ensures that instruments and other study materials are accessible to the population and assists with recruitment, often reaching populations that may be otherwise inaccessible. AASPIRE has benefited from having community partners with active connections to developmental-disabilities programs, both formal and informal self-advocacy groups, and online Autistic community networks. The scientists ensure that the recruitment is being conducted safely and appropriately, obtain any approvals required from institutional review boards (IRBs), and uphold the project's scientific rigor.

The development of accessible instruments and study materials in a CBPR project may include considerations that would not emerge without community input. For example, AASPIRE community partners pointed out that many items on standardized survey measures were incomprehensible to them. Language needed to be direct, specific, and unambiguous; abstract, general, or jargon terms needed concrete examples or definitions. Other measures, such as the standardized Social Responsiveness Scale (Constantino et al. 2003), used for measuring the number and intensity of autistic characteristics, were too offensive to be used at all, and alternatives needed to be found. Qualitative interviews were designed to be administered via e-mail and text chat, as well as in more traditional telephone and in-person forms. There is a very pragmatic reason for this effort: offended, confused, or frustrated research participants are less likely to complete studies or give valid answers.

Although community partners are not asked to become statisticians, they are included, along with the scientists, in discussions surrounding data collection and analysis, at both preliminary and final stages. Scientific questions are posed to the full team: Here is the data; do the results make sense? What might be going on? Sometimes the community has insight that no outsider could access. One of AASPIRE's studies included a measure of online sense of community, a subset of which a nonrandom number of participants declined to answer. Community partners were able to provide insider information that a recent "blowup" of several major online community resources was likely affecting participants' responses on those particular items. Without this insider information, scientists could have easily explained the data as evidence of "autistic deficits." Traditional autism research does not have any mechanism to solicit insider information during data analysis, information that could radically change how data are ultimately interpreted.

During the dissemination phase, findings don't just build on scientific theory and further academic literature but are also used to help the community. Again, the community is involved at every step, from drawing final conclusions about the findings to translating them to the community, the academy, and society in general. Findings may be used to build a subsequent project or to design an intervention. AASPIRE was able to use its pilot data showing health-care disparities for adults on the autism spectrum (Nicolaidis, Raymaker, McDonald, Dern, Boisclair, et al. 2013) to obtain funding for an online tool kit to improve health-care quality and access. Data have also been used from that same pilot study to make a policy case for including people with disabilities as a health-care disparities group and to successfully lobby state government to shift its focus toward reducing health and health-care disparities for individuals on the autism spectrum.

Community involvement during dissemination also helps ensure that the language, content, and conclusions in scientific publications do not further marginalize the community. If individuals on the autism spectrum had been involved in the publication of the University of California daydreaming study, would its findings have been presented differently? Would it still have drawn the same conclusions about the findings and about what individuals on the autism spectrum might imagine? At every stage of the research process, CBPR seeks to mitigate the marginalization of minorities in traditional approaches to science while also providing both scientists and community members with the skills, tools, and understanding to generate systems change.

"Nothing about Us without Us": CBPR, Autistic Communities, and Systems Change

Individuals on the autism spectrum in the United States have traditionally been excluded from autism-policy development and from direct involvement in research. Traditional autism research is conducted *on* autistic subjects, not conducted *with* autistic people. Because of the highly coupled feedback between Autistic communities, scientists, and mainstream society, this exclusion inevitably affects individuals on the autism spectrum. This effect is something Autistic communities have little control over, as complex systems have significant momentum and traditional structures reinforce systemic oppression.

Including members of Autistic communities as full participants in every aspect of autism research disrupts this traditional dynamic without the need for more difficult structural changes. The coupling between Autistic communities, scientists, and mainstream society begins working for individuals on the spectrum instead of against them. Reinforcing feedback, like the loops discussed in the knowledge-production model, produces exponential behavior; whether what is reinforced is beneficial or harmful depends on the content of what is being reinforced. Reinforcing community priorities, respect for personhood, individual and community empowerment, capacity for advocacy, and a positive view of autism may lead to significant social change over time.

CBPR provides a historically effective route to social change for minority communities, whether they are defined by disability or by other indicators of marginalization. AASPIRE has adopted the principles and general framework of CBPR, but it has also improvised in order to accommodate the Autistic community's geographic dispersal and social and communication needs. This experience enables AASPIRE to contribute to the growing field of participatory research, infusing CBPR with insights gleaned from our experience working far outside the social mainstream. Participatory research may not be the only route to systems change for minorities, but the shifts it produces in the knowledge-production system could significantly improve both our scholarship and our society.

NOTE

We capitalize "Autistic" when indicating Autistic community and culture; it is not capitalized when indicating a diagnostic label. We use this convention with respect for the Autistic community.

ACKNOWLEDGMENTS

We thank the AASPIRE team members, including Katherine McDonald, Elesia Ashkenazy, Sebastian Dern, and everyone else we have worked with, past and present, who have greatly influenced the ideas in this chapter. AASPIRE is based at Oregon Health and Science University. AASPIRE collaborates with other academic and community institutions and organizations, including Portland State University, Syracuse University, Autism

Society of Oregon, and the Autistic Self Advocacy Network. AASPIRE's work is funded, in part, through the Oregon Clinical and Translational Research Institute, grant number UL1 RR024140 from the National Center for Research Resources, a component of the National Institutes of Health (NIH) and NIH Roadmap for Medical Research; Portland State University; and the National Institute of Mental Health, award number R34MH092503. The content of this paper is solely the responsibility of the authors and does not necessarily represent the official views of the National Institute of Mental Health or the National Institutes of Health.

REFERENCES

Argyris, C. 1955. "Organizational Leadership and Participative Management." *Journal of Business* 28 (1): 1–7.

Balcazar, F. E., et al. 1998. "Participatory Action Research and People with Disabilities: Principles and Challenges." *Canadian Journal of Rehabilitation* 12 (2): 105–12.

Bhopal, R. 1997. "Is Research into Ethnicity and Health Racist, Unsound, or Important Science?" *British Medical Journal* 314 (7096): 1751–56.

Biever, C. 2007. "Web Removes Social Barriers for Those with Autism." *New Scientist* 2610: 26–27.

Chamak, B. 2008. "Autism and Social Movements: French Parents' Associations and International Autistic Individuals' Organizations." *Sociology of Health and Illness* 30 (1): 76–96.

Chamak, B., et al. 2008. "What Can We Learn about Autism from Autistic Persons?" *Psychotherapy and Psychosomatics* 77 (5): 271–79.

Constantino, J. N., et al. 2003. "Validation of a Brief Quantitative Measure of Autistic Traits: Comparison of the Social Responsiveness Scale with the Autism Diagnostic Interview—Revised." *Journal of Autism and Developmental Disorders* 33 (4): 427–33.

Corbie-Smith, G., S. B. Thomas, and D. M. M. St. George. 2002. "Distrust, Race, and Research." *Archives of Internal Medicine* 162 (21): 2458–63.

Cowen, T. 2009. "Autism as Academic Paradigm." *Chronicle Review.* Accessed December 23, 2011, http://chronicle.com/article/Autism-as-Academic-Paradigm/47033.

Dalton, J. H., M. J. Elias, and A. Wandersman. 2007. *Community Psychology: Linking Individuals and Communities.* Belmont, Calif.: Wadsworth.

Fals-Borda, O., and M. A. Rahman. 1991. *Action and Knowledge: Breaking the Monopoly with Participatory Action Research.* New York: Apex.

Girod, M. n.d. "Ethics in Research." Western Oregon University. Accessed September 7, 2010, http://www.wou.edu/~girodm/research/ethics.html.

Hall, B. L. 1992. "From Margins to Center: The Development and Purpose of Participatory Research." *American Sociologist* 23 (4): 15–28.

Hatch, J. 1993. "Community Research: Partnership in Black Communities." *American Journal of Preventative Medicine* 9 (6): 27–31.

Institute of Medicine. 1997. *Improving Health in the Community: A Role for Performance Monitoring.* Washington, D.C.: National Academy Press.

Israel, B. A., E. Eng, et al. 2005. *Methods in Community-Based Participatory Research for Health.* San Francisco: Wiley.

Israel, B. A., A. J. Schulz, et al. 1998. "Review of Community-Based Research: Assessing Partnership Approaches to Improve Public Health." *Annual Review of Public Health* 19: 173–202.

Jordan, C. 2010. "Evolution of Autism Support and Understanding via the World Wide Web." *Intellectual and Developmental Disabilities* 48 (3): 220–27.

Kaufman, J. 2007. "Campaign on Childhood Mental Illness Succeeds at Being Provocative." *New York Times.* Accessed September 6, 2010, http://www.nytimes.com/2007/12/14/business/media/14adco.html?_r=1&ref=business.

Kennedy, D. P., E. Redcay, and E. Courchesne. 2006. "Failing to Deactivate: Resting Functional Abnormalities in Autism." *Biological Sciences: Neuroscience* 103 (21): 8275–80.

Lendaris, G. 1986. "On Systemness and the Problem Solver: Tutorial Content." *Systems, Man, and Cybernetics* 16 (4): 603–10.

Lewin, K. 1946. "Action Research and Minority Problems." *Journal of Social Issues* 2 (4): 34–46.

Maguire, P. 1996. "Considering More Feminist Participatory Research: What's Congruency Got to Do with It?" *Qualitative Inquiry* 2 (1): 106–18.

McMillan, D. W. 1996. "Sense of Community." *Journal of Community Psychology* 24 (4): 315–25.

McMillan, D. W., and D. M. Chavis. 1986. "Sense of Community: A Definition and Theory." *Journal of Community Psychology* 14 (1): 6–23.

Minkler, M., and N. Wallerstein. 2003. *Community-Based Participatory Research for Health.* San Francisco: Wiley.

Mittelmark, M. B., et al. 1993. "Realistic Outcomes: Lessons from Community-Based Research and Demonstration Programs for the Prevention of Cardiovascular Disease." *Journal of Public Health Policy* 14 (4): 437–62.

Moorman, P. G., et al. 2004. "Racial Differences in Enrolment in a Cancer Genetics Registry." *Cancer Epidemiology, Biomarkers, and Prevention* 13 (8): 1349–54.

Murray, D., and A. Aspinall. 2006. *Getting IT: Using Information Technology to Empower People with Communication Difficulties.* London: Kingsley.

Murthy, V. H., H. M. Krumholz, and C. P. Gross. 2004. "Participation in Cancer Clinical Trials: Race-, Sex-, and Age-Based Disparities." *Journal of the American Medical Association* 291 (22): 2720–26.

National Council on Disability. 1997. "Equality of Opportunity: The Making of the Americans with Disabilities Act." National Council on Disability. Accessed September 6, 2010, http://www.ncd.gov/newsroom/publications/1997/equality.htm.

Ne'eman, A. 2007. "Victory! The End of the Ransom Notes Campaign." Autistic Self Advocacy Network. Accessed September 6, 2010, http://www.autisticadvocacy.org/modules/smartsection/item.php?itemid=23.

Nelson, G., et al. 1998. "'Nothing about Me, without Me': Participatory Action Research with Self-Help/Mutual Aid Organizations for Psychiatric Consumer/ Survivors." *American Journal of Community Psychology* 26 (6): 881–912.

Nicolaidis, C., D. Raymaker, K. McDonald, S. Dern, E. Ashkenazy, et al. 2011. "Collaboration Strategies in Non-traditional CBPR Partnerships: Lessons from an Academic–Community Partnership with Autistic Self-Advocates." *Progress in Community Health Partnerships* 5 (2): 143–50.

Nicolaidis, C., D. Raymaker, K. McDonald, S. Dern, W. C. Boisclair, et al. 2013. "Comparison of Healthcare Experiences in Autistic and Non-autistic Adults: A Cross-Sectional Online Survey Facilitated by an Academic–Community Partnership." *Journal of General Internal Medicine* 28 (7). doi: 10.1007/s11606-012-2262-7.

Oden, K., B. Hernandez, and M. A. Hidalgo. 2010. "Payoffs of Participatory Action Research: Racial and Ethnic Minorities with Disabilities Reflect on Their Research Experiences." *Journal of the Community Development Society* 41 (1): 21–31.

Office of Autism Research Coordination. 2009. "2008 IACC Autism Spectrum Disorder Research Portfolio Analysis Report." Interagency Autism Coordinating Committee. Accessed September 6, 2010, http://iacc.hhs.gov/portfolio-analysis/2008/index.shtml.

Parker, R. 1987. "Acquired Immunodeficiency Syndrome in Urban Brazil." *Medical Anthropology Quarterly* 1 (2): 155–75.

Pearson, H. 2006. "Autistic Brains May Daydream Less." Nature.com, May 8. Accessed September 6, 2010, http://www.nature.com/news/2006/060508/full/news060508-3.html.

Raymaker, D. M. 2006. "Review of 'Daydreaming' Paper." *Asperger Syndrome Live Journal Community*. Blog post. Accessed December 23, 2011, http://asperger.livejournal.com/1236717.html.

Robertson, S. 2007. "Information Technology and the Autistic Culture: Influences, Empowerment, and Progression of IT Usage in Advocacy Initiatives." Paper presented at Autreat, Pennsylvania, Pa.

Sarason, S. B. 1974. *The Psychological Sense of Community: Prospects for a Community Psychology*. San Francisco: Jossey-Bass.

Senge, P. 1990. *The Fifth Discipline: The Art and Practice of the Learning Organization*. New York: Doubleday/Currency.

Sinclair, J. 2005. "Autism Network International: The Development of a Community and Its Culture." Autism Network International. Accessed September 6, 2010, http://www.autreat.com/History_of_ANI.html.

Sterman, J. D. 2000. *Business Dynamics: Systems Thinking and Modeling for a Complex World*. Boston: Irwin/McGraw-Hill.

Steuart, G. W. 1993. "Social and Cultural Perspectives: Community Intervention and Mental Health." *Health Education Quarterly*, suppl. 1: S99–S111.

Susser, M. 1995. "The Tribulations of Trials: Intervention in Communities." *American Journal of Public Health* 85 (2158): 156–58.

Thomas, S. B., and S. C. Quinn. 1991. "The Tuskegee Syphilis Study, 1932 to 1972: Implications for HIV Education and AIDS Risk Education Programs in the Black Community." *American Journal of Public Health* 81 (11): 1498–1505.

Wallerstein, N. 1999. "Power between Evaluator and Community: Research

Relationships within New Mexico's Healthier Communities." *Social Science and Medicine* 49 (1): 39–53.

Wallerstein, N., and B. Duran. 2006. "Using Community-Based Participatory Research to Address Health Disparities." *Health Promotion Practice* 7 (3): 312–24.

Wallis, C. 2009. "'I Am Autism': An Advocacy Video Sparks Protest." *Time*, November 6. Accessed September 6, 2010, http://www.time.com/time/health/article/0,8599,1935959,00.html.

PART III. Diagnosis and Difference in Autism

Capturing Diagnostic Journeys of Life on the Autism Spectrum

Sara Ryan

A utism-spectrum disorders (ASDs) trouble conventional understandings of the concept of diagnosis. As Judy Singer, drawing
on her personal experiences as a person with ASD, suggests, "Whereas
the traditional image of 'diagnosis' is of something reluctantly sought,
dreaded, resisted and imposed from outside, people with 'marginal' neurological differences clamor at the gates, self-diagnosed and demanding
to be let in" (1999, 65). Singer seeks to capture the peculiarity of the medicalization of autism in that, for her, ASD is ontologically linked to personal identity; it is not a condition that people have, but rather an identity
that people are. Yet, for many, including Singer, there is significant delay
in accessing this identity, and diagnosis may not happen until adulthood.
The experiences of those diagnosed with ASD in adulthood have received
little attention in existing research, yet these experiences can challenge
narrowly drawn, stereotypical understandings of autism. In this chapter,
I explore notions of self, identity, and aspects of the life course through
an analysis of the diagnostic journeys undertaken by nineteen people diagnosed with ASD as adults in the United Kingdom.

For some, this journey marks a radical redefinition of self, offering
answers to long-standing social and emotional puzzles, tensions, and difficulties experienced since childhood. For others, diagnosis simply confirms and legitimates an identity they may have already assumed (though
not necessarily disclosed). Actively seeking a diagnosis of ASD in adulthood involves a complex contextual, emotional, relational, and interactive
journey across a wide social terrain. It involves not only health and other
professionals, but family members, friends, and colleagues, as well as an
engagement with the various representations and understandings of autism, including diagnostic criteria, fiction, and autistic autobiographies.

The firsthand accounts presented in the growing number of autistic autobiographies have been the subject of recent academic attention. Studies of gender, sociospatial inclusion, identity and disclosure, communication, culture, and the use and creation of language have all been examined through the lens of personal experience (Davidson 2007a, 2007b, 2008, 2010; Davidson and Henderson 2010). These autobiographical texts provide insight into the constitution of autistic experience and the emergence of an autistic discourse. In so doing, they go some way toward lessening the "one-sidedness" of efforts by people with ASD to fit into mainstream life and enable a greater understanding of the subject—autistic experience of everyday life—by the nonautistic majority population (Davidson and Henderson 2010).

This chapter analyzes data from two qualitative-research projects, in which people with ASD were asked to talk about their experiences. Although people with ASD may prefer the written word over verbal communication, face-to-face interviews offer the possibility of exploring different aspects of participants' experiences, and the use of prompts facilitates the generation of thick description of autistic life (Geertz 1973). Given the predominance of the diagnosis of Asperger Syndrome (AS), rather than autism or ASD, in the sample considered here, it is prudent to touch upon ongoing debates about the distinction between AS and autism (Foster and King 2003; Frith 2004; Matson and Wilkins 2008). This discussion will consider the ambiguity surrounding diagnosis of AS, particularly in relation to adults; the concept of looping (Hacking 2007); and whether the development of a reflexive self is incongruent with an autistic self. (After this discussion, I will use "ASD" nondiscriminately, as an acceptably inclusive term, to include AS.) I will then turn to an exploration of the data and, after describing the methods used, will examine why participants decided to seek diagnosis in adulthood. I follow the process of diagnosis from participants' initial request to GPs for referral, through the diagnostic procedures, to receiving the label. The final, empirical section will look at how participants made sense of their diagnosis. The chapter concludes with a discussion of the power that an "official" diagnosis holds for participants and returns to the question of the reflexive autistic self.

The Emergence of Asperger Syndrome

The American Psychiatric Association's *Diagnostic and Statistical Manual of Mental Disorders (DSM)* contains the criteria for the classification of mental-health disorders. At this writing, the *DSM* is currently in its fourth edition (1994). (A text revision of the fourth edition *[DSM-IV-TR]* was published in 2000.) AS was first included in this manual in 1994; its classification has a peculiarity about it that underlines the ambiguity of the condition, namely, the similarity and overlap of the characteristics of autism and AS, the former of which entered the *DSM* in 1980. Hans Asperger first described the syndrome in Austria in 1944, around the same time that Leo Kanner independently identified "classic autism" (Frith 1991). The creation of the category of AS occurred only decades later, when the condition entered the World Health Organization's *International Classification of Diseases (ICD-10)*, in 1992. The inclusion of AS at this point is commonly held to be due to Lorna Wing's use of Asperger's writing in her case-study work (1981). The reconceptualization of autism as a continuum allowed space for both Kanner's definition of autism and Asperger Syndrome from the early 1980s onward (Eyal et al. 2010).

AS is typically characterized by difficulties with interaction, an obsessive focus on particular interests, and no significant language delay (Frith 1991). These typifications contribute to and help sustain stereotypical, and static, perceptions of AS. Asperger himself described AS as a personality gestalt—a unique human type—admitting infinite variation and nuance (Eyal et al. 2010). There are no standardized diagnostic tools (Silverman 2010), and the interpretation and application of existing diagnostic tools, such as the ADOS (autism diagnostic observation schedule) and the ADI-R (autism diagnostic interview—revised), vary (Woodbury-Smith and Volkmar 2009).

Diagnosis, particularly in adulthood, is further complicated by the reliance on parents' memory, as the *DSM* criteria refer to developmental milestones rarely recorded as they occur (Matson and Wilkins 2008). In addition, the interactive and relational dimensions of autistic experience and of the diagnostic process can create more complications. For example, the proliferation of autistic autobiographies (Lawson 2000; Grandin 1996; Hall 2011; Willey 1999; Slater-Walker and Slater-Walker 2002; Williams 1992), the large number of autism-related forums and Web sites (such as www.wrongplanet.net and www.aspie.com), novels, television documentaries, films, and news items may influence people's self-descriptions during the diagnostic process (Davidson 2007a). The increase in cultural representations of autism have led to concern about a divergence between stereotypical representations and the clinical reality of the condition (Draaisma 2009). At the same time, the increase in autistic autobiography has created a language with which to understand and make sense of ASD (Hacking 2009a).

Returning to questions of classification, Wilbur J. Scott suggests that conditions included in the *DSM* are "always-already-there objects" in the social world, waiting to be identified (1990). This interpretation is overly positivist; I support Ian Hacking's suggestion that the process of classification brings into being alternative types of people (2007). For Hacking, this interactive process involves classification, people, institutions, knowledge, and experts. The classified person interacts with the classification in a "looping process" modifying the original condition.[1] This transformative process in relation to autism has drawn some criticism (Draaisma 2009; McGeer 2009). For example, Victoria McGeer argues that autistics cannot internalize norms related to different ways of being if they are unable to internalize norms more generally; looping involves a susceptibility to "comindedness," that is, a shared understanding of language and interaction, which autistics do not have. Others, taking a more cognitive approach, have questioned how autistic experience can be written or retold with great insight if the authors have a theory-of-mind deficit (Draaisma 2009; Szatmari 2004). Theory of mind is a concept referring to the ability of people to be able to reflect on their own and others' minds, and it is strongly associated with autism research and diagnosis (Baron-Cohen, Leslie, and Frith 1985). Although the concepts of comindedness, theory of mind, and socialization have different disciplinary backgrounds, all three assume shared understandings. Mark Osteen (this volume) raises different questions around narrative representation. For Osteen, quoting Matthew K. Belmonte (2007), autistics are "human, but more so," underlining the mistaken or misplaced emphasis on deficit that is characteristic of representations of autism. In our earlier analysis of this research, Ulla Raisanen and I argued that people with ASD did not internalize norms and values during childhood (Ryan and Raisanen 2008). They didn't develop a generalized other and so were not able, or readily able, to put themselves in the place of others. Some participants attained a level of acceptable or functional performativity, but it often remained conscious work (S. Scott 2009). In effect, the process of socialization was not an effective mechanism for people with ASD. We are judged, or judge people, using a narrowly defined set of criteria that preclude recognition of autistic strengths and abilities.

McGeer suggests that the lack of shared meaning that is character-istic of autism negates the possibility of transformative autistic experi-ence that suggests a looping process (2009). A transformative autistic experience is one in which the autistic self-narrative can both inform and transform how the spectrum is constituted. Exploring the diagnos-tic journeys of people diagnosed with ASD in adulthood will, I hope, contribute to this discussion. It will, at the same time, add to the growing literature disseminating thick description of the phenomenon of autism, advancing new narratives of autism that challenge dominant, deficit-laden constructions through an emphasis on difference and diversity.

Generating Stories

The data discussed here are from two qualitative studies, based in the United Kingdom, focusing on the experiences, support, and information needs of people diagnosed with ASD. The first, funded by the Wellcome Trust, involved interviews with twenty-one participants, and data were collected in 2007. The second, funded by the U.K. government's Depart-ment of Health, extended the original project with a further eighteen interviews; these data were collected in 2010. Both studies were con-ducted by the author, and lay summaries of the findings have been pub-lished online, at Healthtalkonline (2013), with video, audio, and text extracts from the interviews. The analysis presented here focuses on nineteen interviews with people diagnosed with ASD in adulthood. One person was diagnosed with autism, the remainder with AS. Details of the sample are presented in Figure 8.1. The sociodemographic compo-sition of the sample was varied. Occupations of those in paid work in-cluded kitchen assistant, retired scientist, barber, IT consultant, artist, and part-time kennel worker. Five participants were in long-term rela-tionships, and six had children.

Face-to-face interviews were conducted with participants in their own homes or, if they preferred, in a convenient meeting room (such as a hotel meeting room or a room in a community center). One woman was not comfortable interacting face-to-face and so was interviewed using e-mail. Five participants were interviewed with their partners at their express preference. Participants were asked to start by talking about

Characteristics	Number of Participants
Age at Interview	
16–24	1
25–34	5
35–44	8
45–54	1
55–64	2
65+	2
Age at Diagnosis	
16–24	4
25–34	5
35–44	5
45–54	3
55–64	1
65+	1
Ethnicity	
White British	18
Other	1
Gender	
Male	10
Female	9
Employment and Education Status	
In employment or education	13
Not in employment or education	6

FIGURE 8.1. *Demographic details of the subsample of nineteen participants analyzed from two qualitative-research projects that asked participants with autism-spectrum disorder to discuss their experiences*

their experiences, and then an interview schedule was used to explore and probe areas of their accounts. Most participants disliked the broadness of the opening question and requested a less abstract question. The interviews lasted between twenty minutes and three hours and were transcribed verbatim. The data were analyzed thematically using the organizational support of NVivo 2 software in the first study and N8 in the second. The data were open-coded, and then the codes were organized into several categories, including getting a diagnosis, feelings about diagnosis, feeling different, employment experiences, and relationships. A second researcher independently coded two interview transcripts in order to compare the coding structure that was developing. Axial coding was conducted alongside constant comparison of words used, codes, and categories until there was a "fit" between the data analysis and the social reality it represented (Charmaz 2006). Pseudonyms are used in the data extracts presented in the following sections.

Why Seek Diagnosis?

Although participants had varied backgrounds, they all described experiencing difficulties in their lives. Some ostensibly led successful lives with families and long-term careers but talked about consistently struggling with social interaction, expectations, and social norms. Others struggled with education, employment, and relationships and had been involved with mental-health services over the years. Several participants had been misdiagnosed with conditions including personality disorder, schizoid personality, and social anxiety. Others had had more derogatory labels applied to them. None of these labels fits with participants' experiences, and they sought further answers, as evidenced by the following exchange:

> INTERVIEWER: What was it that made you want to get the diagnosis in the first place?
> PARTICIPANT: Well, because I'd got that many labels shoved on me, I wanted the correct label.
> I: What sort of labels?
> P: Well, I've had, I've had "stupid," "thick," "weirdo." I've had all sorts, so I just wanted . . . if they were going to call me weirdo, then obviously I wanted the correct label to go with it, you know. (June, 49)

A few participants explicitly linked their decision to seek diagnosis to the need to access support. For example, Abbey, 36, and Graham, 27, both returned to university and wanted to avoid problems previously experienced in further education. Edward, 83, wanted support to manage his temper more effectively, and David, 44, wanted help with his concentration.

For others, a specific crisis or series of crises motivated them to seek diagnosis. For example, Jonathan, 33, a postman, was taken to court by his employer for hoarding the mail. His mother persuaded him to see a psychologist to "see what was going on in my mind." Three married participants were encouraged to seek diagnosis by their partners because their relationships were reaching a breaking point. Others experienced a gradual buildup of discomfort and difficulty in trying to lead a "normal" life:

> I think it was sort of something that I felt I sort of had to face up to and stop sort of sticking fingers in the ear and pretending it wasn't an issue, which I had more or less always done previously. I had been very sort of adamant everything is fine, everything is normal. I will fit in. I will behave in the manner that is expected, I will do all sorts of things that everyone else does and just pretend that this isn't an issue. And I think on the whole I was reasonably good at that. But it, you know, sort of day in, day out, sort of doing the . . . I think the best way to describe it would be sort of, you know, putting on an act and you know, playing that role, just became sort of mentally exhausting, um, and eventually reached a point when I was working where I just thought, I can't go in this week, no, just not up to it. Not happening. (Robert, 27)

Robert highlights the dramaturgical dimension involved in "trying to fit in," which involves considerable effort (Goffman 1969). This was common among other participants as well and is reflected both within autobiographical literature discussed earlier and analyses of this literature (Davidson 2008, 2010).

The interactive and relational dimensions of the diagnostic journey were very apparent, as family, friends, colleagues, and others played various roles in the process. Although it is not clear whether Jonathan's mother was aware of ASD when she encouraged her son to see a psychologist, many participants talked about people explicitly raising the possibility of diagnosis with them. For example, Susan, 25, was having difficulty learning to drive and was surprised when an aunt responded to this by sending a newspaper cutting about ASD. Joan, 44, described how, "unbeknown to me, my mother had been told about Asperger Syndrome by a friend of hers—because her son had Asperger's—and when she was told about all the symptoms she just . . . she was really certain that I did have this. So we decided that we wouldn't be fobbed off anymore and that we would, um, push for formal diagnosis." The networks of nonmedical others involved in the diagnostic process included friends, relatives, work colleagues, and members of Internet forums. This suggests that the "symptoms" displayed by participants were recognizable as characteristics of ASD, whether the individuals concerned welcomed this recognition or not.

The interactional dimension extended to participants' engagement with existing literature and media (in the form of autistic autobiographies, Web sites, fiction, self-help manuals, blogs, and forums). Most participants talked about "doing research" before seeking a referral. A characteristic of ASD is an ability to intensely focus on particular topics, and the condition became a special interest for several participants who gained an in-depth knowledge of the subject. Indeed, it is difficult to disentangle some of their personal experiences from the reading and research they had done. As Francisco Ortega suggests (this volume), people assimilate the diagnostic categories into their descriptions and practices of the self. Firsthand accounts of others on the spectrum resonated most with participants; there were similarities in the ways in which experiences and stories were retold by participants and the published or online accounts of others' personal experiences. Mary, 43, explicitly contrasted her description of experiencing social life with the description provided by Donna Williams (1992). Tim, 37, described how Clare Sainsbury's description of her school days (2000) mirrored his own almost word for word. Abbey subverts common representations of autism (Davidson and Henderson 2010) in articulating her understanding of and engagement with ASD:

> I remember feeling, I felt very strongly that I know myself really well, and I've been reading all these books, and the ones that make most sense were actually the books written by people with Asperger's or autism themselves, because the ones written by the people that don't, it's like they're describing me from the outside, it's sort of like, if an alien was describing the human race, it, you know, you recognize yourself, but you recognize yourself from a different perspective, you know [laughs], whereas when you read books like by Donna Williams, you know, I totally, even though she's not Asperger's, she's actually kind of autism, but I totally do relate to lots of what she says. It makes so much sense.

Instead of her own experiences being alien, Abbey suggests that non-autistic authors writing about autistic experiences are themselves alien. Alternative representations of autism (such as the presentation of a neurotypical rather than autistic syndrome) are beginning to emerge in academic publications and may signal an important development in the analysis of ASD (Brownlow 2010; Hacking 2009b).

Three participants realized they may be on the autism spectrum while researching autism on behalf of their children. For example, Tim recognized aspects of himself in what he was reading when looking into the possibility of his son being autistic. The autobiographical work he read provided him with the certainty that he, too, was on the spectrum, despite his view that the diagnostic criteria were not an exact fit. He objected to the emphasis within the *DSM* on deficit.

Recognizing "symptoms" of ASD, or being prompted by a family member or friend to explore the possibility of a diagnosis, might not necessarily lead to someone actively seeking diagnosis. However, most participants expressed a strong motivation to be diagnosed, as is illustrated by the following extract:

> I: And what was it that made you think that you wanted to get the diagnosis?
>
> P: I didn't want not to know. I mean, if you have got something that you think is there, I think most people would rather know than just bury their head in the sand, for instance. You know, I thought, well, I would rather know for sure, because . . . in actual fact, I got really concerned about it. I got really worried and paranoid, and I really needed to know, because I was getting really anxious about it. I was thinking, well, if I have . . . because it looked so familiar, looking at all the, you know, the diagnostic criteria and reading people's stories, um, . . . I just, I thought, if I haven't got Asperger Syndrome, then what is wrong with me? (Mary)

This uncertainty and concern about not getting a diagnosis was apparent in the accounts of many participants. In part, this was because the lack of an ASD diagnosis might mean a less desirable alternative explanation. Several people talked about their fear of being diagnosed with a personality disorder or psychopathic tendencies (or, as discussed earlier, they had actually been misdiagnosed with other conditions). This concern about not getting a diagnosis could also be related to the strong desire for order that many participants experienced. For example, Neil, 39, said the "officialness" of the diagnosis related to his focus on exact things; he preferred to be able to say, "I am officially autistic" rather than "I am probably autistic." Other participants expressed a similar desire to obtain "an official stamp" and valued the sense of certainty associated with being able to say what they definitely were rather than what they might be.

Two participants differed in their approach to diagnosis from the rest of the sample. Abbey and Neil each delayed seeking a diagnosis for several years. Abbey read about ASD twenty years earlier and said, "It didn't really bother me. I just thought—as teachers had told me I was too quiet—so I just thought they don't like, society as a whole doesn't like, this type of personality I've got. So they decided to make it a disorder." She sought a diagnosis only recently, after experiencing difficulties returning to university. She explains her understanding of ASD: "It's a difference like being black or like being gay. People don't have to have a diagnosis to tell them that they're gay. They can, you know, they can understand that about themselves. So to me it's sort of like that. . . . Diagnosis is only necessary if you need some support, which I needed at college. So I mean I, I, the fact that I've, because lots of people have said to me, 'That's wonderful, you've got a diagnosis, do you feel you know yourself better now?' It's like, no. I [laughs], I already knew myself." The pediatrician who diagnosed Neil's son made it clear that Neil was also on the spectrum. He delayed seeking a diagnosis for himself for eight years. Although the unofficial diagnosis helped Neil (and his wife) make sense of some aspects of his behavior, he sought a diagnosis only when he began to experience more difficulties as he grew older. Abbey's and Neil's experiences may reflect a large number of self-diagnosed adults, and highlight how the salience of having a diagnosis of ASD varies across the life course and can involve an element of choice and autonomy.

The Process of Diagnosis

It is clear that the majority of participants had realized, decided, or at least hoped that they were on the spectrum before they approached their GPs to ask for referral. The response of GPs to their request could ease or obstruct their diagnostic journey. An individual GP's receptiveness, in turn, depended on his or her knowledge of ASD and a broader under-standing of the difficulties that patients may have experienced over the years. Some GPs were supportive: "So I went to my GP, whose husband happened to have an interest in autism, and she looked at my medical history and said in her opinion there was a very high probability I was on the spectrum and that getting a formal diagnosis, in her opinion, would help me and open up access to help for my self-harm" (Trisha, 42). Others described dismay at their GP's attitude toward their request. Some older participants described how their GP couldn't understand why they would want a diagnosis:

> I think they virtually say, "Well, you've lived with it up to now; you can live with it a bit longer." And I'm thinking, well, maybe yes, but maybe no. I do think, no matter what age you are, I do think you deserve an answer and shouldn't be allowed to go through the rest of your life having to live, just live with it and get on with it. (June)

> Although the GP had said, he had said to me, "Why do you need a diagnosis? There is no treatment." But, I mean, I just backed my wife's view on the diagnosis and, for me, I also thought that I would rather be an Asperger than be wrong, weird, with no known cause. (Richard, 58)

The reluctance of some GPs to refer participants suggests a lack of aware-ness of the function and meaning of a diagnosis to participants, a func-tion that appears to have been understood by those lay others who en-couraged participants to seek diagnosis.

Once referred, the diagnostic process varied among participants but included a lengthy interview or interviews with consultants who had various backgrounds, including medicine, psychology, or psychiatry. Several participants were asked to nominate other family members, who were interviewed independently to provide further detail about the participant's childhood. Many participants were also asked to complete detailed questionnaires. There were few consistent accounts of the di-agnostic process among participants. A few reflected on the subjective nature of the process, either through their own agency or the agency of the clinician. For example, David said, "It's also true that actually a lot of psychiatrists operating out there in the NHS [National Health Service] don't really know the strict criteria of conditions laid down in *DSM*. I mean, they will not give you a diagnosis when actually really you do meet the *DSM* criteria, because they're working based on their own experience and what was, what they were trained at rather than what's in the latest diagnostic manual." Graham remembered "having a bit of a sweat about it" as he worried about not answering the questions on the questionnaire "as if I had AS." A few female participants felt that their gender influenced their GP's judgment. They felt that because the majority of people diagnosed with autism are male, as women, their concerns were not taken seriously. Jenny talked about the "subtlety" of ASD and was told by the first consultant that she couldn't be on the spectrum because she was interacting too well. This is consistent with autobiographical literature and the analyses of such accounts (Davidson 2007a, 2007b).

Many participants described the experience of receiving the diagnosis and framed this in different ways; the diagnosis of ASD was something they were "given," something they "had," or something that facilitated access to a new identity; they "were" autistic. Richard, for example, assumed an autistic identity and presented himself as "being an Aspie" or, as he described earlier, "being an Asperger," a different type of being. Mary also assumed an autistic identity and located herself at a point on a spectrum, using statistics to support the legitimacy of that position: "She [the consultant] said I was 95 percent, because, which is stupid, because it says, because they can't work in 100 percent, so I had to only be 95 percent." Several participants talked about being given an "official diagnosis," and they interpreted the diagnosis as something they "had" rather than something they "were."

The emphasis on "official diagnosis" was a common theme in the analysis.[2] An official or "formal" diagnosis (that is, one obtained through the U.K. NHS) was perceived to be more acceptable and authoritative—less potentially "questionable"—than one gained through other diagnostic centers, such as the National Autistic Society Lorna Wing Centre for Autism. Further, such official diagnosis also facilitates access to support and services, including financial allowances such as Disability Living Allowance, as the following extracts illustrate:

Well, first, I think, the, the woman in the, the woman at the college, the disability coordinator. She, even when I got this diagnosis, she didn't really truly believe me, because it was a private diagnosis. She thought the NHS wasn't going—because I get an NHS bursary for the course—she didn't think it was a real one, she didn't think it was proper. She didn't really believe that I had Asperger's Syndrome. (Abbey)

So, so, yes, and then we had to try and get a diagnosis, which was not easy. We got it on the NHS. We did at one point consider going private, because, you know, you do have to wait such a long time, but it's very, very expensive to do it private and also, you know, we wanted it to be done properly. It's more official if it's done on the NHS than if it's done privately, because not all private diagnoses are accepted, so we wanted to do it the proper way. (Jenny, 21)

Susie, 34, received a diagnosis within the NHS but didn't receive confirmation in writing and said that people don't take her diagnosis seriously as a result. Some participants offered to produce written evidence of diagnosis during their interview, and June later sent a copy of her own accord in the post, highlighting how important documentation was for them.

Consequences and Meaning of Diagnosis

For some participants, the medical diagnosis represented a radical redefinition of the self (Davidson and Orsini, this volume). They were able to make sense of difficult experiences in their lives commonly involving social interaction, relationships, education, and employment. This sensemaking is, arguably, particularly significant to people who struggle to understand the norms and values that are an integral part of mainstream society. Several participants also described a sense of relief:

I: So what did you think when you actually received the diagnosis?
P: Well, relief! I thought, that is it! When I first went over to the clinical psychologist, he asked me a list of diagnostic questions. And [snaps fingers] somebody understands what I mean. Yes, I do constantly misread people. I have got a habit, a long history

of misreading people. Not knowing quite what people's mo-
tives are, unless it is very obvious, if it is absolutely blindingly
obvious. . . . But I, yes, when I had to go back again the second
time to see the clinical psychologist and he said, "Yes, you have
certainly got Asperger's. In my opinion you have got Asperger
Syndrome." Ho! At last! Somebody bloody understands and it
just fitted into place. (Peter, 65)

When I received the diagnosis, I was very, very happy. Um, because
it, I was really relieved. It was just so good to know that I wasn't, I
was not a psychopath, no, I was, because, you know, I know I'm not,
but it's kind of like [two-second pause] what, what other thing could
I have if it wasn't Asperger's? . . . And to have Asperger's Syndrome,
because I don't think for me, that's not a problem at all. . . . I was relieved. Um, you see, but it's just kind of something you're born with,
and it's, it's not like you're mad or anything. It just, um, can make
you a little bit different. (Jenny)

Other participants were more measured in their response to receiving
the diagnosis. They had gained a fuller understanding from the research
they had done and, as David said, the diagnosis was "just official confirmation of something, in my own mind, I knew to be the case already."
Similarly, Graham, 26, said, "I had decided that even if they said I wasn't
autistic, I had decided that I was." He described how "it doesn't change
who you are, because it is who you are," but at the same time he felt
"more defined as a person." He elaborated: "I mean it is what it is, it's
Asperger's Syndrome. It's not something, it's not something that you
can catch. You know, you can't cure it, you can't catch it, and it's just
part of your personality, it's part of who you are. It's like saying, I don't
know, I'm left-handed, I'm right-handed. I kick a ball on the left foot or
I do things in a certain way. It's part of who you are. It's how you work.
How you operate as a person. That's what Asperger's Syndrome is." The
relational and interactional dimensions of the diagnostic journey make
it difficult to unpack exactly how participants felt about the diagnosis. It
wasn't clear whether they were happy to be autistic, glad to have something to help them understand their lives and feel less alone; or relieved
to not have another condition, such as personality disorder or psychosis, that they felt was worse. Michael, 26, illustrates the complexity by

describing how he experienced relief to get the diagnosis because it helped him to make sense of his life but how, at the same time, he didn't want to be autistic: "Well there are very few good things about autism; it's ruined my life and I never wanted to be autistic, and if I had a choice to not be autistic, I never would. . . . I just, I really can't say anything much positive, particularly positive, about autism. It's ruined my life as far as I can tell, and it's ruined a lot of lives of people I've met who have been autistic." A few people expressed sadness at finding out that they would not ever "be fixed," but these feelings were mixed, again, with relief about knowing what the problem was: "But I think right before the diagnosis I sort of started feeling a bit, 'Oh god, what if I have got it? I mean, ah, that is it. That is it. I have got it. I have got Asperger's. I have got autism. Oh my god' kind of thing. But, mostly it was a relief. It was just a big 'Thank god I know what I have got'" (Caroline, 25). A few participants talked about the significance of being able to access support following diagnosis in a way that helped them to negotiate particular areas of social life, such as that involved with further education. As Robert said, "I think that certainly the most positive outcome of it all—apart from my own sanity, of course—is the fact that you have this little magic piece of paper that says, yes, please, can you sort of treat this person a little differently."

Accessing a "new" autistic identity, with an array of literature to draw upon and learn from, led several participants to think about ways of changing their behavior and learning ways of fitting in more effectively. Richard, for example, embarked on a "project of the self" following diagnosis (Giddens 1991). He learned about appropriate body language from self-help books and was starting to work on developing empathy. Although he had been to relationship counseling with his wife on a few occasions in the past and was aware that his wife found his behavior frustrating, and often upsetting, it wasn't until he started to read about autism that he began to understand the impact of his behavior and obsessive focus on others. Other participants, rather than embarking on a "project of the self," felt that their new identity allowed them a legitimate excuse for avoiding situations that made them feel uncomfortable. As Neil said, "It suddenly goes from being something that you can fix, to something you can't fix. You can only try and cope with it."

ASD remained a special interest for many participants who enjoyed interacting online with other "Aspies" and reading about autism. The transformative effect of this research was apparent within some accounts. For example, Michael described how "I was only diagnosed three years ago. And I'd gone through a lot of different mental health problems prior to this. I didn't really know what was wrong with me. And while I suppose the diagnostic criteria when I saw them fit me perfectly, the actual experience of it all, it took me much longer and much more time to understand exactly what it's like to be autistic, I suppose. It's not immediately obvious, and so in this regard I suppose I've been influenced very much by what I've read on the topic." Here, the salience of looping is apparent. The "looseness" of the diagnostic criteria, combined with the autobiographical (and other) literature, allows people, once diagnosed, to make their own sense of who they are, within the space offered by an autistic identity. The ways in which existing literature, and more interactional spaces such as Internet forums, feeds back into participants' perceptions of self have been considered (Davidson 2007b, 2008). Earlier extracts from the data illustrate how some participants related autobiographical writings to their own experiences. For example, Michael openly acknowledges the ways in which his reading has helped shape his autistic identity.

Participants also reflected on the implications of being diagnosed later in life, and on how different their lives could have been if ASD had been classified earlier. Mary commented, "People didn't know about it before 1994. People thought I was mentally ill or emotionally frail." For Peter, "If somebody younger was seen and assessed, screened, and somebody would say, 'Well, look, don't do anything drastic, we will help you to make the most of it, to make the most of your life. And you will live a profitable and productive life, and we are not going to mollycoddle you, but we will be there to keep an eye on you from afar, as it were, you know, to make sure you are not going to get yourself into serious difficulties,' and my life would have been completely different." There has been little focus to date on the experiences of people diagnosed with ASD in adulthood, and an increasingly significant gap in research on ageing and ASD remains.

Conclusion

This chapter began with a discussion of how ASDs seem to subvert conventional understandings of diagnosis. Although there is no cure for ASD (and not everyone would welcome it if there were), a diagnosis offers potential access to an autistic identity and culture. This identity was formalized only after the classification of ASD in the *DSM* in 1980 (and of AS in the 1990s), which means that many older people, like Peter, Edward, and Richard, have lived a large part of their lives without access to a fuller understanding of their differences. They grew up being told, for example, that they were "weird" or "stupid." Being able to access an alternative explanation for the difficulties they experienced, and finding out that other people have similar experiences, was a source of significant relief and comfort to them. The analysis presented here highlights the contextual, relational, and emotional dimensions to getting a diagnosis of ASD in adulthood and the meaning diagnosis has in real-life contexts. Of course, the doors to the autistic community or communities are not guarded by health professionals, and it could be the case that many people end their diagnostic journeys at the point of finding out about ASD for themselves. They may remain contentedly self-diagnosed throughout their lives, and so are absent from studies such as this one. Others, like Abbey and Neil, may remain self-diagnosed until a particular event leads them to seek a medical diagnosis. The analysis here, however, underlines the power and importance that a diagnosis has for many on the spectrum.

This is apparent when considering the distinction many participants made between an official diagnosis—that is, one given within the context of the NHS—and diagnoses obtained through private health-care provision. Most participants didn't focus on the distinction between self-diagnosis and "doctor diagnosis" but were concerned, rather, with the perceived legitimacy and thus acceptability of different diagnostic sources (Brownlow 2006). This emphasis underlines the contested dimension of ASD. The lack of a universal diagnostic tool and the infinite variation and nuance inherent in ASD mean that access to the diagnosis can be uncertain and the diagnosis itself highly prized. This is particularly the case for women; as I have noted, GPs may be less likely to recognize characteristics in women because the majority of people diagnosed with ASD are male. Most participants wanted the confirmation that they were autistic. Thinking that they might be was not only insufficient for their own sense of self but also would not be convincing for other people and institutions across a wide social terrain.

The role played by GPs as gatekeepers to the diagnostic process is clearly significant. Some GPs foreclosed on the possibility of referral for diagnosis without understanding the difficulties that participants, and in some cases other family members, were facing. A greater understanding about the significance and meaning of a diagnosis of ASD to people at different stages across the life course is needed. Further research exploring ageing and ASD would also offer important insights. Engagement with experiential accounts that both describe and constitute autistic experience offers a way of developing a deeper understanding of autistic lifeworlds. As Joyce Davidson suggests, authors of autistic autobiographies offer "access to and act as navigational guides through their own 'alien' environments" (2010, 306). Concern about a divergence between stereotypical representations and clinical reality (Draaisma 2009) risks the dismissal of firsthand accounts as anecdotal and an overemphasis on very rigid diagnostic criteria. There is, or at least should be, space for both scientific and experiential knowledge in understandings and constructions of autism.

The diagnostic journeys explored here offer some support for the concept of looping. Diagnosis is a dialogic process (Cimini 2010) involving interaction, interpretation, negotiation, change, and, sometimes, tension. Participants' understandings of and engagement with ASD were informed by their interaction with a wide range of people, texts, and spaces, such as the Internet. Although people may attempt to fit within a set of criteria that describe both the symptoms and deficits deemed as constituting ASD, these criteria, paradoxically, can appear to have little subsequent authority in organizing their lives (Davidson 2007b).

McGeer has argued that autistic self-narratives could not transform autistic experiences, because autistics cannot be co-minded (2009). The stories retold here have coherence and a reflexive dimension that may appear at odds with some popular and clinical representations of "the autistic self." Participants interact with existing literature and knowledge about ASD, changing how they talk and think about themselves in the process. They learn about autism and, in some cases, contribute to the body of autistic self-narratives through blogging or taking part in research. Whether they are co-minded with other autistic people or remain differently minded, the experience of being autistic appears to be transformative and dynamic. The problem or tension is the persistence of neurotypical frameworks of understanding autism that are not easily translatable into the terms and experiences of autistic lifeworlds.

In this chapter, an examination of these often hidden, insider stories, focusing on how the diagnostic process during adulthood transforms participants' own subjectivities, enriches narrowly drawn and limited understandings of autism.

NOTES

1. Both Scott's and Hacking's interpretations are of particular interest when considering AS because of the proposed removal of the condition from the next edition of the *DSM*. Clinical uncertainty surrounding diagnoses of AS, together with the overlap with some diagnostic criteria for autism and AS, as well as other manifestations of ASD such as high-functioning autism, has long generated discussion about whether AS and autism should be considered separate conditions. It may be that, in the longer term, the proposed removal will lead to a greater acceptance of all people simply identified as being "on the spectrum."

2. A recent exchange between the author and a psychiatrist highlights the contested nature of ASD diagnosis, particularly in relation to adults. This individual had visited the project Web site and questioned the composition of the sample, suggesting that some of the participants were eccentric people rather than people with ASD. He cautioned that we should not ask people whether they have been diagnosed with autism, but who diagnosed them. This personal exchange adds weight to the contested dimension of ASD, particularly in adults.

REFERENCES

American Psychiatric Association. 1994. *DSM-IV: Diagnostic and Statistical Manual of Mental Disorders.* 4th ed. Arlington, Va.: American Psychiatric Association.

Baron-Cohen, S., A. M. Leslie, and U. Frith. 1985. "Does the Autistic Child Have a 'Theory of Mind'?" *Cognition* 21 (1): 37–46.

Belmonte, M. K. 2007. "Human, but More So: What the Autistic Brain Tells Us about the Process of Narrative." In *Autism and Representation*, edited by M. Osteen, 166–80. New York: Routledge.

Brownlow, C. 2006. "The Construction of the Autistic Individual: Investigations into Online Discussion Groups." PhD diss., University of Brighton, U.K.

———. 2010. "Representing Autism: The Construction of 'NT Syndrome.'" *Journal of Medical Humanities* 31 (3): 243–55.

Charmaz, K. 2006. *Constructing Grounded Theory: A Practical Guide through Qualitative Analysis.* London: Sage.

Cimini, N. 2010. "Struggles over the Meaning of Down's Syndrome: A 'Dialogic' Interpretation." *Health* 14 (4): 398–414.

Davidson, J. 2007a. "'In a World of Her Own . . .': Representing Alienation and Emotion in the Lives and Writings of Women with Autism." *Gender, Place, and Culture* 14 (6): 659–77.

———. 2007b. "'More Labels Than a Jam Jar': The Gendered Dynamics for Diagnosis for Girls and Women with Autism." In *Contesting Illness: Processes and Practices*, edited by P. Moss and K. Teghtsoonian, 239–58. Toronto, Ont.: University of Toronto Press.

——. 2008. "Autistic Culture Online: Virtual Communication and Cultural Expression on the Spectrum." *Social and Cultural Geography* 9 (7): 791–806.

——. 2010. "'It Cuts Both Ways': A Relational Approach to Access and Accommodation for Autism." *Social Science and Medicine* 70 (2): 305–12.

Davidson, J., and V. L. Henderson. 2010. "'Coming Out' on the Spectrum: Autism, Identity, and Disclosure." *Social and Cultural Geography* 11 (2): 155–70.

Draaisma, D. 2009. "Stereotypes of Autism." *Philosophical Transactions of the Royal Society* 364 (1522): 1475–80.

Eyal, G., et al. 2010. *The Autism Matrix: The Social Origins of the Autism Epidemic.* Cambridge: Polity.

Foster, B., and B. H. King. 2003. "Asperger Syndrome: To Be or Not to Be?" *Current Opinions in Paediatrics* 15 (5): 491–94.

Frith, U. 1991. "Autistic Psychopathy in Childhood." In *Autism and Asperger Syndrome*, edited by U. Frith, 37–92. Cambridge: Cambridge University Press.

——. 2004. "Emanuel Miller Lecture: Confusions and Controversies about Asperger Syndrome." *Journal of Child Psychology and Psychiatry* 45 (4): 672–86.

Geertz, C. 1973. *An Interpretation of Cultures.* New York: Basic Books.

Giddens, A. 1991. *Modernity and Self-Identity: Self and Society in the Late Modern Age.* Cambridge: Polity.

Goffman, E. 1969. *The Presentation of Self in Everyday Life.* Harmondsworth, U.K.: Penguin.

Grandin, T. 1996. *Thinking in Pictures: And Other Reports from My Life with Autism.* New York: Vintage.

Hacking, I. 2007. "Kinds of People, Moving Targets." *Proceedings of the British Academy* 151: 285–318.

——. 2009a. "Autistic Autobiographies." *Philosophical Transactions of the Royal Society* 364: 1467–73.

——. 2009b. "Humans, Aliens, and Autism." *Daedalus* 138 (3): 44–59.

Hall, K. 2011. *Asperger Syndrome, the Universe, and Everything.* London: Kingsley.

Healthtalkonline. 2013. Accessed April 30, 2013, http://www.healthtalkonline.org/

Lawson, W. 2000. *Life behind Glass: A Personal Account of Autism Spectrum Disorder.* London: Kingsley.

Matson, J. L., and J. Wilkins. 2008. "Nosology and Diagnosis of Asperger's Syndrome." *Research in Autism Spectrum Disorders* 2 (2): 288–300.

McGeer, V. 2009. "The Thought and Talk of Individuals with Autism: Reflections on Ian Hacking." *Metaphilosophy* 40 (3–4): 517–30.

Ryan, S., and U. Raisanen. 2008. "'It's Like You Are Just a Spectator in This Thing': Experiencing Social Life the 'Aspie' Way." *Emotion, Space, and Society* 1 (2): 135–43.

Sainsbury, C. 2000. *The Martian in the Playground.* London: Sage.

Scott, S. 2009. *Making Sense of Everyday Life.* Cambridge: Polity.

Scott, W. J. 1990. "PTSD in DSM-III: A Case in the Politics of Diagnosis and Disease." *Social Problems* 37 (3): 294.

Silverman, C. 2010. "Autism's Prosaic Technologies." Paper presented at "Critical Autism Studies: Enabling Inclusion, Defending Difference," University of Ottawa, September 24–25.

Singer, J. 1999. "'Why Can't You Be Normal for Once in Your Life?' From a 'Problem with No Name' to the Emergence of a New Category of Difference." In *Disability Discourse*, edited by M. Corker and S. French, 59–67. Buckingham, U.K.: Open University Press.

Slater-Walker, G., and C. Slater-Walker. 2002. *An Asperger Marriage*. London: Kingsley.

Szatmari, P. 2004. *A Mind Apart: Understanding Children with Autism and Asperger Syndrome*. New York: Guilford.

Willey, L. H. 1999. *Pretending to Be Normal: Living with Asperger's Syndrome*. London: Kingsley.

Williams, D. 1992. *Nobody, Nowhere: The Remarkable Autobiography of an Autistic Girl*. London: Kingsley.

Wing, L. 1981. "Asperger's Syndrome: A Clinical Account." *Psychological Medicine* 11 (1): 115–30.

Woodbury-Smith, M., and F. Volkmar. 2009. "Asperger Syndrome." *European Child and Adolescent Psychiatry* 18 (1): 2–11.

World Health Organization. 1992. *ICD-10: International Statistical Classification of Diseases and Related Health Problems*. 10th rev. Geneva: World Health Organization.

Divided or Opposed?

The Level-of-Functioning Arguments in Autism-Related Political Discourse in Canada

Dana Lee Baker and Lila Walsh

Autism exists on a spectrum. Though ongoing debate among autism-policy stakeholders surrounds the question of whether the "D" in "ASD" should be "difference" or "disorder," replaced with "conditions," or dropped entirely, the designation "spectrum" tends currently to inspire less discursive interest.[1] The latter designation, which has also been used, for example, with fetal alcohol syndrome, signifies diversity of experience. One of the most influential sources of definitions of neurological differences is the American Psychiatric Association's *Diagnostic and Statistical Manual of Mental Disorders (DSM)*, in which autism has been included as a distinct category since 1980. Each time the *DSM* has been revised, autism has been reconstructed, in part because of increased understanding of autism within the medical and psychiatric community and in part in response to concerns brought forth by autistics, individuals with autism, and other stakeholders. By the time the *DSM-IV* was released, in 1994, autism had been expanded into a spectrum including Rett disorder, childhood disintegrative disorder, and pervasive developmental disorder not otherwise specified (PDD-NOS). At the time of this writing, the fifth edition of the manual is under development and is expected to include revised definitions of autism-spectrum disorders. General agreement exists on the basic principle that the way of being called autistic varies in near-infinite degrees. Use of the spectrum concept becomes complicated once one begins to actually describe what the term specifically involves. In particular, the tendency to describe one end as so-called low-functioning autism (typically understood as coincident with mental retardation) and the other as high-functioning autism (described by many as similar, if not identical, to Asperger Syndrome) raises some proverbial eyebrows.[2] Like all attempts to measure nonphysical human characteristics, efforts to rank essential characteristics of autism along a one-dimensional measurement scheme prove complicated and are at risk of becoming subjective to the point of meaninglessness. Nevertheless, position on the spectrum and, by extension, description as either high- or low-functioning serve as identifying elements used by both individuals with autism and other issue stakeholders (that is, anyone with an active interest or political stake surrounding a given public challenge, such as parents, family members, friends, and professionals).

In policy contexts, spectrums have the power to create conundrums. This is a characteristic of the larger political environment in which autism politics takes place, including most efforts to create, implement, and evaluate policy targeting disability-related issues (such as the disability-policy subsystem). First of all, despite increasing (if sometimes begrudging) recognition of the role that social and political infrastructures play in the creation of disability, the design of most disability policy still turns on the identification of a particular individual as (more or less permanently) having a disability or not (Burns et al. 2004; Hertz-Picciotto and Delwiche 2009). The degree to which this represents a failure of imagination on the part of policy makers or deliberate discrimination on the part of some issue stakeholders remains largely unclear. This reality can be difficult to match to the concept of a spectrum, in that it requires established definitions and agreed-upon cutoff points with regard to what constitutes having a disability. Spectrums also mismatch with current policy infrastructures because of the tendency toward death by diffusion (Baker 2011; Lanham 2006). When an issue becomes overly inclusive—at least in the imagination of the general public—successfully asserting a need for targeted policy becomes more difficult (Wheelan and Malkiel 2010; Weimar and Vining 2010). One reason for this is that the broader category eventually includes many individuals who have few or no significant difficulties with activities of daily living (Moloney 2010; Murray 2012). Finally, and most importantly for the purposes of this chapter, the existence of a spectrum (or even a multilevel taxonomy) creates divisions among autism-policy stakeholders. Such divisions could ultimately lead to circumstances in which forward progress in autism-related policy slows down substantially.

In this chapter, we examine the degree to which conceptions of the needs and interests of so-called low- and high-functioning individuals with autism are set in tension with one another in Canadian political discourse. Autism is the fastest-growing developmental disability in North America; examining political discourse surrounding the spectrum would also be useful at international or comparative levels. The choice here to isolate Canadian political discourse, however, is a methodological decision. Political discourse on autism in Canadian government has been abundant, and it promises to continue to be topical. For example, acts to amend the Canada Health Act to ensure that the cost of behavioral treatments for autistic persons is covered by the health-care insurance plan of every province and to establish a national strategy for autism-spectrum disorders were introduced into the Forty-First Parliament in June 2011. Canadian political discourse provides ample ground for research on the ways in which the autistic spectrum is perceived and discussed in a particular geographical and sociocultural context.

The core research question of this chapter is this: How is the concept of the autism spectrum employed in the political discourse of a modern democracy? To address this question, we examine Canadian political discourse about autism that has taken place at the national level of government in recent parliaments. Consideration of this question is not only of academic interest to both policy and disability studies but also worth the attention of other diverse issue stakeholders, especially as they struggle to work with one another as partners in the development of good policy (albeit with different foci and concerns) rather than as competing adversaries in this endeavor (Van Horn, Baumer, and Gormley 2001; Woshinsky 2007).

In this chapter, we briefly introduce the politics of the disability-policy subsystem, considering how it specifically relates to autism, before moving on to discuss the historical development of autism as a public concern. It is this history that informs the reader as to the conceptual development of autism as a spectrum. To this end, we review the three aspects of prevalence, etiology, and changes in perception of autism as a core element of identity over time. These historical aspects not only highlight the ways in which autism-related policy is an illustrative lens through which to examine disability-policy design, they also provide a useful structure when examining autism political discourse. A sample of Canadian parliamentary documents was reviewed for references to autism, and we present here examples of those references and implications pertaining to the autism spectrum found in the sampled discourse. Of particular interest is the potential for division among autism-issue stakeholders along the spectrum. This was not found in the sampled discourse, however. Spectrum-related divisions (if in existence) may not yet be salient at the national level of discourse. This and other emerging patterns associated with the three historical aspects of autism are discussed in the "Findings and Discussion" section of the chapter.

Political Discourse and the Disability-Policy Subsystem

As is common in any policy subsystem, disability policy incorporates a plethora of issues and goals. From the perspective of some in disability studies, taking a condition-specific look at disability policy does not constitute an appropriate, respectful approach to examining disability policy and politics (see, for example, Olkin and Pledger 2003). This position largely represents a reaction to essentialist or so-called medical models of disability, which, by and large, discuss individual conditions from the perspective of the deficits associated with them (Areheart 2008; Hahn and Belt 2004; Harris 2001; Russell 1998). From the perspective of public policy, however, policy issues can be bounded to quite specific conditions or circumstances, given active political attention and sufficient stakeholder interest in creating such linkages, without necessarily condoning or contributing to essentialist, deficit-oriented interpretations of disability.

Disability is a relativistic concept, one that at least partly relies on time and place for definition. In the case of autism, there was tremendous increase in the observed incidence and prevalence of autism across the globe during the late 1990s and the early twenty-first century (Feinberg and Vacca 2000; Fombonne 2003). In response, attention to and interest in autism-related policy grew dramatically. The concept of a spectrum, however (with the potential for competing inclusionary and exclusionary components), has the capacity to complicate policy development and implementation. For all of these reasons, autism-related policy provides an excellent context for examining the evolution of disability-policy design at the turn of the millennium.

Autism-Related Politics

The disability-policy subsystem is inherently multifaceted and comprises divergent agendas. These agendas can be generally categorized as pertaining to establishing and protecting rights, providing care-based services, supporting searches for cures, and promoting the celebration of difference (Baker 2011). These general categories have shaped the history of autism-related policy, especially as it fits into the larger category of disability policy generally. However, with regard to the conception of a spectrum specifically, a basic understanding of three aspects of the history of autism as a public issue is fundamental to appreciating public and political discourse. These aspects include prevalence, etiology, and diagnosis-related identity.

Prevalence

Conventional wisdom about autism once held that it was a relatively rare condition affecting about 1 in every 10,000 individuals (Feinberg and Vacca 2000; Grinker 2008). The condition was not specifically identified in any known culture until the mid-twentieth century, when it was nearly simultaneously, but separately, identified by Leo Kanner and Hans Asperger (Bursztyn 2007). As a result, as recently as twenty years ago, members of the general public and in fact many professionals, including physicians, teachers, and social workers, went their entire lives without once (consciously, at least) encountering an individual with autism (Grinker 2008; Strathearn 2009). At the end of the first decade of the twenty-first century, it is unusual *not* to encounter a person with autism.

The change in experience and awareness came about as a result of a dramatic increase in the recorded incidence of autism beginning in the 1990s. As of 2010, prevalence rates for autism were estimated to be approximately 1 in 110 children, with about 80 percent of those being male (Lord and Bishop 2010). In addition, incidence has not yet reached a plateau (Hertz-Picciotto and Delwiche 2009), and some organizations, such as Autism Speaks, publicize even higher rates. Debate continues as to whether the observed increase represents socially constructed or physical-biological change in the human experience (Gernsbacher et al. 2010; King and Bearman 2009; Liu, King, and Bearman 2010).

In the context of public policy and, in particular, demand for public programs, increased incidence matters (Baker 2011). As a result of this stunning increase, the issue of prevalence (and incidence) of autism emerged as a political issue in itself. The issue of incidence relates strongly to the concept of a spectrum, especially with regard to the relative distribution of the increase across the spectrum. Furthermore, as we will discuss, rise in incidence kindled and fueled interest in other autism-related policy issues.

Etiology

Interest in the etiology of autism followed quickly on the heels of reports of increased incidence. In particular, use of the phrase "autism epidemic" provoked attention and concern as it raised the specter of biological or environmental contagion (Bumiller 2009; Fombonne 2001; Gernsbacher et al. 2010). Even in the absence of epidemic language and, more basically, of a conception of autism as a public problem to be solved, it is hardly surprising that such a dramatic change in the (perceived) composition of the population achieved a measure of public attention. The strong desire to understand the causes or origin of a condition affecting the population at increasing rates is a natural development in the evolution of autism policy.

Emerging consensus holds that the set of behaviors called autism likely results from several different (and possibly disparate) conditions (Feinstein 2010). Heated debates continue, however, as to the relative role of factors such as genetics, prenatal conditions, environmental factors, changes in diagnostic standards, and special education and health-policy design in explaining autism prevalence (Currenti 2010; Strathearn 2009). Both the consensus and the debate serve to politicize discussion of the autism spectrum.

Another etiology-related issue playing a leading role in autism-related political discourse involves the assertion that vaccines either cause or trigger autism (given genetic susceptibility; Murray 2012). For the most part, the identified culprits are either the measles, mumps, and rubella (MMR) vaccine or the presence of thimerosal as a preservative in any vaccine. Despite increasingly emphatic agreement among most medical researchers and physicians that autism does not result from exposure to vaccines, arguments making this connection continue to manifest in political and public discourse (Offit 2010; Omer et al. 2009). Individuals, including celebrities such as Jenny McCarthy, and organizations such as SafeMinds remain convinced that vaccines play a role in the emergence of autism and engage actively in autism-related politics (Kaufman 2010; Kirby 2006). They also understand themselves to be confronting a conspiracy that protects large corporations selling vaccines, and they work hard to protect members of the scientific community supporting their cause, such as widely discredited British physician Andrew Wakefield (Offit 2010).

Identity and Diagnosis

The concept of identity has personal qualities and communal attachments imbued in it (Hahn and Belt 2004). An individual's own cognitive and emotive views as someone with a disability, as well as in relation to a disabled minority community, are distinct from but related to the concept of formal diagnosis (Bumiller 2009; Kielhofner 2005). Identity and diagnosis represent highly politicized issues across the disability-policy subsystem. In part, this results from the fact that access to services and other disability-oriented public programs tends to be limited to those formally diagnosed with an identified disability. Increasingly, however, political conversation surrounding diagnosis involves more affirming aspects of identity (Hahn and Belt 2004; Kielhofner 2005). In other words, disability and disability-specific communities and cultures rely upon the existence of identifiable and relatively firm boundaries around what constitutes an individual with a (particular) disability. Such discourse is further politicized by frequent disagreement between experiential and scientific knowledge with regard to disability (Brownlow, O'Dell, and Taylor 2006). Autism is no exception to this general rule. In fact, because autism exists in the category of so-called invisible disabilities lacking readily identifiable biological markers with challenges surrounding identification and diagnosis, autism-related identity politics has the potential to become particularly heated. This is especially true in the context of a spectrum.

Autism is and always has been a behavior-based diagnosis. In other words, evidence of autism in any particular definition relies exclusively upon external interpretation of someone's behavior (Armstrong 2010; Bumiller 2009). Such inherent subjectivity complicates both the politics of assigning services to those diagnosed with autism and the cohesive composition of groups formed around a common diagnosis (Lord and Bishop 2010). Furthermore, until quite recently (and particularly prior to the advent of the Internet), it was commonly assumed that individuals with autism could not effectively speak for themselves (Brownlow, O'Dell, and Taylor 2006). In recent years, the challenging of this assumption by prominent individuals with autism has inspired political discourse about the spectrum and the relatively dominant role that so-called high-functioning individuals may be playing in the public articulation of autistic identity. In light of this, a key focus in our examination of political discourse is whether the concept of a spectrum is associated with division or tension among autism-issue stakeholders. In other words, is there evidence of level-of-functioning policy arguments?

This issue is complicated further by the fact that, as discussed earlier, the definition and diagnostic criteria of autism have changed over time. In fact, some researchers attribute much, if not all, of the observed increase in autism to changes in diagnostic criteria over time (King and Bearman 2009; Liu, King, and Bearman 2010). In addition, changes in eligibility for services, such as access to special education, often follow or mirror diagnostic criteria. Autism will likely be redefined again in the forthcoming fifth edition of the *Diagnostic and Statistical Manual (DSM)*, arguably the most influential source of technical definitions of neurological conditions (Lord and Bishop 2010). Proposed changes to the *DSM* (which were expected to be released in 2013) include the elimination of Asperger Syndrome as a separate disorder and its full incorporation into the autism spectrum, thereby creating a single diagnostic autism category (Ghaziuddin 2010). Such a change will likely fuel increased political debate surrounding issues of identity and diagnosis.

Even in the context of an established and unchanging definition, diagnosis can become a politically complicated event. In the case of Down syndrome, such complications arise in association with the issue of genetic testing, which pregnant women are encouraged to undergo and after which they are sometimes subtly counseled to abort their fetus if the test is positive (Bumiller 2009). This is particularly the case if multiple policy arenas are involved in the implementation of policies designed to address the needs of the target population. For example, in the United States, the term "educational autism" was created in order to qualify students not necessarily formally diagnosed with autism for special education services under the Individuals with Disabilities Education Act. Furthermore, diagnostic processes, though purporting to be objective, are prone to sociocultural influences and faddishness (Young 2010). If one diagnosis is currently more popular or accepted than another, it can assume a self-perpetuating quality in the public consciousness.

Generational and life-span effects also contribute to the political energy surrounding identity and diagnosis in autism-related politics (Baker 2011). Young people growing up diagnosed as having autism today face a far different (and, to some degree, less discriminatory) world than that faced by earlier generations. As a result, they (or their parents) approach the diagnosis of autism much differently, having access to multiple and expanded contexts for comprehending autism, than their past counterparts did. For example, prior to the 1980s, "pathological mothering" was thought to be at the root of autism, but over the last few decades autism has been recast as having different social, environmental, and biological explanations (Bumiller 2009). Furthermore, because identity tends to become more complex and multifaceted over the course of a lifetime, including such aspects as professional identity, group affiliations, political leanings, generation affiliations, and more complex family roles, identification as a person with autism or with a larger community of individuals with autism may be of different importance to those who are just starting out as independent adults as opposed to those who are older, with other established personal and professional ties. Finally, over the last several decades, much political energy has been invested in the effort to divest the identification as an individual with a disability of its shame. In the context of autism-related politics, work in this direction has been done using both disability-specific and pandisability approaches (Robertson and Ne'eman 2008). Although much work remains to be done in promoting acceptance and understanding of individuals with disabilities, older individuals with disabilities tend to experience more shame than members of younger generations because of the generally increased acceptance of individuals with disabilities across democratic societies in the modern era (Grinker 2008).

Method

This chapter examines how the concept of the autism spectrum is employed in Canadian political discourse, with specific interest in the degree to which the articulation of the interests of so-called low- and high-functioning individuals with autism are set in tension with one another. A sample of discourse was obtained by searching the electronic parliamentary archives for the term *autism* in records of debates or committee discussion occurring in the Thirty-Sixth through Fortieth Parliaments, from September 1997 through March 2011. Examination of recent parliaments makes the most sense, as this is the time period during which autism emerged as a relatively high-profile political issue. Sifting archives on the basis of a single term, such as *autism,* is tremendously effective in capturing the range of political discourse when such topics are specific and controversial. For the purposes of this study, only documents available in English were included.

The initial search returned 15,616 documents; limiting this search to documents containing the phrase "autism spectrum" reduced that number to 9,472. Because conversations about autism sometimes separate the two words (for instance, when a speaker just mentions "the spectrum"), the more encompassing document set was the population relevant to the study. In order to limit the sample size to discussion focused more specifically on the autism spectrum, the documents were sorted using the "relevance" feature available on the parliamentary Web site.[3] A sample of 50 unique documents was selected based on appearance on the relevance list.

Once the document sample had been selected, references to the autism spectrum were located and cataloged using Concordance content-analysis software. Frequency of use of the terms in documents was noted in order to gain a (rudimentary) sense of how the concept has been used over time. Type of document and speaker were also recorded for the purposes of gaining a clearer understanding of the context in which the concept was employed. All overt references to the autism spectrum were then examined for emerging themes, and we extracted particularly notable quotations that shed light on the meaning and use of the autism spectrum in Canadian political discourse.

Findings and Discussion

The majority of the sampled documents contained at least one reference to "spectrum." Because the conception of a spectrum can create challenges in implementing targeted policy, we were particularly interested in evidence of manifestations of tensions around the spectrum concept.

For the most part, however, discussion of the spectrum did not exhibit level-of-functioning tensions or arguments. In other words, the spectrum was not used to create or reinforce division within autism-policy stakeholders' discussions (or, for that matter, within the disability-policy subsystem at large). Most frequently these references to the spectrum were descriptive, used to indicate the neurological difference(s) included within the diagnostic category of autism-spectrum disorder. Especially in later sampled documents, "autism spectrum" or the acronym "ASD" was routinely employed instead of simply "autism." Intriguingly, some spoke of autism and autism-spectrum disorders as separate categories. For example, during the proceedings of the Standing Committee on Social Affairs, Science, and Technology on November 2, 2006, it was noted that particular researchers "are two of the world leaders in the field of autism and autism spectrum disorder." Such categorical distinctions were uncommon, however.

One subject brought up occasionally, where there was some suggestion of friction, was the disparity in the provision of services (or the potential for such disparities). For example, during discussion of the Standing Senate Committee on Social Affairs, Science, and Technology on November 9, 2006, it was asserted that "there is a myth out there that children with higher functioning autism or Asperger Syndrome require fewer services because they have better abilities. I deal a lot with children and adolescents with Asperger and they are difficult individuals to deal with." The contention was that services should not be secured or awarded merely on the basis of where individuals with autism fall on the spectrum. Although finite resources will always elicit vying for fair shares, disparity in services is not necessarily an argument aimed (intentionally or not) at creating division. However, additional specific research into service disparity would prove useful to unpack the fuller meanings behind such references.

On the whole, however, next to no evidence of use of the spectrum concept for the purposes of creating divisions among autism-issue stakeholders was found in the Canadian political discourse analyzed. In fact, if anything, emphasis was deliberately placed on the similarities and political issues common across the spectrum. For example, on December 9, 2010, before the Subcommittee on Neurological Disease of the Standing Committee on Health the executive director of Autism Speaks Canada explained:

Despite its heterogeneity, there are commonalities that are faced by Canadian families with a loved one who is on the autism spectrum. There are lengthy wait lists to receive a diagnosis, sometimes up to two years, depending on where you live in Canada—two years, just to get a piece of paper that says your child has autism so that you then have the privilege of sitting on a wait list for even longer for treatment. If you have personal wealth, you could access a privately funded diagnosis, which will cost you between $2,000 and $4,000, depending on where you live in Canada.

Such references echoed concerns particularly prevalent in the early sampled discourse—of disparities and distinction not across the spectrum but across the country. For example, in one of the earlier documents in the sample, a debate of the Senate on June 8, 2006, Senator Trenholme Counsell stated, "Indeed, we can hope that the Prime Minister will call upon premiers to direct the several departments in their governments— health, education, community and social services—to be more proactive, more generous and more inclusive with respect to autism spectrum disorder. . . . We can state that nothing less than equality of services across the land will meet the Canadian ideal." Regional disparities appeared of more concern than the existence of or potential for disparities across the autism spectrum.

Whether this finding demonstrates an absence of division on the national scale or simply a lack of awareness of spectrum-related divisions remains unclear. Substantial discussion surrounding the autism-specific aspects of politics (discussed earlier in this chapter) was found in references to the spectrum. Examination of references in the sampled documents reveals intriguing suggestions of emerging patterns connected to the three aspects of autism policy history discussed earlier in this chapter.

As we have mentioned, concerns and discussions relating to prevalence (and incidence) of autism are generally understood to be the central and driving public concern about autism during the late twentieth and early twenty-first centuries. The sampled Canadian political discourse was thoroughly infused with mentions of increased (perceived) rates of autism in the Canadian and global populations. Discourse surrounding the need to direct efforts toward improved understandings of the range of individuals with autism and their characteristics emerged early and continued throughout the entire sampled discourse. For example, during a debate of the Senate on June 15, 2006, Senator Wilbert Keon claimed that "collectively, we must ensure that all children affected by autism and Autism Spectrum Disorder, as well as their families, have an opportunity to fully participate in Canadian society, but we will only get there when we do enough research to know what we are dealing with. . . . This may require some patience along the way." Knowing the number of individuals with autism was assumed key to "know[ing] what we are dealing with." Importantly, this comment illustrates that autism was approached in predominantly essentialist terms. Essentialist understandings of disability place the responsibility for the difference in human functionality within the individual or his or her family (Baker 2011). More social and public-level concerns in the sampled discourse were typically implicitly limited to the challenges and expenses associated with the construction and provision of public services for individuals with autism and their families.

One of the points frequently (and often forcefully) made in autism discourse referencing the spectrum was the change in diagnostic criteria over time. For example, on November 9, 2006, before the Standing Senate Committee on Social Affairs, Science, and Technology, Karen Cohen, the associate executive director of the Canadian Psychological Association, testified, "We heard about rising incidence and I have heard figures around one in 166 and so on, but generally—please feel free to disagree—that rise is attributed to the much broader definition of autism spectrum disorder rather than only autism: more systematic assessments in the community rather than an actual rise in new cases." As Member of Parliament Lois Brown explained during a House of Commons debate on October 9, 2009, "Canadian and international studies show that autism spectrum disorders are more prevalent than previously believed. . . . However, this should be considered in the context of improved diagnostic techniques, better reporting and a broader definition of autism." In the same debate, Member of Parliament Gerald Keddy made a similar point: "Evidencing Canadian and international studies show that autism spectrum disorders, or ASD, are more common than previously believed. . . . We should remember this in the context of improved diagnostic techniques, better reporting and a broader definition of autism. . . . It is also recognized that adults with autism also have a need for support throughout their life." From the perspective

of autism-related policy and politics, the utility of this assertion can be
relatively difficult to understand unless it is meant to quell the potential panic inspired by the suggestion of an epidemic. After all, from the
perspective of public programs, the challenges surrounding the growth
in incidence or prevalence exist regardless of the cause of the growth in
the population (demand for public programs is, in any case, demand).
However, such discussion can be important from the standpoint of the
(potential) politicization of the spectrum, as one implication of such
statements is that diagnostic criteria have expanded to include individuals who in previous eras would have lived out their lives without becoming the focus of disability policy.

Later documents included some discourse on relative prevalence across
the spectrum. This discussion took place in the context of a larger conversation about creating a national surveillance system designed to gain
a better picture of the population of individuals with autism in Canada.
For example, during a discussion of the Subcommittee on Neurological
Disease of the Standing Committee on Health of the House of Commons
on December 14, 2010, Kim Elmslie, director general for the Center for
Chronic Disease Prevention and Control, explained the need for a surveillance system as follows:

> The lack of complete and reliable epidemiologic data on autism
> spectrum disorders in Canada resulted in the identification of the
> need for a national surveillance system that would be equipped
> to fill information gaps and provide reliable information in three
> areas. First is the prevalence of autism spectrum disorders: how
> common are these disorders, and how do they differ in prevalence
> across the country? Second is to describe the population of children
> with autism spectrum disorders. Third is to understand changes in
> prevalence of these disorders over time.

Developing a comprehensive description of the population of children
with autism-spectrum disorders implies a goal of discerning how individuals with autism are distributed across the spectrum. Though not stated
explicitly in this piece of discourse, the third area mentioned opens the
question of the degree to which the spectrum is being expanded to include individuals not traditionally considered to have a disability (understood as, for example, a major life impairment). It is clear from all these

examples of discourse that the prevalence of autism, with particular focus on the (perceived) expanded incidence, is central in the organization of political discourse on the autism spectrum.

The sampled documents contained relatively little discussion about etiology in references to the autism spectrum. One etiology-related implication for public policy found in the discourse regarded tensions surrounding finding an appropriate policy home for autism-related policy. Significant expansion of the disability-policy subsystem occurred in Canada during the twentieth century, with initial growth seen during the Great Depression, additional momentum in the 1960s, and, finally, a fully emergent rights-based disability-policy focus in public policy in the last decades of the century. However, a strong tendency to connect disability policy to more traditional areas of policy (such as education, social welfare, or health) continues. Making this connection is perceived as being complicated in the case of autism-related policy partly because of fuzzy etiology.

Uncertainty about etiology contributed to difficulties positioning needs related to autism in conventional policy subsystems as well as determining the appropriate level of government for policy leadership and development. For example, as Member of Parliament Dean Del Mastro stated during a House of Commons debate on February 14, 2007, "'This does not mean the federal government has no interest in the issue of autism spectrum disorder. Quite the contrary . . . as demonstrated by the announcement on November 21 of the five new initiatives aimed at laying the foundation for a national strategy on autism spectrum disorder, Canada's new government is clearly committed to helping individuals with autism and their families. . . . However, while autism spectrum disorder and treatments for the disorder are serious concerns, the Canada Health Act is not the appropriate vehicle to address these issues." Many who debated this position sought to characterize autism as a disease. Efforts to articulate autism in this way are found in other societies, including the United States and Great Britain, often through discussion of autism as an epidemic (Jaarsma and Welin 2011; Kras 2009). Although it is not always necessary for the etiology of a disease to be understood before creating policy solutions in the health-policy subsystem, a level of consensus around theories of etiology simplifies health-related policy development.

As a result of this high level of uncertainty with regard to the nature and origin of autism, confining autism-related issues to health policy or even attaining a general agreement that health-policy makers should take the lead in addressing public challenges attributed to autism, such as the funding of treatment and qualifying individuals for public provisions of services, was often presented in the sampled discourse as neither possible nor desirable. For example, during a debate in the Senate later that year (on May 1, 2007), Senator St. Germain argued, "With respect to health, one of the difficulties with autism spectrum disorder is that it covers more than one field. It is not only a question of health. They [children with ASD] go to doctors and clinics, but many things would come under the social service umbrella or even the education umbrella. Also, many costs relate to the fact that many of these young people require one parent to stay at home. It is extremely difficult for both parents to work." Although in this instance it is likely that the spectrum was mentioned purely by way of definition, the existence of a spectrum supports the potential for diversity of policy and (public) program needs, including involvement of more than one of the conventional democratic public subsystems. As the president of Autism Society Canada, Jo-Lynn Fenton, explained to the Standing Senate Committee on Social Affairs, Science, and Technology on November 23, 2006, "Because of the spectrum nature of ASD, a cookie-cutter approach will not meet the needs of our diverse community." The typical policy goal in such discourse is the creation or maintenance of a variety of services for individuals with autism. As Dr. Blake Woodside, chair of the board of the Canadian Psychiatric Association, discussed during the proceedings of the Standing Senate Committee on Social Affairs, Science, and Technology on November 6, 2006, "Because autism spectrum disorders affect individuals so differently it is unlikely that there is one recipe or intervention that will be the magic solution for all affected individuals. . . . As is the case with most clinical care, we need a flexible approach because different people need different services." So, although the etiology of autism was not often referenced in discourse on the autism spectrum, the implications of an indeterminate etiology, such as the difficulty in finding an appropriate policy home and in proposing effective programs and policies, were exhibited in the discourse.

The sampled discourse included discussion about identity and diagnosis. This discussion was almost exclusively related to the goal of figuring out the appropriate target population for programs and services.

Also, discussion about the spectrum was typically used to emphasize the individuality of people with autism rather than as a source of individual, group, or political identity in itself. For example, during the proceedings of the Standing Senate Committee on Social Affairs, Science, and Technology on November 8, 2006, Mary Ann Chambers, minister of Children and Youth Services for the province of Ontario, explained: "Autism spectrum disorders, ASD, range in severity, starting from quite mild, almost indistinguishable. There are lawyers practising in this province who have ASD at the milder end. It goes to the very severe, where kids tear their homes apart and beat up their parents when they are asleep. I have photographs showing where they injure themselves badly. There are also parents who speak about autism from the perspective that these kids simply learn differently. We concluded that no two kids with autism spectrum disorder are alike." This focus on individuality supports the construction of a diversity based understanding of autism-related politics and policy while still stopping short of presenting autism (or disability generally) as a fundamental element of diversity in society or the polis. Put another way, there is evidence of increased recognition of individual neurological differences, and the role autism plays in these differences, but there is not an expression of neurodiversity—a perspective that neurological differences can be understood as a source of communal identity similar to the way differences associated with other politicized identities of race or gender, for example, are viewed (Baker 2011). It is perhaps not surprising to see a lack of neurodiversity in public discourse. Although its roots lie in autism activism, it is a still relatively novel concept that is not widely articulated.

Similarly, during a House of Commons debate on December 7, 2006, Member of Parliament Steven Fletcher said, "While we know that many people with autism are not disabled by the impact of the disorder, but live regular, everyday lives, we also know that autism spectrum disorders can affect people in many very difficult ways, sometimes isolating them as a result of compulsive behaviour and speech disorders that close them off from their families, friends, teachers, neighbours, and society as a whole." Later, Dr. Laurent Mottron articulated a similar sentiment at the December 14, 2010, meeting of the Subcommittee on Neurological Disease of the Standing Committee on Health, saying, "As a doctor-scientist and head of the Centre d'excellence en troubles envahissants du développement at the Université de Montréal, I would like to take five minutes to defend the idea that, in Canada, we are making a mistake right now by offering services based on diagnosis rather than on the level of suffering and on the level of adaptive deficiency." What is markedly clear from this last piece of discourse is that the spectrum as associated with diagnosis revolves around creation of and access to services rather than identity per se.

Particularly intriguing pieces of discourse used discussion of the spectrum to illustrate autism as a noncohesive condition. For example, Member of Parliament Glenn Thibeault explained on November 23, 2009, "The term autism is used quite generally to describe a wide spectrum of symptoms. . . . Since children's severity of symptoms can vary so widely, professionals have been using the term autism spectrum disorder, or ASD, to emphasize this variance." The next day, during a debate in the House of Commons, Gail Wilkinson, of FEAT (Families for Early Autism Treatment), stated, "I want to mention briefly what autism is, just in case anybody has questions. . . . Autism is often called autism spectrum disorder because it actually is a spectrum of symptoms. . . . The current thinking about autism is that it is a disorder in how the brain processes information." There are more precise definitions of autism, including that it is a neurological condition specifically involving sensory, communication, and social differences (Fombonne 2003). However, the point to note here is that Wilkinson's consideration of autism as a collection of different—and possibly disparate—causes for similar symptoms encompasses the possibility of effectively removing the potential for social or political identity rooted in autism if symptoms are in fact found to be similar expressions of fundamentally different neurological differences.

Articulation of a boundary for the diagnosis was also discussed in the sampled documents. For example, during proceedings of the Standing Committee on Social Affairs, Science, and Technology on November 2, 2006, the acting director general of the Intergovernmental Affairs Directorate, Health Canada, made the point that "other developmental disorders that are not within the autism spectrum also pose the same types of difficulties for the children and their families. . . . How do you define where you draw the boundaries?" In the same discussion, she also asked about a target population for a policy: "What about pervasive developmental disorder? It does not fall within that spectrum, but often parents use similar types of treatments. For intensive behavioural intervention, they face the same types of funding challenges as parents of autism, so why look only at autism? Why not broaden it at least to developmental disorders?" A spectrum requires boundaries, which, as suggested in the foregoing discussion, could hinder the development of effective disability policy helpful for the population at large. Spectrums require established definitions of what they encompass and agreed-upon cutoff points. The tension between the inclination toward inclusion, creating the potential for "death by diffusion," and exclusionary components, as expressed in the need for boundaries, can challenge the development of a targeted policy (Murray 2012).

This potential for death by diffusion was especially articulated in later documents. For example, during testimony before the Subcommittee on Neurological Disease of the Standing Committee on Health on December 14, 2010, Dr. Laurent Mottron stated, "There is such a range in the autism spectrum in the DSM-V, which finds that there is a single category, but that there are so many modifiers in the table that providing a single service, specifically the ABA method, based on the diagnosis, makes absolutely no sense." Such discussion is, in part, a reaction to a sustained and organized attempt led by organizations such as FEAT to achieve the basic policy goal of providing applied behavior analysis (ABA) or intensive behavioral intervention (IBI) to all children with autism. Disability-based identity remains frequently misunderstood or unnoticed by both professionals and members of the general population (except possibly for the most famous example of Deaf culture, in which the deaf community has been largely successful in being recognized as a linguistic and cultural minority; Kras 2009; Ladd 2003; Padden and Humphries 2006; Robertson and Ne'eman 2008). Furthermore, many with disabilities were offended by or indifferent to the suggestion of disability-based identity, perceiving in some cases an all-too-convenient excuse for failure to invest in cure-oriented research (see, for example, Mitchell 2007). Nevertheless, some prominent members of the population of adults with autism embrace identities connected publicly or privately to autism (Kras 2009; Baker 2011). Such an identity would be expected to be much easier to embrace for those who have experienced at least some positive results of their differences, such as the ability to turn unique characteristics into gainful employment. The common assumption is that this circumstance is more frequently experienced by individuals understood as being on the so-called higher-functioning end of the autism spectrum.

Finally, the possibility of coming off the spectrum entirely—that is, becoming overtly indistinguishable from neurologically typical peers— was also brought up in the sampled documents. On December 9, 2010, the executive director of Autism Speaks Canada said, "I'd also like to talk about coming off the spectrum: recovery. The word 'cure' even comes up at times. I just want to say that people are writing books about it. Researchers, neurologists, doctors, service providers, and autism organizations are talking about it and acknowledging it." The question of cure constitutes a sticky wicket for both public and personal identity rooted in disability. The need for cure is often articulated in the currency of suffering. For example, on February 9, 2005, Member of Parliament James Moore introduced a petition by saying, "Mr. Speaker, in the second petition that I am pleased to present, the petitioners cite children suffering from autism spectrum disorder as being among the weakest and most vulnerable citizens in Canadian society. . . . The petitioners believe that until a cure is found, children with autism can benefit from the provision of intensive behavioural intervention therapy treatment based on the principles of applied behavioural analysis." Similarly, on November 23, 2005, Member of Parliament Scott Reid described a petition as follows: "In the preamble the petitioners give a lengthy explanation of how early intervention treatment can assist in ensuring that children will not be trapped permanently in this terrible disease, but only if intervention occurs early enough. . . . That requires that the *Canada Health Act* be amended in order that autism spectrum disorder early intervention treatment is covered." As the case *Auton (Guardian ad litem of) v. British Columbia (Attorney General)* (2004), in which the Supreme Court ultimately determined—to many activists' dismay—that ABA-IBI did not qualify for universal funding and that provinces should independently decide whether to fund ABA, made its way up to and awaited a decision from the Supreme Court of Canada, such introductions of petitions became common. The most striking shared characteristics of these petitions were the emphasis on early treatment (which is hardly surprising, given that they were often led by FEAT) and the description of autism as a disease.

Conclusion

The story of self-conscious autism-related politics, particularly with regard to issues relating to neurodiversity, is still in its infancy. This supports the assertion commonly made by activists and in some autism-related scholarship (see, for example, Grinker 2008; and Eyal et al. 2010) that autism-related politics still considers the issue primarily to be a medical one focused on a nebulously defined epidemic. As was pointed out during proceedings of the Standing Committee on Social Affairs, Science, and Technology on November 2, 2006, "We have only recently begun to identify autistic spectrum disorders as a real category of disorders." Although much progress has been made even in the short time since this statement was made with regard to understanding autism as a complex social issue involving a diversity of policy agendas, the implications of the use of spectrum-related language in political discourse surrounding autism will likely become clearer over time because of autism's continued topical relevance in public and political discourse.

As this sample of discourse illustrates, the desire to more fully understand the observed increase in incidence persists. The distribution of incidence across the spectrum, and the related debate as to whether its increase represents a biological change or an expanded social understanding of the human experience, will further underscore the importance of the spectrum concept in autism-related discourse. The sampled discourse also spotlights how the concept of a spectrum relates to the many issues of diagnosis and identity presently being discussed in the disability-policy subsystem and in larger political discourse. The articulation of the need for spectrum boundaries, the strong relationship between diagnosis and access to public services, and the observed tendency in the discourse to emphasize the individuality of people with autism (rather than to emphasize group or political identity) all imply a need for a richer understanding between spectrum-related language and autism policy. As Member of Parliament Jim Maloway pointed out during a House of Commons debate on October 29, 2010, "A number of years ago I think people were simply not aware of the problem [ASD] and tended to ignore it. The recognition that we have to be proactive is coming to the forefront in this country." A key factor affecting this conversation is, of course, that the prolonged and ongoing effort to reintegrate individuals with disabilities into society—typically demonstrated through policies of deinstitutionalization—necessarily includes more complicated and sophisticated policy designs (Eyal et al. 2010).

The finding that political discourse employing the concept of the autism spectrum appears to have been little used to divide or create division is encouraging. There was some reference to the spectrum when discussing disparities in services, but it was unclear whether such discussion is provoking division-of-resources arguments (how the resource pie should be allocated) or arguments for increased all-around resources for autism (how much bigger the resource pie should be). Overall, however, there is little evidence of level-of-functioning arguments being used to create division among autism-issue stakeholders. In spite of this, optimism surrounding this finding should be cautious. It is not clear whether there is an absence of spectrum-related division or whether, given the presence of both different understandings of autism and discomfort with the boundaries of the spectrum in the sampled documents, such division among stakeholders is not sufficiently salient in macro-level Canadian political discourse.

Finally, it is worth noting that the sampled discourse included no overt discussion of neurodiversity. This is not entirely surprising, as a search of the entire parliamentary record of debates and committee discussion for the time period analyzed returned only twenty-three references to neurodiversity. It also highlights the reality that a more inclusive definition of neurodiversity—even given its support of diversity and its increased reflectiveness of individuals' experiences and sense of identity—can nevertheless make securing a rights-based position on the formal government agendas more challenging. The discourse examined in this study suggests that discussion of the spectrum is not connected, in the minds of most people, to discussion of neurodiversity specifically nor, arguably, to issues related to disability as an element of diversity more generally. The concept of a spectrum of conditions or a spectrum of functioning ostensibly has great potential to galvanize a neurodiverse perspective as time goes on, however. As the history of autism policy continues to unfold, watching the articulation of disability diversity—particularly in the context of neurological differences—is likely to be fascinatingly challenging and complex.

NOTES

1. In this chapter, *autism* is used as shorthand to describe all of the autism spectrum, including Asperger Syndrome and pervasive developmental disorder not otherwise specified. This is done only in the interest of brevity and linguistic coherence. The usage is in keeping with the *DSM-IV* (expected to be issued in the fifth edition in 2013) and with the use of the term in both the general academic literature surrounding autism and most organizations focused on autism.

2. Academic discussion of the politics of neurological difference is challenged by differing preferences, meanings, and sensitivities surrounding the language used to identify both individuals and groups (Halmari 2010). The references to the spectrum as a continuum that are made in this chapter refer to how individuals are typically categorized and are not intended as a reliable or necessarily meaningful description of capability or capacity. Furthermore, for the most part, this chapter employs people-first language unless overtly discussing autism (or disability generally) as a deliberately embraced element of political or social identity. Disability-first language is also used as found in the context of cited documents or when referencing social or political movements.

3. A random sampling strategy was also considered. However, because the goal of the study was to examine a specific discourse constituting a rare population in the context of all political discourse taking place in four different parliaments, a purposive sampling strategy was ultimately deemed more appropriate to the study.

REFERENCES

American Psychiatric Association. 1994. *DSM-IV: Diagnostic and Statistical Manual of Mental Disorders.* 4th ed. Arlington, Va.: American Psychiatric Association.

Areheart, B. A. 2008. "When Disability Isn't 'Just Right': The Entrenchment of the Medical Model of Disability and the Goldilocks Dilemma." *Indiana Law Journal* 83 (1): 181–232.

Armstrong, T. 2010. *Neurodiversity: Discovering the Extraordinary Gifts of Autism, ADHD, Dyslexia, and Other Brain Differences.* Cambridge, Mass.: Da Capo Lifelong.

Baker, D. L. 2011. *The Politics of Neurodiversity: Why Public Policy Matters.* Denver, Colo.: Rienner.

Brownlow, C., L. O'Dell, and S. J. Taylor. 2006. "Constructing an Autistic Identity: AS Voices Online." *Mental Retardation* 44 (5): 315–21.

Bumiller, K. 2009. "The Geneticization of Autism: From New Reproductive Technologies to the Conception of Genetic Normalcy." *Signs: Journal of Women and Culture in Society* 34 (4): 875–99.

Burns, B. J., et al. 2004. "Mental Health Need and Access to Mental Health Services by Youths Involved with Child Welfare: A National Survey." *Journal of the American Academy of Child and Adolescent Psychiatry* 43 (8): 960–70.

Bursztyn, A. M., ed. 2007. *The Praeger Handbook of Special Education.* Westport, Conn.: Praeger.

Currenti, S. A. 2010. "Understanding and Determining the Etiology of Autism." *Cellular and Molecular Neurobiology* 30 (2): 161–71.

Eyal, G., et al. 2010. *The Autism Matrix: The Social Origins of the Autism Epidemic.* Cambridge: Polity.

Feinberg, E., and J. Vacca. 2000. "The Drama and Trauma of Creating Policies on Autism." *Focus on Autism and Other Developmental Disabilities* 15 (3): 130–37.

Feinstein, A. 2010. *A History of Autism: Conversations with the Pioneers.* Hoboken, N.J.: Wiley-Blackwell.

Fombonne, E. 2001. "Is There an Autism Epidemic?" *Pediatrics* 107 (2): 411–12.

———. 2003. "The Prevalence of Autism." *Journal of the American Medical Association* 289 (1): 87–89.

Gernsbacher, M. A., et al. 2010. "Three Reasons Not to Believe in an Autism Epidemic." *Current Directions in Psychological Science* 14 (2): 55–58.

Ghaziuddin, M. 2010. "Brief Report: Should the DSM V Drop Asperger Syndrome?" *Journal of Autism and Developmental Disorders* 40 (9): 1146–48.

Grinker, R. R. 2008. *Unstrange Minds: Remapping the World of Autism.* New York: Basic Books.

Hahn, H. D., and T. L. Belt. 2004. "Disability Identity and Attitudes toward Cure in a Sample of Disability Activists." *Journal of Health and Social Behavior* 51 (4): 453–64.

Halmari, H. 2010. "Political Correctness, Euphemism, and Language Change: The Case of 'People First.'" *Journal of Pragmatics* 43 (3): 828–40.

Harris, J. 2001. "One Principle and Three Fallacies of Disability Studies." *Journal of Medical Ethics* 27 (6): 283–87.

Hertz-Picciotto, I., and L. Delwiche. 2009. "The Rise of Autism and the Role of Age at Diagnosis." *Epidemiology* 20 (1): 84–90.

Jaarsma, P., and S. Welin. 2011. "Autism as a Natural Human Variation: Reflections on the Claims of the Neurodiversity Movement." *Health Care Analysis,* February, 1–18.

Kaufman, S. R. 2010. "Regarding the Rise in Autism: Vaccine Safety Doubt, Conditions of Inquiry, and the Shape of Freedom." *Ethos* 38 (1): 8–32.

Kielhofner, G. 2005. "Rethinking Disability and What to Do about It: Disability Studies and Its Implications for Occupational Therapy." *American Journal of Occupational Therapy* 59 (5): 487–96.

King, M., and P. S. Bearman. 2009. "Diagnostic Change and the Increased Prevalence of Autism." *International Journal of Epidemiology* 38 (5): 1224–34.

Kirby, D. 2006. *Evidence of Harm: Mercury in Vaccines and the Autism Epidemic: A Medical Controversy.* New York: St. Martin's.

Kras, J. F. 2009. "The 'Ransom Notes' Affair: When the Neurodiversity Movement Came of Age." *Disability Studies Quarterly* 30 (1).

Ladd, P. 2003. *Understanding Deaf Culture: In Search of Deafhood.* Clevedon, U.K.: Multilingual Matters.

Lanham, R. L. 2006. "Borders and Boundaries: The Ends of Public Administration." *Administrative Theory and Praxis* 28 (4): 602–9.

Liu, K., M. King, and P. S. Bearman. 2010. "Social Influence and the Autism Epidemic." *American Journal of Sociology* 115 (5): 1387–434.

Lord, C., and S. L. Bishop. 2010. "Autism Spectrum Disorders: Diagnosis, Prevalence, and Services for Children and Families." *Social Policy Report* 24 (2): 1–20.

Mitchell, J. 2007. "Neurodiversity: Just Say No." Personal Web site. Accessed April 29, 2013, http://www.jonathans-stories.com/non-fiction/neurodiv.html.

Moloney, P. 2010. "'How Can a Chord Be Weird if It Expresses Your Soul?' Some Critical Reflections on the Diagnosis of Aspergers Syndrome." *Disability and Society* 25 (2): 135–48.

Murray, S. 2012. *Autism.* New York: Routledge.

Offit, P. 2010. *Autism's False Prophets: Bad Science, Risky Medicine, and the Search for a Cure.* New York: Columbia University Press.

Olkin, R., and C. Pledger. 2003. "Can Psychology and Disability Studies Join Hands?" *American Psychologist* 58 (4): 296–304.

Omer, S. B., et al. 2009. "Vaccine Refusal, Mandatory Immunization, and the Risks of Vaccine-Preventable Diseases." *New England Journal of Medicine* 360 (19): 1981–88.

Padden, C. A., and T. L. Humphries. 2006. *Inside Deaf Culture.* Cambridge, Mass.: Harvard University Press.

Robertson, S., and A. Ne'eman. 2008. "Autistic Acceptance, the College Campus, and Technology: Growth of Neurodiversity in Society and Academia." *Disability Studies Quarterly* 28 (4).

Russell, M. 1998. *Beyond Ramps: Disability at the End of the Social Contract.* Monroe, Maine: Common Courage.

Strathearn, L. 2009. "The Elusive Etiology of Autism: Nature or Nurture?" *Frontiers in Behavioral Neuroscience* 3 (11): 1–3.

Van Horn, C. E., D. C. Baumer, and W. T. Gormley. 2001. *Politics and Public Policy.* Washington, D.C.: CQ Press.

Weimar, D., and A. R. Vining. 2010. *Policy Analysis: Concepts and Practices.* 4th ed. New York: Longman.

Wheelan, C., and B. G. Malkiel. 2010. *Naked Economics: Undressing the Dismal Science.* New York: Norton.

Woshinsky, O. 2007. *Explaining Politics: Culture, Institutions, and Political Behavior.* New York: Routledge.

Young, G. 2010. "Trends in Psychological/Psychiatric Injury and Law: Continuing Education, Practice Comments, and Recommendations." *Psychological Injury and the Law* 3 (4): 323–55.

Autism and Social Movements in France

A Comparative Perspective

Brigitte Chamak and Beatrice Bonniau

S ocial movements in the field of health have emerged to challenge health-care access and quality of care, as well as to advocate for broader social change (Brown and Zavestoski 2004). Scholars interested in health-related social movements explore the dynamics that propel actors to mobilize collectively around health issues, and they examine, as well, the links between health-related and other social movements that are organized around cleavages such as race, gender, and class, among others (Barnett and Steuernagel 2007).

This chapter provides a comparative perspective on autism advocacy using insights gleaned from the study of health-related social movements. In the field of autism advocacy and activism, there are deep divisions between parents' groups and autistic persons' organizations (sometimes referred to in the U.S. context as "self-advocates") about how to best represent autism and advocate for autistic people. In addition, these actors clash over views about the fundamental nature of autism. Given these factors, autism advocacy incorporates all of the characteristics of an embodied health movement (EHM), one of the three types of health-related social movements identified by Phil Brown and Stephen Zavestoski (Orsini 2008). EHMs are typically organized around conditions for which scientific agreement on etiology, diagnosis, and treatment has not been reached (Brown and Zavestoski 2004).

Until recently, only parents' associations expressed their grievances and challenged representations of autism, mainly by adopting a biomedical model of autism. These parent-led associations, many of which promote a deficit-model of autism, are assuming an increasingly important role in shaping public policy in the field of autism (Chamak 2008a). Today, however, newly formed associations of autistic individuals are taking parents' associations to task for speaking on their behalf, and are challenging the medical model of autism (Chamak 2008a; Ne'eman 2006; Orsini 2008; Ortega 2009; Silverman 2008; Sinclair 2005).

In recent decades, the medical definition of autism has also changed. The widening of the diagnostic criteria for autism introduced in the early 1990s in the international and American classifications of diseases redefined boundaries between normality and abnormality (Chamak 2008a; Eyal et al. 2010; Grinker 2007; Hacking 2002; Nadesan 2005; Silverman 2008). By including verbal persons in the autism category, the classifications enabled more people to fit the diagnosis of autism.

Autistic self-advocates begin from the premise that autistic adults are able to communicate to others what autism is like from the inside (Dekker 1999). Several published autobiographical and other firsthand accounts by persons with autism-spectrum disorder (ASD) provide valuable insights into both the nature and the subjective experience of autism (Chamak 2008b; Hacking 2007; Murray, this volume; Peeters 2002). People who recognize themselves as autistic have begun to campaign against being labeled as suffering from a mental disease, shifting the discourse from victim blaming to system blaming (Chamak 2008a). The success of these groups' mobilization efforts rests in part on changes brought about in the way their potential members view not only their life situation but also themselves. At the international level, the historical dynamics of this mobilization show that the people concerned refuse the representation of autism as a disease and criticize a society in which autism is understood solely according to a deficit model (Chamak 2008a, 2010; Murray, this volume). The first association of autistic persons, Autism Network International (ANI), set up in 1991 in the United States, defends the idea that autism is neither a disease nor a disability, but a different mode of cognitive functioning.

The neurodiversity concept, which rallies individuals who view autistics as having a different mode of cognitive functioning, was first developed by Judy Singer, an Australian whose mother and daughter have Asperger Syndrome and who is on the spectrum herself. She argued, "The key significance of the 'autistic spectrum' lies in its call for and anticipation of a politics of neurological diversity, or neurodiversity. The 'neurologically different' represent a new addition to the familiar political categories of class/gender/race and will augment the insights of the social model of disability" (1999, 64). In the foreword to the edited collection *Women from Another Planet* (Miller 2003), Singer asserted, "We are the first wave of a new liberation movement, a very late wave, and a big one, just when you thought the storm of identity politics, with its different minorities jockeying for recognition, was surely over. We are part of the ground swell [sic] of what I want to call neurological liberation" (xii). The neurodiversity concept has spread successfully via the Internet, as is illustrated by accounts of autistic persons (Meyerding 1998; Ne'eman 2006; Nelson 2004) and through the development of the Web site neurodiversity.com. The autism-rights movement adopts the neurodiversity concept and encourages both autistic and nonautistic people to accept autism as a variation in functioning rather than a mental disorder to be cured.

The aim of this chapter is to analyze the different forms of activism among autistic persons in a variety of contexts, and especially to explore the particularities of the French case as compared with movement organizing based mainly at the international level. The disability movement and awareness of the significance of gender dynamics in autism are not as developed in France as they are elsewhere (Chamak 2010), and this context influences the form of activism. In a previous work, one of the chapter's authors has identified differences between the international movement and the French one, as the latter does not refer to neurodiversity and rejects the idea of an autistic community (Chamak 2010).

In preparing this chapter, we analyzed firsthand accounts written by autistic persons, including twenty-nine autobiographies (which are indicated in the References list with an asterisk) and twenty-five accounts published in edited collections (such as Sinclair 1992) or posted online (for example, see Dekker 1999; Meyerding 1998; Ne'eman 2006; Shelly 2004; Sinclair 1993, 2005). Discourse produced from Web sites, newsletters, and publications and colloquia from advocacy associations, particularly ANI, ASAN (the Autistic Self-Advocacy Network), and Aspies for Freedom, was also analyzed. For the French case, we focused on Satedi, the only association that exists in France for autistics. Satedi has French, Belgian, and Canadian members. In addition to analysis of the Web site and forum exchanges, fifteen in-depth interviews were conducted with French, Belgian, and Canadian respondents diagnosed as autistic or as having Asperger Syndrome. Unlike the international movement, Satedi does not challenge the medical and deficit models. It does challenge, however, the definition of autism as a mental disease. A comparison of the international autism-rights movement with the French case allows us to demonstrate the heterogeneity of movements for autistic people and illustrates the need to examine how historical and cultural factors influence the ways social movements express their grievances and challenge society and the state.

Autism Advocacy at the International Level: The Emergence of an Autistic Community

By publishing autobiographical books in which they give their personal view of what it is like to be autistic, the American Temple Grandin (and Scariano 1986) and the Australian Donna Williams (1992) took part in the development of an identity politics around autism, allowing other people to recognize themselves in their accounts (Chamak 2008a). Temple Grandin and Donna Williams were the first ones to express themselves through the medium of autobiography and have been followed by other autistic authors including the Swede Gunilla Gerland (1997) and the Americans Liane Holliday Willey (1999) and Edgar Schneider (1999).

The self-advocacy movement developed in the North American context when Jim Sinclair and other autistic persons participated in the Autism Society of America national conference in 1991 and decided to found ANI, an association interested in stimulating autism self-advocacy, autistic peer support, and empowerment. Sinclair, Williams, and Kathy Grant cofounded ANI, which has grown from a small group to an international community (Sinclair 2010). Sinclair has played a leading role in organizing the movement and developing the idea that being autistic means being different and different does not necessarily mean defective: "Being autistic does not mean being inhuman. But it does mean being alien. It means that what is normal for other people is not normal for me, and what is normal for me is not normal for other people. . . . But my personhood is intact. My selfhood is undamaged. I find great value and meaning in my life, and I have no wish to be cured of being myself. If you would help me, don't try to change me to fit your world" (1992, 295). Sinclair's presentation at the International Conference on Autism, a joint conference of the Autism Society of America and the Autism Society of Canada, held in July 1993 in Toronto, directly challenged the "autism as tragedy" narrative and drew a lot of attention to ANI (Sinclair 1993). It led to a dramatic increase of exchanges on the online parents' forum created by the Autism Society of America, the only public forum about autism at that time. Although some people strongly disagreed with Sinclair's presentation, most of the responses were positive (Sinclair 2005). Autistic persons became particularly active on the forum, and parents launched attacks against these interventions. In response to these attacks, ANI decided to create an autistic cyberspace. At that time, there were not yet any public Internet sites such as Yahoo! Groups to host e-mail forums. ANI had to use a Listserv on an academic server. In 1994, ANI launched its own forum, and in 1996 the Autism Network International Listserv (ANI-L) moved to its current home on the Syracuse University server. The influence of ANI increased and blazed a trail for autistic people from other countries to found national movements themselves (Dekker 1999; Shelly 2004; Sinclair 2005).

In previous research, one of the chapter's authors analyzed the historical dynamics of ANI (Chamak 2008a). Findings revealed that its members share certain values and have developed their own terminology, using the names "neurotypical" (NT, or "normie") for a nonautistic person, "aspie" to refer to a person diagnosed with Asperger Syndrome, "autie" to refer to a person diagnosed with autism, and "cousin" to refer to a nonautistic person who has some other significant social and communication differences (Sinclair 2005). Members have their own set phrases and in-jokes, each of which is part of an autistic culture that facilitates the mobilization of a collective identity. Certain testimonies of autistic persons show that this movement enables them to share experiences, to avoid loneliness, and to develop a more positive view of their condition (Lawson 2005; Newport 2001; Schneider 2003). ANI challenges representations of autism by contesting negative cultural representations of autism and celebrates an alternative collective identity based on abilities rather than deficiencies.

Not only does ANI take a leading role in bringing together and representing autistic people, it also structures different social spaces, such as a space for collective learning (in the form of a forum, a newsletter, and conferences). When Sinclair, Williams, and Grant decided that their "mission was to advocate for civil rights and self-determination for all autistic people" (Sinclair 2005), they set boundaries between private autistic connections and exchanges with parents and nonautistic people. Distinguishing "us" from "them," the forum has been subdivided into an "AC" section for messages of interest to autistic people and cousins, and a "Parents' Auxiliary" (PA) section for messages about parenting. Sinclair (2005) explained that the idea of an exclusively "autistic space" was a guiding theme when ANI members decided to create their own autistic conference, in 1996, called Autreat. Most Autreat attendees live in North America, but people also come from Australia, Finland, Israel, Japan, New Zealand, Norway, and other countries (Dekker 1999; Shelly 2004; Sinclair 2005). ANI and Autreat conferences enabled autistic persons from different countries, including Martijn Dekker in the Netherlands and Sola Shelly in Israel, to set up new online communities and associations around the world.

Shelly, one of the founders of the Autistic Community of Israel (ACI), explained at an Autreat meeting in 2004 that she had been formally diagnosed and is also the mother of an autistic adult. In her view, "Autistic culture expresses the special way that autistic people perceive the physical, emotional and social world" (2004). She was surprised to learn that much of the writing about autistic culture was produced by female authors, and she quoted from the book *Women from Another Planet? Our Lives in the Universe of Autism* (2003), an anthology initiated and edited by Jean Kearns Miller. This book focuses on the interplay between the roles of women in society and their characteristics as auties or aspies (Shelly 2004). It provides a framework for advocacy as well as recommendations for the development of positive autistic identities. Building on insights provided by this book, Kristin Bumiller analyzed the broader implications of grassroots autism-rights activism for women and for the feminist movement and showed that gender identity matters for the experience of autism (2008). Girls are much less likely to be diagnosed and to gain access to services, especially if they are not on the severe end of the spectrum (Davidson 2007). Conversely, males with autism are more likely to be stereotyped as violent. Females might receive more encouragement than males to develop the kinds of social skills that render them better able to compensate for the problems that they have. However, being better able to compensate for a problem does not mean one does not have the problem (Dekker 1999). As a group whose identity is based on difficulties conforming to social norms, autistic people are likely targets for social discrimination, and resistance toward this discrimination is essential for participation in society (Bumiller 2008).

At the international level, the autism-rights movement, which includes organizations such as ANI, ASAN, and Aspies for Freedom, has contributed to building a positive collective identity for autistic people and has been pivotal in mobilizing against discrimination ("Autism Rights Movement" 2013). The valuing of genuinely autistic traits and persons comes with certain risks, however, and may be coupled with a devaluation of nonautistic characteristics and individuals. For example, the Institute for the Study of the Neurologically Typical, the satirical Web site created by Muskie, a high-functioning autistic woman, defines "neurotypical syndrome as a neurobiological disorder characterized by preoccupation with social concerns, delusions of superiority, and obsession with conformity" (Muskie 1998–2002). The negative picture of nonautistic people mirrors the more familiar devaluation of autistic people encountered throughout popular culture. At times, the strategy fuels conflict between nonautistic and autistic persons, as well as among autistic persons, because the descriptions of nonautistic persons are caricatured: "Neurotypical individuals often assume that their experience of the world is either the only one, or the only correct one. NTs find it difficult to be alone. NTs are often intolerant of seemingly minor differences in others. When in groups NTs are socially and behaviorally rigid, and frequently insist upon the performance of dysfunctional, destructive, and even impossible rituals as a way of maintaining group identity. NTs find it difficult to communicate directly, and have a much higher incidence of lying as compared to persons on the autistic spectrum" (Muskie 1998–2002).

Analysis of forum exchanges on the Aspies for Freedom Web site (http://www.aspiesforfreedom.com) suggests that certain autistic persons may actually use these negative descriptions, but not in a metaphorical way. Some of them believe quite firmly that as autistic persons, they are genuinely superior to nonautistics. For example, Fistfullo1337 wrote in an Aspies for Freedom forum on April 4, 2007, "I have never suffered from this gift, I cherish it, nourish it, make it so I have solace in knowing that I am biologically superior to NTs, you should do [sic]." In the same forum, Scandy007 wrote on September 2, 2010, "Autistic people and people with Asperger's are a mental evolution of humankind with (possibly) the highest natural intelligence there is." One might interpret these characterizations and excessive generalizations as just as inappropriate as negative depictions of autistic persons.

The Internet has played a crucial role in the emergence of the autistic community by facilitating exchanges and promoting positive self-identification for autistics. As Martijn Dekker explains, the Internet is, for many autistics, what sign language is for deaf people (1999). Dekker set up a mailing-list server on his computer in the Netherlands called Independent Living on the Autistic Spectrum (InLv). In 1997, Dekker traveled to the United States, where he met several autistic persons and concluded that autistic communication appears to occur without much protocol and in a direct way, with less nonverbal communication. Joyce Davidson explored the distinctive styles of autistic communication and referred to the Wittgensteinian concepts of "language games" and "family resemblances": "You might not be able to say exactly what these features are, but you tend to recognize them when you see them" (Wittgenstein 1988, 66). The notion of shared experiential background led Davidson to argue that a place on the spectrum could constitute membership of an autistic "form of life," "a shared background and cultural association among members who tend to respond to and communicate about situations in certain ways rather than others" (2008, 794).

Ari Ne'eman, the president of ASAN, has been active in the autistic culture and disability-rights movements for a number of years. On the ASAN Web site, Ne'eman explains: "Society has developed a tendency to examine things from the point of view of a bell curve. How far away am I from normal? What can I do to fit in better? But what is on the top of the bell curve? The answer is mediocrity. That is the fate of American society if we insist upon pathologizing difference and seek to 'cure' it. The person who is socially isolated because he views the world in a different light may use that difference in perception to invent something revolutionary" (2006). On December 16, 2009, President Barack Obama announced that Ne'eman would be appointed to the National Council of Disability, a federal agency charged with advising Congress and the president on disability-policy issues. In April 2010, he was appointed as a public member to the Interagency Autism Coordinating Committee, a federal advisory committee that coordinates all efforts within the Department of Health and Human Services concerning autism. The fact that a proponent of autistic culture is a member of this committee might be taken to suggest that the highest political authorities in the United States are open to recognizing the existence of an "autistic community."

The French-Speaking Association:
The Notion of a Community Is Rejected

The lone association of autistic persons in France, Satedi, was set up in December 2003, twelve years after ANI. At the outset, Satedi was closely related to Autisme France, a parents' association, and it adopted the claims and positions of that association. Currently, Satedi has distanced itself from the parent association and has acquired more autonomy, but its aims remain different from those encountered in the international context. Whereas the international movement campaigns against the biomedical model of autism, Satedi has accepted the definition of autism as a neurodevelopmental disease. In the French context, the persistence of psychoanalytical interpretations of autism in the professional milieu may influence Satedi's adoption of the neurological hypothesis. The analysis of forum exchanges, Web site content, and interviews with French autistic persons suggests that most Satedi members have internalized the notion of disability and the definition of autism as a dysfunction of the brain. In the forum of the Satedi Web site (http://www.satedi.net) on October 15, 2010, Yoyo wrote, "I know well that it is a disability without curing. There are those who were born deaf or blind, we were born autistic." For Kikuta, "If I had to put a name on my problem, I would have defined it as a dysfunction of the brain" (April 2, 2010); and Gib explained, "My memory is very selective and I do not understand its functioning. All is complicated. It is not easy to have a queer brain" (December 24, 2008).

Satedi's main aims are to help autistic persons and their families and to influence autism research and government autism policy. It explicitly does not associate with the broader international autism-rights movement. The leaders of Satedi reject the notion of community; nor do they refer to the notion of neurodiversity. Exchanges on the forum illustrate the differences between French and Canadian members of Satedi, with the latter referencing the notions of community and neurodiversity and expressing hostility to the notion of disability. In July 2009, when Dorry and Idlem (both pseudonyms), from the Canadian province of Quebec, intervened to promote the neurodiversity concept and refused the definition of autism as a disability, some French participants responded that they preferred the label "disability" rather than the stigma of having a psychiatric disease. The adoption of the notion of disability is also a means to get services and help. In December 1996, autism was officially recognized as a disability by law in France. Changing the status of autism from a psychiatric disease to a disability enabled autistic persons to be granted rights and to receive disability benefits provided by the 1975 disability law (and now by a 2005 law for the equality of rights of disabled persons).

Idlem argued in July 2009 in the Satedi forum, "Autism is not a disability. Autism tends to be viewed as a disease only because people refer to and so help to construct it as a disease." According to Idlem, "The autistic persons are closer to the better way of evolution than the NTs." When Idlem defined autism as a "racial advantage" (August 11, 2009) the president of Satedi, who moderated the forum, intervened and threatened to exclude Idlem from the forum (August 14). The president was hostile to the notion of community. During a presentation at a seminar, "How to Classify/Declassify without Stigmatizing?" (2010), he explained that he viewed the concept of neurodiversity as a product of "folklore." He disagreed with Idlem's idea that autism should be seen as an advantage rather than a disability. Another French member, Samoju, responded to Idlem in August 2009: "If autism is a racial advantage, why do you exchange in a forum for people who describe their difficulties?"

The leaders of Satedi have staked out a moderate position, one that enables them to be taken seriously by professionals, parents, and political authorities, many of whom often consult them about autism. They participated in the elaboration of the Plan Autisme (2008–2010), a government program that aimed to improve services for autistic persons by offering earlier diagnosis, better integration in school for autistic children, and services for autistic adults. The National Ethics Advisory Committee called on Satedi for opinions on ethical issues regarding autism. Two Satedi members were invited to participate in the working group for the elaboration of guidelines for professionals concerning therapies and services for autistic persons. Had Satedi embraced the concept of neurodiversity and the notion of an autistic "community," its autistic members would likely have been excluded from the discussions with professionals, parents, and political authorities. Interviews with parents, professionals, and autistic persons evidence this drastic difference from other countries such as the United States, Australia, and Sweden (Chamak 2005).

Sociocultural and Political Differences

In order to understand the differences between the ideas and claims of the international movement and those of the French movement, it is important to analyze aspects of the historical, political, and sociocultural context in France. The French system is characterized by a partnership between the state and the parent associations and by historical and cultural features, such as the long-standing opposition toward communitarianism (Saunders 2008). The French model contrasts with the American model, in which communities play a crucial role in social organization (Donzelot 2003). With reference to the universalistic ideas of the Enlightenment, French society accords priority to universal rights over communal bonds and particularistic values. The French model favors "universalism," which treats all citizens in the same manner, and rejects "particularism," according to which people are to be treated differently based on the group to which they belong (Etzioni 2004). Proponents argue that disabled persons are better served by a model of universalism than by a civil rights or "minority group" approach (Bickenbach et al. 1999).

The French preference for universalism and its resistance toward cultural diversity inhibits public recognition of groups, minorities, and communities, although not completely. The French Constitution (one nation, one language, one state) proclaims that "France is an indivisible, secular, democratic and social Republic" that "shall guarantee equality before the law of all citizens without distinction according to origin, race, or religion. It shall respect all beliefs." This principle is not always applied, however, because gender, ethnic origin, and disability are often used as grounds for discrimination.

Anticommunitarianism is enforced by state institutions, including the High Council for Integration (Haut conseil à l'intégration), established in 1998, and the High Authority for the Struggle against Discrimination and for Equality (Haute autorité de lutte contre les discriminations et pour l'egalité [HALDE]). The legal setting for this institutional activity is provided by two laws: the 1901 law on associations and the 1905 law on the separation of church and state. The Observatoire du communautarisme was established in August 2003 and has adopted the anticommunitarian goal of defending the republic and the universalism of republican citizenship against the particularism of identities attached to all forms of communitarianism. It opposes long-lasting as well as more recent communitarianist identity campaigns, ranging from Breton regionalism to gender-based community campaigns (Saunders 2008).

Modern-day Anglo-American communitarianism began in the 1970s and 1980s in reaction to John Rawls's book *A Theory of Justice* (1971). Its proponents question the universalistic claims of liberal theory, critique notions of individualism, and advocate the social nature of the self (Sandel 1981; Walzer 1983). Community is closely associated with symbolic boundary construction. In the United States, community can be a symbol for egalitarianism, the quest for a place where every individual is recognized as an equal member of the community. The idea of community is ubiquitous and versatile. It is a potentially powerful idea for crafting diverse political projects (Collins 2009). French anticommunitarianism opposes "a political order that must view individuals first of all through the communitarian prism that is assigned to them" (Saunders 2008, 166).

Unlike in the United States, Canada, or other European countries, in France social movements demanding autonomy for disabled people eschew the language of civil rights (Galli and Ravaud 2000). Civil-society forces rally around the management of specialized structures directed by parent associations. This method of organization enables delegation of public services to the associations managing structures set up for disabled people and constitutes the foundation of the partnership between the state and the associations. In some cases, the institutionalization of the relationships between the state and the associations has taken on personalized forms, with circulation taking place between services of the state and associations. For instance, high-ranking civil servants join the boards of associations, and some administrators of associations become civil servants (Barral 2007).

Recently, the French government labeled autism the "Great National Cause for 2012." This label gave the French parents' associations the benefit of free publicity for campaigns on public TV and radio channels, and enabled them to raise awareness of their demands. They present the situation of autism in France as a scandal (as is illustrated by numerous articles in the French newspapers), criticize the persistence of psychoanalytical frameworks associated with certain French psychiatrists, and highlight the need for access to free behavioral treatments.

However, the parents' associations do not always adopt positions considered satisfactory by those most directly concerned: autistic people. Regarding the differences between the parents' associations and those representing autistic persons, Juanne Clarke and Gudrun van Amerom noted, "Organizations, sometimes called charities, certainly have more power and economic suasion than diagnosed individuals. Their construction of problems clearly represents a more powerful perspective than do the blogs of one or even many individuals. Moreover, in order to exist and to justify their continued existence, charities constantly have to seek financial support by claiming to be helping those in need" (2007, 772).

In their recent book *The Autism Matrix*, Gil Eyal and colleagues argue that the new institutional matrix (community treatment, special education, and early-intervention programs), following the deinstitutionalization of mental retardation, signaled a massive change in the social organization of expertise: "It was pushed forward by challenges to psychiatry from relatively marginal groups—special educators, occupational therapists, behavioural psychologists, activist social scientists identified with the anti-psychiatric movement—and parents" (2010, 4). In the United States, the National Association for Retarded Children played a crucial role, and so did the National Society for Autistic Children—both parents' groups. All of these groups sought to undermine the dominance of the psychiatric profession, which had ignored or belittled their expertise in the past. In the new network of expertise, parents were recognized as credible experts.

At the international level, the aims of the autistic rights movement are very different from those of the parents' associations, because they aim to deconstruct the notion of disability and the deficit model. In their review and critique of models of disability, Jerome Bickenbach and colleagues argue that although disability movements were correct to criticize the medical model for turning a socially constructed disadvantage into a problem with a person's body or mind, they suggest that the extreme position those movements advocate is equally problematic. They conclude that "the politics of disablement will be torn by an internal struggle between two antagonistic political strategies. The first characterizes disabled people as a social minority group who must seek out their basic civil rights and fight against discrimination in order to correct the injustices of the past and the present. The second insists that disablement is a universal human phenomenon that has been systematically ignored with dire and unjust social consequences" (1999, 1178–79).

In France, the autistic rights movement is almost absent, because the cultural influence, especially the hostility to communitarianism, prevails among French autistic persons (Chamak 2010). The deficit model is relatively well accepted, and the distance from the international trend favors relations with the state, parents, and professionals. The radical discourse produced at the international level by some autistic persons, such as Amy Nelson (2004), is badly received in France. If reference to the brain is widespread in France, as in other countries, the notion of an "autistic community" is flatly rejected by political authorities and professionals, as well as autistic persons themselves.

Neurodiversity and the Brain

In November 2004, Amy Nelson, one of the founders of Aspies for Freedom, drafted a proposal that the autistic community be considered a social minority group by the United Nations. From her point of view, this move "could help to end discrimination for those who have this neurological difference." For Kathleen Seidel, who owns and operates the Web site neurodiversity.com, diagnosis is an aid, because "we could make sense out of things that had been inexplicable to us; we felt validated. I encountered the word neurodiversity, and it just sang to me. I thought, 'What a beautiful word that encompasses the reality that God has many different ways to build a brain'" (quoted in Solomon 2008).

Such references to the brain and differences regarding cerebral functioning are widespread in the recent discourse of autistic persons, as well as in society at large. The neurodiversity concept and reference to the brain are used by the autism-rights movement to construct a collective identity redefining autism as a difference and not as a disease. A symposium entitled "Personhood in a Neurobiological Age: Brain, Self, and Society," held in London in 2010, questioned, "To what extent is neuroscience reshaping our understanding of human beings? To what extent are people going to recognize themselves in brain language?" Alain Ehrenberg answered by saying, first, that "neuroscience does not change anything about our concept of person, either descriptive or normative," and second, that "if people are moving towards recognizing themselves in their brain, this will be a social process, not a biological truth that everybody will eventually recognize as a truth based on proof established on an empirical basis coming from the laboratory. This claim means it will be learned: these are not neurobiological facts that are at stake, but their transformations into social and moral references to act in social life. From this perspective, this recognition is a new language game" (2010). Many authors (including Ehrenberg 2004; Ortega 2009; and Vidal 2009) emphasized the present-day diffusion of neuroscientific concepts beyond the laboratory and their penetration in society. Discourse about the brain and its illustration using brain imaging influence the way we talk about ourselves. Researchers in the social sciences and humanities have investigated the role of neurological vocabulary in the elaboration of identities (Ortega, this volume) and have found that the widespread use of brain metaphors and analogies is changing the way people understand their own subjectivities (Hacking 2007). The functioning of the brain is used as an explanation for the functioning of the person, as is illustrated by Jane Meyerding. When she discovered she was autistic, she thought, "It's my brain that doesn't fit" (2003). She describes herself as being "differently brained" (1998). This is the new language adopted by some advocates for autistic persons.

Conclusion

The neurodiversity concept has helped to shape for autistic persons a collective identity, "a perception of a shared status which may be imagined rather than experienced directly" (Polletta and Jasper 2001, 285). Beyond recruitment, identity work is crucial to sustaining solidarity and commitment (Polletta and Jasper 2001). The question of collective identity is central when studying social movements. Indeed, a social-movement process is in place when collective identities that go beyond specific campaigns and initiatives develop. Collective identity is a process that is strongly associated with recognition and the creation of connectedness (Diani and Bison 2004). How is collective identity constructed in the course of mobilization? How are common interests defined? How has an autistic culture developed within such a community? Who is accepted in the group? Who is not? At the international level, an autistic community emerged from a group including those with Asperger Syndrome, autistic persons, and "cousins." Nonautistic people can participate, but decision-making power and organizational leadership rest in the hands of autistic people. ANI is aligned with the disability-rights movement, whereas Satedi is not. The French-speaking association has accepted the notion of disability and the biomedical model. It favored the constitution of a network but not a community, a concept that has a negative connotation for French people. The collective identity of French autistic persons is focused on sharing experiences but not on using the neurodiversity concept. Activists may define their identities in different ways, depending on the strategic situation. In the context of massive contemporary changes, refocusing attention on contested perspectives of community organization sheds light on how people organize themselves and others for diverse political ends.

REFERENCES

Titles preceded by an asterisk are firsthand accounts of autism analyzed by the authors.

"The Autism Rights Movement." 2013. Autism Spectrum Disorders Fact Sheet. Synapse: Reconnecting Lives. Accessed April 30, 2013, http://www.autism-help .org/points-autism-rights-movement.htm.

Barnett, I., and G. Steuernagel. 2007. "U.S. Health Social Movements and Public Policy: Autism and Alzheimer's." Paper presented at the annual meeting of the Midwest Political Science Association, Chicago, Illinois, April 12, 2007.

Barral, C. 2007. "'Disabled Persons' Associations in France." *Scandinavia Journal of Disability Research* 9 (3–4): 214–36.

*Barron, J., and S. Barron. 1992. *There's a Boy in Here*. New York: Simon & Schuster.

Bickenbach, J., et al. 1999. "Models of Disablement, Universalism, and the International Classification of Impairments, Disabilities, and Handicaps." *Social Science and Medicine* 48 (9): 1173–87.

*Bouissac, J. 2002. *Qui j'aurai été . . . Journal d'un adolescent autiste*. Colmar, France: Les Editions d'Alsace.

Brown, P., and S. Zavestoski. 2004. "Social Movements in Health: An Introduction." *Sociology of Health and Illness* 26 (6): 679–94.

Bumiller, K. 2008. "Quirky Citizens: Autism, Gender, and Reimagining Disability." *Signs: Journal of Women in Culture and Society* 33 (4): 967–91.

Chamak, B. 2005. "Les transformations des représentations de l'autisme et de sa prise en charge en France: Le rôle des associations." *Nouveau malaise dans la civilisation: Cahiers de recherche sociologique* 41: 171–92.

———. 2008a. "Autism and Social Movements: French Parents' Associations and International Autistic Individuals' Organisations." *Sociology of Health and Illness* 30 (1): 76–96.

———. 2008b. "What Can We Learn about Autism from Autistic Persons?" *Psychotherapy and Psychosomatics* 77 (5): 271–79.

———. 2010. "Autism, Disability, and Social Movements." *Alter: European Journal of Disability Research* 4 (2): 103–15.

Clarke, J., and G. van Amerom. 2007. "'Surplus Suffering': Differences between

Organizational Understandings of Asperger's Syndrome and Those People Who Claim the 'Disorder.'" *Disability and Society* 22 (7): 761–76.

Collins, P. H. 2009. "The New Politics of Community." *American Sociological Review* 75 (1): 7–30.

Davidson, J. 2007. "'More Labels Than a Jam Jar . . .': The Gendered Dynamics of Diagnosis for Girls and Women with Autism." In *Contesting Illness*, edited by P. Moss and K. Teghtsoonian, 239–58. Toronto, Ont.: University of Toronto Press.

———. 2008. "Autistic Culture Online: Virtual Communication and Cultural Expression on the Spectrum." *Social and Cultural Geography* 9 (7): 791–806.

Dekker, M. 1999. "In Our Own Terms: Emerging Autistic Culture." Paper presented at the National Autistic Society Cyber Conference, "Autism 99," November.

Diani, M., and I. Bison. 2004. "Organizations, Coalitions, and Movements." *Theory and Society* 33 (3–4): 281–309.

Donzelot, J. 2003. *Faire société: La politique de la ville aux Etats-Unis et en France.* Paris: Seuil.

Ehrenberg, A. 2004. "Le sujet cérébral." *Esprit* 309: 130–55.

———. 2010. "Does Neuroscience Change Something in the Concept of Personhood?" Paper presented at the symposium "Personhood in a Neurobiological Age: Brain, Self, and Society," London, September 13, 2010.

Etzioni, A. 2004. *From Empire to Community: A New Approach to International Relations.* New York: Palgrave Macmillan.

Eyal, G., et al. 2010. *The Autism Matrix: The Social Origins of the Autism Epidemic.* Cambridge: Polity.

Galli, C., and J. F. Ravaud. 2000. "L'association vivre debout: Une histoire d'autogestion." In *L'institution du handicap: Le rôle des associations*, edited by C. Barral et al., 325–35. Rennes, France: Presses Universitaires de Rennes.

*Gerland, G. 1997. *A Real Person: Life on the Outside.* London: Souvenir.

*———. 2000. *Finding Out about Asperger Syndrome, High Functioning Autism, and PDD.* London: Kingsley.

*Grandin, T. 1995. *Thinking in Pictures: And Other Reports from My Life with Autism.* New York: Doubleday.

*———. 2005. *Animals in Translation: Using the Mysteries of Autism to Decode Animal Behavior.* New York: Simon & Schuster.

*Grandin, T., and M. M. Scariano. 1986. *Emergence: Labeled Autistic.* Novato, Calif.: Arena.

Grinker, R. R. 2007. *Unstrange Minds: Remapping the World of Autism.* Cambridge, Mass.: Basic Books.

Hacking, I. 2002. *Historical Ontology.* Cambridge, Mass.: Harvard University Press.

———. 2007. "Kinds of People: Moving Targets." *Proceedings of the British Academy* 151: 285–318.

*Lawson, W. 2005. *Life behind Glass. A Personal Account of Autism Spectrum Disorder.* London: Kingsley.

*McKean, T. 2001. *Soon Will Come the Light: A View from Inside the Autism Puzzle.* Arlington, Tex.: Future Horizons.

Meyerding, J. 1998. "Thoughts on Finding Myself Differently Brained." Personal blog. Accessed November 26, 2010, http://www.autreat.com/jane.html.

———. 2003. "AS Paradox: Rational Anger." In Miller, *Women from Another Planet?* 99–101.

*Miller, J. K. 2003. *Women from Another Planet? Our Lives in the Universe of Autism.* Bloomington, Ind.: 1st Books.

*Mukhopadhyay, T. R. 2003. *The Mind Tree: A Miraculous Child Breaks the Silence of Autism.* New York: Arcade.

*Murray, D. 2006. *Coming Out Asperger: Diagnosis, Disclosure, and Self-Confidence.* London: Kingsley.

Muskie. 1998–2002. "What Is NT?" Institute for the Study of the Neurologically Typical. Accessed April 30, 2013, http://isnt.autistics.org.

Nadesan, M. 2005. *Constructing Autism: Unravelling the "Truth" and Understanding the Social.* London: Routledge.

*Nazeer, K. 2006. *Send in the Idiots: Stories from the Other Side of Autism.* New York: Bloomsbury.

Ne'eman, A. 2006. "Difference Is Not a Disease." Autistic Self Advocacy Network. Accessed May 11, 2011, http://nyln.org/Clearinghouse/Documents/Difference%20is%20NOT%20Disease.pdf.

Nelson, A. 2004. "Declaration from the Autism Community That They Are a Minority Group." Personal blog. Accessed May 11, 2011, http://amynelsonblog.blogspot.com/2004/11/declaration-from-autism-community-that.html.

*Newport, J. 2001. *Your Life Is Not a Label: A Guide to Living Fully with Autism and Asperger's Syndrome for Parents, Professionals, and You!* Arlington, Tex.: Future Horizons.

*O'Neill, J. L. 1998. *Through the Eyes of Aliens: A Book about Autistic People.* London: Kingsley.

Orsini, M. 2008. "Political Economies of Hope: Mapping the Contested Terrain of Autism Activism." Paper prepared for the annual meeting of the Canadian Political Science Association, Vancouver, British Columbia, June 4–6.

Ortega, F. 2009. "The Cerebral Subject and the Challenge of Neurodiversity." *Biosocieties* 4 (4): 425–45.

Peeters, T. 2002. "We Teach People with Autism: But What Have I Learned from Them?" *Good Autism Practice* 3 (2): 10–20.

"Personhood in a Neurobiological Age: Brain, Self, and Society." 2010. Symposium. London School of Economics and Political Science, London, September 13. http://www.lse.ac.uk/collections/brainSelfSociety/.

Polletta, F., and J. Jasper. 2001. "Collective Identity and Social Movements." *Annual Review of Sociology* 27: 283–305.

*Prince-Hughes, D. 2002. *Aquamarine Blue: Personal Stories of College Students with Autism.* Athens: Ohio University Press / Swallow Press.

Rawls, J. 1971. *A Theory of Justice.* Cambridge, Mass.: Harvard University Press.

Sandel, M. 1981. *Liberalism and the Limits of Justice.* Cambridge: Cambridge University Press.

Saunders, D. 2008. "Anticommunautarisme and the Government of Religious Difference." *Economy and Society* 37 (2): 151–71.

*Schneider, E. 1999. *Discovering My Autism—Apologia pro vita sua (with Apologies to Cardinal Newman).* London: Kingsley.

*————. 2003. *Living the Good Life with Autism.* London: Kingsley.

*Segar, M. 1997. *Coping: A Survival Guide for People with Asperger Syndrome.* Nottingham, U.K.: Early Years Diagnostic Centre.

Shelly, S. 2004. "Women from Another Planet? Feminism and AC Awareness." Presentation at Autreat conference "Making Connections," June 28–July 4, Pennsylvania. Accessed June 2011, http://www.solashelly.org/Women.pdf.

*Shore, S. 2003. *Beyond the Wall: Personal Experiences with Autism and Asperger Syndrome.* Shawnee Mission, Kans.: Autism Asperger.

Silverman, C. 2008. "Critical Review: Fieldwork on Another Planet: Social Science Perspectives on the Autism Spectrum." *Biosocieties* 3 (3): 325–41.

Sinclair, J. 1992. "Bridging the Gaps: An Inside-Out View of Autism." In *High-Functioning Individuals with Autism,* edited by E. Schopler and G. B. Mesibov, 294–302. New York: Plenum.

————. 1993. "Don't Mourn for Us." *Our Voice* (newsletter of Autism Network International) 1 (3). Accessed May 2011, http://www.autisticrightsmovementuk .org/pages/jimsinclair01.pdf.

————. 2005. "Autism Network International: The Development of a Community and Its Culture." Autism Network International. Accessed July 2010, http:// www.autreat.com/History_of_ANI.html.

————. 2010. "Being Autistic Together." *Disability Studies Quarterly* 30 (1). Accessed May 2010, http://www.dsq-sds.org/article/view/1075/1248.

Singer, J. 1999. "Why Can't You Be Normal for Once in Your Life? From a 'Problem with No Name' to the Emergence of a New Category of Difference." In *Disability Discourse,* edited by M. Corker and S. French, 59–67. Buckingham, U.K.: Open University Press.

Solomon, A. 2008. "The Autism Rights Movement." *New York Magazine,* May 25. Accessed May 2011, http://nymag.com/news/features/47225/.

*Tammet, D. 2006. *Born on a Blue Day: Inside the Extraordinary Mind of an Autistic Savant.* London: Hodder & Stoughton.

*————. 2009. *Embracing the Wide Sky: A Tour across the Horizons of the Mind.* London: Hodder & Stoughton.

Vidal, F. 2009. "Brainhood, Anthropological Figure of Modernity." *History of the Human Sciences* 22 (1): 5–36.

Walzer, M. 1983. *Spheres of Justice: A Defence of Pluralism and Equality.* Oxford: Blackwell.

*Willey, L. H. 1999. *Pretending to Be Normal: Living with Asperger's Syndrome.* London: Kingsley.

*————. 2001. *Asperger Syndrome in the Family: Redefining Normal.* London: Kingsley.

*————. 2003. *Asperger Syndrome in Adolescence: Living with the Ups, the Downs, and Things In Between.* London: Kingsley.

*Williams, D. 1992. *Nobody Nowhere: The Extraordinary Autobiography of an Autistic.* New York: Avon.

*————. 1994. *Somebody Somewhere: Breaking Free from the World of Autism.* New York: Times Books.

*————. 1998. *Autism and Sensing: The Unlost Instinct.* London: Kingsley.

*————. 2004. *Autism: An Inside-Out Approach.* London: Kingsley.

Wittgenstein, L. 1988. *Philosophical Investigations.* Oxford: Blackwell.

PART IV. Cultural Productions and
Representations of Autism

Narrating Autism

Mark Osteen

The rapidly rising tide of autism diagnoses has brought with it a large collection of autism stories. Despite the widely divergent abilities of persons with autism, however, many of these stories are strikingly similar. In this chapter, I outline a set of rules that these stories follow and that have threatened to collapse autism's diversity into a menu of formulas. But these formulas constitute only one aspect of what I call "the narrative problem of autism." A second element lies in the nature of autism itself. Because autistic people often tend to think less linearly than neurotypical folks, and because their habits and preferences may strike neurotypicals as repetitive or inexplicable, nonfiction books by and about autistic people frequently display a tension between the demands of narrative cohesion and the obligation to tell the truth. As a result, most nonfiction autism books maintain a conflicted relationship with narrative, often either lapsing into convention or eschewing narrative cohesion altogether. Perhaps, I suggest, the written word is an unsuitable medium through which to portray autistic lives. Instead, visual media, because of their flexibility in capturing the human experience of time and their capacity to render atypical states of consciousness, offer a more adequate means to narrate autism.

Following the Rules

Before the current flood of autism stories arrived, the best-known depiction of an autistic person was in Barry Levinson's Oscar-winning 1988 film *Rain Man,* in which Dustin Hoffman plays Raymond Babbitt, an autistic adult who has lived for many years in an institution. Hoffman's closely observed performance and Ron Bass's script create an engaging tale. But the film also established a number of stereotypes about autistic people that have hardened into formulas. In one scene, as Raymond prepares to leave a diner with his brother, Charlie, we learn that Raymond has memorized half of a town's phone book in a single night and can instantly count the toothpicks that fall from a jar. These abilities have yielded *Rule #1: The autistic person must be a savant.* This rule has been followed slavishly in most cinematic portrayals of autistic persons, from 1994's *Silent Fall* (featuring a young autistic boy with extraordinary echolalia) to the 2005 film *Mozart and the Whale*; it even marks, to some degree, the otherwise compelling 2010 biopic about Temple Grandin, as well as popular books such as Daniel Tammet's *Born on a Blue Day* (2006). It is likely that only a small percentage of autistic persons exhibit savantlike abilities; but even if, as one recent study suggests, a higher percentage of autistic people possess such extraordinary skills, the main problem here is not inaccuracy. Rather, it is the implication that, as Anthony Baker has noted, autistic people are valuable *only* if they are geniuses (2008, 236; see also Hacking 2010, 642; Happé and Frith 2009, 1346).[1]

In the scene cited from *Rain Man*, Raymond is first "othered" by certain aspects of his condition, such as his rigid insistence that he must have syrup for his waffles; then he is rendered strange in the opposite way—that is, depicted as superhuman—by his savant abilities. But despite his trying moments (such as when Charlie attempts to get him on a plane), Raymond is generally portrayed as endearing and unintentionally funny ("'Course, I'm an excellent driver," he maintains, though he has never taken the wheel). Humor can be an indispensable tool for maintaining one's sanity in life with autism, but portrayals of autistic people as lovable eccentrics do them no favors, because they imply that such people may not need long-term support or therapies. Such depictions barely hint at autism's linguistic problems, behavioral difficulties, and sensory issues. Out of these stories also comes *Rule #2: The autistic must be charmingly quirky but not too severely disabled.*[2]

Raymond's brother is selfish and arrogant and, until late in the film, uses Raymond mostly as a means to obtain what he believes to be his rightful inheritance. We are meant to condemn Charlie for using his brother as a tool. Yet the film does the same thing, for Rain Man is less a character than a device to humanize Charlie. In stories like this one, autistic people chiefly serve as what disability theorists David Mitchell and Sharon Snyder call a "narrative prosthesis": a "crutch on which . . . [to] lean for . . . representational power, disruptive potential, and social critique" (2001, 17). Such autistic persons exist only to reflect the values or growth of the neurotypical characters. This pattern yields *Rule #3: The autistic person must be a catalyst to advance, or a yardstick to measure, the moral progress of nonautistic characters.*[3]

While pretending to bring us close to their autistic characters, these formulaic narratives actually dehumanize them by depicting them as freaks or turning them into instruments for the humanization of others. Instead of exploring autistic agency or presence, they pander to the needs of the majority audience, which, it seems, wants the autistic person to be something or someone else—a savant, a witty oddball, or a tool. Ultimately, then, these stories cater to the hidden desire that, as I suggest further in this chapter, may actually underlie their misrepresentations: that autism and autistic people vanish completely. Thus, in *Rain Man*, Raymond is first made strange, and then humanized, only to be taken back to the institution, where he will become invisible once again.

The explosion of autism books has included several novels narrated by young people who, like Charlie Babbitt, have autistic brothers. All of them follow Rule #3 to a tee. For example, Eli Gottlieb's *The Boy Who Went Away* recounts thirteen-year-old narrator Denny Graubart's final summer with his autistic older brother, Fad, humorously conveying Denny's resentment at being the brother of what he calls an "authentic genetic fuckup" (1997, 142). But what Denny most despises is that his brother is "almost me": that Fad embodies *Denny's* feelings of inadequacy and alienation (2). Fad is the boy who goes away, but in a sense he is never really there except as an instrument to measure Denny's growth. An autistic sibling plays an equally symbolic role in Martha Witt's Southern gothic *Broken as Things Are* (2004), where adolescent female narrator Morgan-Lee develops a quasi-incestuous relationship with her autistic brother, Ginx, who comes to represent perverse sexual desire and family dysfunction. A kind of reverse prosthesis, he stands for a disability that Morgan-Lee must overcome. Marisa Silver's novel *The God of War* (2008) supplies a similar situation. Its teenage protagonist, Ares, truly cares about his autistic brother, Malcolm, and understands him better than anyone else. But Ares is haunted by guilt over an incident, years earlier, in which he dropped Malcolm on his head and thus, he wrongly believes, caused his brother's disability. His need to protect Malcolm eventually precipitates a violent confrontation that leads to Ares's escape and Malcolm's disappearance from his life. Again, the autistic brother exists mostly as his sibling's yardstick and catalyst, rather than as a complex human character; in all three cases, the autistic character ultimately disappears.

Novels about the parents of autistic kids have followed the same rules. For instance, *Daniel Isn't Talking* (2006), by Marti Leimbach (herself the mother of an autistic child), centers on Melanie, whose three-year-old autistic son, Daniel, eventually makes implausibly rapid improvement via a mixture of applied behavioral analysis (ABA) and play therapy. Though Leimbach accurately, and at times touchingly, portrays Daniel's behaviors and Melanie's fears, she tethers this material to a trite, predictable story in which Daniel's progress toward recovery (with the help of a miraculously astute therapist who also becomes Melanie's lover) is merely a crutch with which Melanie limps to a better life. In addition to epitomizing Rule #3, this novel exemplifies a fourth rule, which obtains whenever Rule #1 does not, and which also governs most nonfiction autism narratives: *Rule #4: The autistic person must experience a miraculous cure.* This rule at least makes explicit the subtext hidden in the other rules: autism (and people with autism) must be erased.

Each of these novels is stymied by one aspect of the narrative problem of autism: how to portray autistic persons without lapsing into the conventions I've outlined. None of them, however, is narrated by the autistic person. Two other recent novels present relatively "high-functioning" autistic narrators (that functioning level may be a necessity, given that an entirely nonverbal or intellectually impaired narrator would present seemingly insurmountable challenges to storytelling). Yet the two differ radically in their presentation of autistic selfhood.

Elizabeth Moon's near-future novel *The Speed of Dark* (2003) offers a twist on Rule #4. Protagonist Lou Arrendale works as a computer specialist; though socially awkward, he is a competent fencer and is generally successful and contented. So it is difficult to accept when, given the chance to undergo an operation that would eliminate his autism, Lou agrees to be normalized. His decision invokes the disability-versus-difference controversy that rages in today's autism community: Should autistic people be taught to act like others, or should they embrace their differences as intrinsic elements of their identities?[4] Lou maintains that he is not ashamed of his autistic self but decides to have the operation in order to enhance his personal, professional, and social development. It is disheartening, however, that Lou employs his autistic agency to choose *not* to be autistic; once again, the autistic character exists only to be ultimately erased.

Whereas Lou wants to be someone else, Christopher Boone, the teenage narrator of Mark Haddon's best-selling novel *The Curious Incident of the Dog in the Night-Time* (2003), is quite pleased with himself just as he is. And why not? He is pictorially imaginative, self-aware, and observant enough to be a fairly good detective. Haddon's novel juxtaposes chapters of linear narrative with digressions in which Christopher explains his inner world. Alternately static and dynamic, at once stringently focused and sprawling, the novel successfully depicts Christopher both in neurotypical terms and in his own, autistic terms. Indeed, the novel's greatest triumph is Haddon's rendering of Christopher's mental world via drawings, math problems, maps, lists, and, in one very effective scene, a chaotic barrage of signs that illustrates his disorientation in a noisy train station (170).

Yet Haddon does not really break the rules: Christopher's mathematical gifts mirror Rule #1, his eccentricities conform largely to Rule #2, and he serves partly as a yardstick for his parents' behavior and a catalyst for their emotional problems (Rule #3). But although Christopher discovers unknown abilities, defeats his fears, and passes his A-levels, *Curious Incident* is not a recovery story. Christopher remains autistic, and his development occurs through, not in spite of, his condition. Not only is he still present at novel's end, he is also stronger, more confident, and more assertive. At once disabled and gifted, unusual and typical, definitively himself yet capable of growth, Christopher is one of us. The novel portrays autism as just another way of being human. Moreover, in refusing to wipe out its autistic character, *Curious Incident* succeeds where virtually every other autism novel has failed.

Why are the rules so pervasive? James T. Fisher argues that autism cure stories resemble the Protestant tales of the redeemed self that are deeply embedded in Western consciousness, with religious conversion transposed into recovery from the disorder (Fisher 2008, 51–52). The heroic-parent story (as exemplified in Leimbach's novel) is, further, a variation on what medical sociologist Arthur Frank terms the "restitution narrative," whereby a patient is cured through someone else's expertise (1995, 79). In both genres, the agent of change is an external power, and the patient remains subordinated, passive, or invisible. As Stephen Shore suggests, these stories are versions of the "castle parable," in which neurotypicals rescue the autistic person trapped behind walls by slowly gaining his or her trust and then leading that person out of the castle (2003, ix–x). Such narratives reassure neurotypical people of our "normality," letting us feel good about ourselves for caring, meanwhile reinforcing the ethos of individualism and conversion: "You only have to *want* to overcome a disability and, with hard work, you can do it!"

Purportedly nonfictional narratives of autism are equally subject to these formulas. Thus, one popular autism narrative depicts evil corporations and government institutions colluding with malicious or incompetent doctors to inject children with autism-causing vaccines. Luckily, the story goes, a few heroic parents, such as Jenny McCarthy (most often described as a "former *Playboy* model"), save their children by subjecting them to all manner of dubious treatments, as a prelude to wiping out the autism scourge forever (see McCarthy 2007).[5] Once again, these stories are not really about autism but about people trying to eliminate it. Indeed, the ghost of Bruno Bettelheim lurks behind these narratives, which, like his notorious theory that autism is caused by uncaring mothers, focus not on autistic people but on their parents (1967). Heroism, after all, is but the flip side of demonization.

These tales may seem preferable to older stories of parent-blame, hopelessness, and stigma; but they, too, perpetuate misleading ideas about autism's causes and "cures," presenting it as an unmitigated curse from which parents must rescue their children, thereby adding to the guilt of family members whose autistic loved ones don't recover and diverting attention and resources from other research and services. Because such stories dominate the marketplace, alternate narratives— both those of the majority who don't recover and those of a growing minority of autistic people who object to the idea that they are sick and need to be cured—may go unheard.

Sibling memoirs provide an essential perspective. The best of them show how living with autism requires adjusting one's expectations and one's definitions of normality, and demonstrate how those adjustments enable one to accept oneself and one's sibling as both similar to and different from others. (A recent fine and varied collection of sibling stories is Cumberland and Mills 2011.) Yet even these books struggle to avoid Rules #3 and #4.

A case in point is Karl Taro Greenfeld's bracingly honest and well-written *Boy Alone* (2009), which tells of life with his severely autistic older brother, Noah, who was already the subject of three memoirs by their father.[6] The title refers as much to Karl as to Noah: partly because of his brother, Karl has lived much of his life as a self-exile, struggling with drug abuse and experiencing problems with intimacy. The book implies, indeed, that Karl and Noah are mirror images. But Noah is such a difficult brother that perhaps Karl can be forgiven for perpetrating an authorial trick: for some fifty pages, he portrays Noah as a "high-functioning" adult—a man capable of speaking clearly and even of starting a romance—before jolting us back to reality with a list of Noah's medical interventions and a picture of Noah's actual grim adulthood. One may feel betrayed that Karl couldn't resist presenting a fictional cure story that parallels his own rehabilitation. Yet this alternate-world tale does capture the mixed feelings he holds for the brother about whom he writes: "He remains the center of my life. I hate him for that" (331).

The vast majority of parent memoirs adhere to the four rules, but mostly to Rules #3 and #4. There are far too many to discuss them all here. But that scarcely matters, for most of them are alike: recovery stories touting a specific therapy or therapies. In this vein are Catherine Maurice's *Let Me Hear Your Voice* (1993), featuring ABA/Lovaas therapy; Annabel Stehli's *The Sound of a Miracle* (1991), auditory training; Jenny McCarthy's *Louder Than Words* (2007), diet and heavy-metal detoxification; and Russell Martin's *Out of Silence* (1994), facilitated communication. *How I Saved My Child from Autism and Became a Better Person* could be their one-size-fits-all title. Such books also seem designed to absolve the parent by singling out a scapegoat. Well-intended though they are, they fuel the misconception of autism-spectrum disorders as a set of temporary problems that can be remedied by undaunted parents who discover a magic bullet. In these narratives, Rules #3 and #4 converge in an unhealthy marriage of myths.

Even some of the better recent accounts of life with an autistic child fall prey to the tyranny of the recovery story. For example, Dan E. Burns's 2009 memoir *Saving Ben* movingly describes his pursuit of appropriate therapies for his severely autistic son Ben (meanwhile, Dan comes out as gay and copes with a mentally ill ex-wife; he pushes a lot of hot buttons!). Other parents of autistic children will surely empathize with his vividly portrayed frustration, anger, elation, and fear; yet even these parents may raise eyebrows at his readiness to try anything under the sun, no matter how implausible, and at his belief that only *he* can save Ben. Though his love for Ben is palpable, the book presents recovery as the be-all and end-all of their relationship. It is less about Ben than about Dan and, even at the end, when we learn that the young adult Ben remains significantly disabled, his father is still trying to save him (154). Having shaped his material to fit Rule #4, he has nothing left to say when Ben remains in his "castle."

Stasis or Chaos

Other nonfiction books reveal that the narrative problem of autism transcends questions of formula by exposing challenges peculiar to autism. First, because of the notorious autistic love of routine, family members may feel that they live in the movie *Groundhog Day* (1993), in which every day is like every other day. How do you craft a tale about events or people that never change? In other cases, autism strikes family members as a series of constant, inexplicable explosions of chaos that produce a life of perpetual interruption. How does one forge a cohesive narrative about continual disruption? As Irene Rose notes, the need for narrative cohesiveness conflicts with the narrative content (2008, 45). As soon as chaos or interruption is given narrative order, it ceases to be chaos or interruption. Autism thus seems uniquely resistant to narrative, and tensions between narrative order and disruption—whether figured as relentless repetition or as outbreaks of chaos—characterize virtually all nonfiction autism stories, particularly parent memoirs. As I discovered while writing my own memoir (Osteen 2010), autism seems uniquely resistant to narrative.

A handful of parent memoirs have dared to break Rule #4. Each author seeks a method—be it denial, indignation, or stoic acceptance—to deal with his or her initial grief, rage, and guilt. Each one also seeks a path between the feeling that autism is a terrible demon and the more elusive sense that it may also be a gift. Most important for my purposes here, they all grapple with the conflict between autism as it is lived and autism as it can be narrated, by seeking a strategy to depict stasis or disruption. Because I have discussed three such books in my introduction to *Autism and Representation* (Osteen 2008, 20–22), I'll merely sketch my analysis here.

Robert Hughes's *Running with Walker* (2003) candidly recounts his son Walker's difficult behaviors and his own depression, anger, and feelings of inadequacy. Though Hughes describes Walker as "low-functioning" (15), he successfully portrays the joie de vivre that renders Walker a fascinating character and lovable son and brother. The book nicely balances the highlights and lowlights of life with autism, but it remains a series of episodes, its rhythm as uneven as Walker's characteristic pace.

Kate Rankin's *Growing Up Severely Autistic: They Call Me Gabriel* (2000) displays a similar problem. Rankin's understated style reflects the truth that her son Gabriel's eccentricities require no rhetorical flourishes, for he may be the most seriously impaired child yet depicted in a parent memoir: at age seventeen he is not toilet-trained, doesn't speak, engages in no typical play, possesses no social or academic skills, climbs compulsively, runs away, and destroys furniture. But though Rankin's son is unforgettable, the book never gains narrative momentum, just as Gabriel never changes. He resists treatment both clinically and narratively.

Charlotte Moore portrays the challenges of living with *two* autistic sons in *George and Sam* (2004). Rather than extolling a specific therapy, she sensibly notes that the audio integration therapy that benefited George had no effect on Sam, and that dietary interventions that did nothing for George helped Sam immensely. Humorous and down-to-earth, Moore's book isn't a story but a set of essays on issues such as education, food, imagination, and diagnostics. Unfortunately, her attempt to reach a wide audience also leads to the troubling conclusion that autistic people's most valuable quality is to "provide a yardstick for neurotypical moral behavior" (222). Even in Moore's savvy and generally enlightened book, Rule #3 rears its head.

Two other recent parent memoirs deliberately eschew the desire to tell a book-length story, yet each one sacrifices something important in the process. In *The Only Boy in the World* (2006), Michael Blastland, rather than relating a tale of recovery, thoughtfully explores theory of mind, obsessions, sensory issues, and social interactions and raises intriguing, if unresolvable, questions about our definitions of the human.[7] In often sparkling prose, Blastland details pivotal episodes in his life with his son, Joe—the boy's suddenly blocking access to a water slide; his being hit by a car (miraculously avoiding injury); his striking a crying baby—and provides a brilliantly apt oxymoron for his feelings after such incidents: "seething pity" (166). Blastland explicitly addresses the problems with Rule #3 yet also adheres to it, asserting near the end of the book that "one of the greatest aids to self-understanding is the differences in others who give us something to compare": his own self-understanding, not Joe's (194–95). Blastland also transforms the theory-of-mind deficit from a tendency into a monolithic Truth, declaring that Joe has no conception of others' thoughts and intentions, and representing his son's world as an alien domain of arbitrary actions performed by mysterious beings. But time and again (it's not clear whether this is intentional), Blastland reveals the limitations of *his own* theory of mind. For example, after contending that Joe cannot recognize his own emotions, he recalls his son telling him that he was "pee," that is, happy (122). Tenaciously adhering to his theory despite evidence to the contrary and sacrificing narrative connection for local coherence, Blastland proves that Joe is his father's son. Indeed, he does not solve the narrative problems of autism so much as exemplify them.

In *Weather Reports from the Autism Front* (2008), James C. Wilson writes about his adult son, Sam, while insightfully considering key issues such as cure, self-injury, socializing, and medications. Though working primarily from a neurodiversity standpoint—for example, recognizing that self-injurious behaviors are a form of "embodied language" and acknowledging the validity of many autistic bloggers' resistance to medication—Wilson also remains skeptical about certain emerging neurodiversity dogmas (73). It's not hard to see why: Sam, an intelligent man with well-developed interests and even some friends, nonetheless bangs his head, occasionally hits others, and displays disabling rigidities. As his father writes, "Sometimes . . . the decision to medicate is not a matter of choice," and "when your autistic child begins banging his head on the wall, neurodiversity theory doesn't provide much comfort" (154, 23–24). Nor does Sam's father try to solve the narrative problem of autism: rather than a cohesive story, the book is presented a series of "reports" whose repetitiveness sometimes mirrors Sam's perseverations.

Despite their flaws, these memoirs prove that a once-invisible segment—the more severely impaired autistic people who do not "recover" and whose stories don't make neurotypical readers feel warm and fuzzy—has emerged. Yet they also expose the problem: no cure, no story. Having abandoned the recovery narrative, they grope for a central thread, thereby embodying the difficulties of narrating autism.

One extraordinary sibling memoir, however, illustrates a possible solution. Paul Karasik and Judy Karasik's *The Ride Together* (2003) juxtaposes Paul's graphic vignettes with his sister Judy's more conventional account to create a moving portrait of life with their autistic brother David in the 1950s and 1960s. Paul's comic strips trenchantly illustrate the world according to David, who habitually reenacts entire memorized television shows, most notably *Superman*. Paul also beautifully demonstrates how he learned to respect David's echolalia and eruptions. At a Three Stooges film festival, Paul is initially mortified by David's shouts of "Moe, Larry, cheese!" Then the Stooges' world spills into the theater, causing a pie fight and general mayhem. Back in "reality," David walks out, but his departure provides an opportunity for Paul to flirt with a pretty theater worker. The vignette ends with the brothers gleefully shouting in unison, "Moe, Larry, Cheese!!" (125–31). Through such incidents, Paul learns to accept his brother as a kind of Lord of Misrule, a "hole blown through ordinary behavior," as Judy puts it (139). Rarely has the radiant chaos of life with autism been better captured.

Judy more quietly dramatizes her efforts to understand David. When an investigation reveals that David has been abused in a residential placement, Judy agonizingly reassesses her responsibilities. But after their ride together from his new facility, David asks about the upcoming holidays and gives her a kiss. Only later does she realize that while she thought she was reassuring David, he was actually reassuring *her*, telling her not to feel guilty about leaving him. That night she watches *Rain Man* as David sleeps beside her. The film that once moved her now leaves her cold: "I couldn't be with the movie . . . that I had used to make a neat package out of David, and be with David at the same time" (151). Like the Stooges, David breaks out of the box into which others place him. He refuses to disappear.

The Karasiks show that their brother is not just a disorder or a patient but a complex, creative human being who can't be fully captured by the label of "autism." They appreciate David not as a yardstick for their own growth but as a mix of abilities and disabilities like other humans. And like Wilson, though not explicitly, the Karasiks suggest that autism is not an individual disorder but a family condition that responds to and generates interpersonal dynamics not so different from those in ordinary families (Wilson 2008, 185). (This is also a major theme in the movie *The Sandwich Kid*, which I discuss later in the chapter.) Each story, indeed, illustrates how other family members "become autistic" and are forced to learn empathy—the ability to perceive the world as another sees it—in order to inhabit the worlds their autistic loved ones create. Most importantly for my purposes here, the Karasiks' book's mixed media brilliantly portray both chaos and stasis while permitting the authors to produce and stick to a narrative line.

Local Coherence

Several essays in *Autism and Representation* offer novel ways of reframing autism's relation to narrative consciousness and imagination. Each one highlights the notion of "local coherence." Bruce Mills, for example, explicates Ralph Waldo Emerson's and Samuel Taylor Coleridge's analyses of the unifying ("esemplastic") power of the imagination and demonstrates how these ideas inform contemporary clinical accounts of autistic deficits in theory of mind and central coherence. But rather than viewing these traits as impairments, Mills proposes, we may find in the work of autistic creators Jessy Park and Temple Grandin an art of local coherence that displays an imagination "defined by close attention to mechanical or physical patterns not psychological or social rules" (2008, 126). Attention to local coherence, he concludes, enables us to expand our definition of creativity and to nurture a richer idea of human possibility.

Matthew K. Belmonte similarly argues that the theory of mind and executive dysfunctions often named as core impairments in autism may be more accurately viewed as disruptions of narrative organization—a penchant to perceive the world in parts rather than as a connected whole. Threatened by the chaos this perceptual style generates, autistic people must work harder to construct a theory of reality than do neurotypical persons. But humans have always employed narrative as a defense against chaos. Viewed in this light, Belmonte concludes, autistic people are prototypes for a universal human struggle to craft narrative meaning from the menacing surround: they are human, but more so (2008, 166–79).

What about autistic people themselves? How do they narrate their lives? Given Belmonte's conclusions, one would expect narrative to present an insurmountable problem for autistic authors. One might even assume that anybody who can write her or his life has, by definition, recovered. Autistic authors thus encounter a dilemma: how to represent their lives as both autistic *and* akin to those of other humans. Complicating this problem is the fact that, as G. Thomas Couser points out (and as

I myself experienced as I sought publication for my memoir), publishers generally consider disability to be "depressing" unless it is harnessed to a tale of triumph or cure (Couser 2000, 308).[8] Not surprisingly, then, many autistics' autobiographies follow Rules #1 and #4. Yet they also display a creativity that is genuinely autistic: locally, rather than glob ally, coherent.

The first two such books, Temple Grandin and Margaret Scariano's *Emergence: Labeled Autistic* (1986) and Donna Williams's *Nobody Nowhere* (1992), exemplify these patterns. Grandin's story is framed by Bernard Rimland's foreword, stating that she has "recovered," earned a PhD in animal science, and now travels the world lecturing on autism (1986, 5, 7). She would appear to be a living embodiment of Rules #1 and #4. The book itself, however, is more ambiguous. For example, Grandin's obsessive reiteration of images of doors and tunnels (rendered vividly in the recent biopic about her [*Temple Grandin* 2010]) indicates a mind wedded to repetition. And though Grandin recognizes that her autism has caused her great difficulties, she also suggests that her obsession with cattle chutes enabled her to construct a psychic or developmental tunnel through which to enter the neurotypical world. In other words, autism helped her generate the tropes and objects that permitted her "emergence" from it. In fact, Grandin's narrative suggests that she didn't emerge from autism so much as *merge with* it, crafting a self from within autism that let her keep one foot on each side of the threshold. Her autism cannot be separated from her creativity.

Like Grandin's book, Donna Williams's *Nobody Nowhere* contains a preface that praises Williams's "transition from autism to near-normalcy" (Rimland 1992, ix). Yet her own voice and viewpoint—blunt, headlong, self-obsessed but unreflective—clearly bespeak an *autistic* consciousness that rarely generalizes or condenses, shows little interest in others, and possesses a weak grasp of narrative connection or global coherence. Whereas Grandin is obsessed with doors, Williams uses repeated images of mirrors and shadows, as young Donna repeatedly attaches herself to and imitates particular friends while hiding behind two imaginary alter egos—soft-hearted, sunny Carol and prickly, controlling Willie— each embodying shards of her "fractured" identity (1992, 56, 209, 95, 102). Donna emerges only when she incorporates her alternate selves. Yet throughout her episodic story, Williams sustains one theme: the desire to integrate her intensely private world with that of others. Like *Emergence*, then, *Nobody Nowhere* tells two stories at once: a narrative of normalization and a counternarrative of creativity emerging from within autism.

In some respects, Grandin's and Williams's self-portraits resemble classic bildungsroman protagonists, who battle oppressive authorities and endure degrading love affairs yet borrow from positive role models to synthesize a coherent identity and discover a vocation, which is manifest by their authorship of the books we are reading.[9] But shaping an identity is far more difficult for these autistic authors, because their perceptions arrive in bits and pieces. Thus, they resort to strategies of bricolage— echolalia, imitation, fixations, alter egos—to construct a self by assembling spare parts (Grandin's second autobiography thus also describes itself as a set of "reports" [1995]). As Belmonte suggests, these autistics, like David Karasik, anchor themselves in the chaotic sea of sensation by battening upon stray flotsam. Perhaps autistic creativity and identity are paradoxically synthesized through an arduous process of self-effacement (as is also indicated by the many interpolated texts in *Emergence*), yielding an emergence that is also submergence. The authors don't exactly disappear; instead, they exist on two planes simultaneously—both the autistic and the neurotypical. The books, therefore, send mixed signals to autistic readers: we are autistic and have written books, so you can too— but only if the story is framed as a recovery or emergence tale. The inner narrative of consolidation may be lost within the formulaic framework.

How does one render an autistic consciousness when the demands of narrative seem to violate its essence? Kamran Nazeer's *Send in the Idiots* (2006) embodies another possible answer: tell not one story but several, and in each one present the author as both reporter and subject. Nazeer tracks the lives of four former classmates (who, like him, were diagnosed with autism as children), inserting digressions about conversation, sociability, and autistic consciousness, to achieve an unorthodox but effective blend of narrative and interpretation, empathetic involvement and authorial distance. This hybrid strategy lets him resist the recovery narrative; moreover, through investigating and inhabiting the lives of other autistic adults, he discovers his own hybrid adult identity, one that is sometimes autistic, sometimes neurotypical. Rather than reifying autism, Nazeer proves that it can be many different things and that an autistic person may be just as contradictory as any other human.

The fact that these authors have written at all is crucial, not just because they can serve as models for other aspiring autistic authors but also because the process of writing their lives has helped them to *compose* those lives—to transform their authorial selves into gateways through which neurotypical readers may pass to reconsider conventional notions of selfhood and agency and thus become their empathetic collaborators. The books serve both as doors into the room of autistic consciousness and as mirrors in which to see our neurotypical selves *as* them. As such, they typify the universal human struggle to create coherence from the blooming, buzzing confusion of unfiltered reality. They are human, but more so.

They Don't Count Toothpicks

To some degree, the narrative problems I have outlined lie in the nature of writing itself. Although twentieth- and twenty-first-century authors have pushed the limits of chronology and linear storytelling, writing seems inevitably harnessed to a linear mode of consumption: even when we jump around while reading (as new technologies encourage us to do), we ultimately must read one word after another. Such a medium may not fit autistic people, who tend to think, as the books by Haddon, Grandin, and Williams demonstrate, in focused bursts of concentration or, as the title of Grandin's second book states, "in pictures" rather than in words (1995). Hence, visual media such as comics and the cinema may be more suitable than writing for capturing autism accurately and authentically. Indeed, although narrative, for a century now, has been the primary mode in which movies are presented, that wasn't always the case. As Tom Gunning, among others, has demonstrated, very early movies were often more about spectacle than story; as part of what he calls a "cinema of attractions," they prided themselves chiefly on the "ability to *show* something," particularly the "magical possibilities of the cinema" (1990, 57, 58). They offered a "rhetoric of display for the viewer rather than fashioning a process of narration" (Gunning 2006, 35). Such a rhetoric of display might merely represent autistic people as freaks; but an innovative filmmaker might employ the "magical possibilities of cinema" to render autistic consciousness visually. One can imagine a filmmaker doing so through devices such as jump cuts, flashbacks, dissolves (that is, the superimposition of images), montage sequences, and freeze frames; by breaking the fourth wall, as Paul Karasik does in his graphic panels; or by way of sonic or visual manipulations (amplification or color saturation and the like), double exposures (as in the Temple Grandin biopic), and so forth. Liberated from the need to tell a linear story, a cinema of autistic attractions might emancipate autism from the fetters of verbal narration.

Unfortunately, most mainstream fiction films "about" autism have used rhetorics of display mostly to invite audiences to regard autistic persons as freakish "attractions." Few have even tried to represent autistic consciousness through imaginative cinematic techniques, and most have ended up resorting to the rules I have outlined. Indeed, as Anthony Baker (2008) and Stuart Murray (2008) have shown, fiction films purportedly about autism seldom are: they rarely grant autistic people agency or full humanity. The hazards for nonfiction films are slightly different. One peril is exemplified by Keri Bowers's *The Sandwich Kid* (2007), which uses interviews to train the spotlight on the siblings of people with intellectual disabilities. The siblings' candid responses furnish invaluable perspectives on life as a "sandwich kid" (one caught in the middle), but the interview format eventually becomes repetitive. Untethered from a narrative anchor, the film drifts, prompting Bowers to insert herself and lecture us about what we're supposed to be learning. She ultimately blocks our view of her autistic subjects.

A few of cinema's spectacular visual devices are employed imaginatively, however, in *George* (2000), a documentary directed by Henry Corra and Grahame Weinbren, with help from the title character, Corra's then-twelve-year-old autistic son (the film was shot mostly in 1995). Eschewing narrative in favor of associative connections, *George* splices together interviews with friends and family and George's experiments with his new camcorder. In one sequence, cellist Tom Cora (he spells his name differently than his brother), George's uncle, compares George's thinking to musical improvisation, and the film is indeed structured as a kind of free-form jazz composition. Henry Corra also allows his son to assist in making the film. We witness George determining which questions to ask interviewees, and we watch him at the editing console, giggling in delight as he creates jump cuts so that interviewees repeat gestures and phrases—for example, a classmate's self-description as a "psycho idiot"—again and again. The filmmakers also employ freeze frames and still photographs to portray George's peculiar temporal sense. Perhaps most important, in presenting George's obsessions with airplanes, geography, and meteorology nonlinearly, the film combines repetition with disruption in a fashion that captures the boy's view of the world. In some respects, the film is about its own creation—both by Henry (as in an early scene in which Henry learns that HBO no longer wants to broadcast the film because George "isn't autistic enough") and by George. But it is most of all about the making of George himself as at once a subject (through interviewees' statements about him and through the camera's eye) and an auteur. In creating and viewing the film, Henry, George, and viewers *compose* George's identity. Like Grandin's and Williams's autobiographies, then, *George* reflects an authentically autistic local coherence through strategies of bricolage and self-reflexivity. If George's self-presentation remains mediated by neurotypical adults, the film nevertheless shows that visual and multisensory media hold great promise as means of transforming the narrative problem of autism into an advantage. However, we still await the emergence of a mature autistic filmmaker talented enough to fully control the reins of representation and narrate autism from the inside.

Until that time, a couple of recent nonfiction autism films by neurotypical filmmakers exemplify other successful ways to negotiate the narrative problems of autism. Although neither of these films is particularly innovative in its visual style, and though both gesture toward narrative formulas, they ultimately subvert them, sacrificing the global coherence of a single narrative thread for the local coherence of illuminating individual moments. Lizzie Gottlieb's documentary *Today's Man* (2006) introduces us to her twenty-something Asperger brother Nicky, as he seeks independence from his parents and tries to keep a job. Articulate, possessed of a phenomenal memory (though the film breaks Rule #1 by not emphasizing Nicky's savantlike skills), and understanding his condition quite well, Nicky is also socially inept and rigid, insisting on watching his favorite television shows (he loves *Mister Rogers' Neighborhood* and the afternoon soaps) every day without fail. At his first job, he tells his supervisor that the many African Americans in his workplace make him believe he is in Harlem instead of on Wall Street. Clueless about racial sensitivities, Nicky does not grasp why this remark might offend; he loses the job when he departs midday to watch his beloved TV programs. Before long, he obtains another position as a receptionist at a theater company. The job suits his genial personality and meticulous organizational abilities, and he briefly thrives. But soon Nicky, unaware of social proprieties most people would instinctively grasp, receives a reprimand for opening a coworker's mail. And when customers call to cancel tickets for a show that is receiving poor reviews, Nicky blithely concurs with them that the show is awful. He is fired the next day. *Today's Man* reminds us that the line between "high-functioning" and "low-functioning" is blurry: though smart and charming, Nicky seems destined to reside in his parents' apartment for the foreseeable future. He eventually finds companionship in an Asperger support group, but there's no recovery in the offing and there are no spectacular scenes; instead, we witness a struggling young adult who happens to be autistic.

Autism: The Musical (2007) traces the attempt by Elaine Hall, the mother of a nonverbal autistic boy, to stage a musical in which the roles will be played by autistic children. Each child—Lexi, a talented singer with severe echolalia; Henry, obsessed with dinosaurs; Adam, who experiences violent tantrums; Wyatt, terrified of bullies and unable to make friends—is briefly spotlighted, and each child's parents recount the toll that autism has taken on their lives and marriages. At first the film seems merely to mobilize yet another tired formula—the hoary "let's put on a show" device—with the promise of a trumped-up, triumphant conclusion (the title of Hall's enterprise, *The Miracle Project*, underlines that expectation). But the musical is less a setup for a climactic conclusion than a vehicle to dramatize the small gains each child makes along the way. We never see the full show, nor do the children magically overcome their disorders: at the premiere, some forget their lines, and others can't remember where to stand, sing off-key, or stim. Also, as the film proceeds, we grasp how tedious Henry's dinosaur lectures become, share Lexi's frustration over her inability to form original sentences, and witness how parents such as Rosanne, Adam's angry mother, refract their children's traits. Yet we embrace the children because of their differences and come to appreciate and celebrate the less showy victories each one achieves. Most of all, we understand that they are, in many respects, just ordinary kids.

Both films invoke narrative conventions—a young man overcomes adversity to find a job; a group of children put aside their problems to stage a hit show—only to overturn them. Sacrificing catharsis or cure, these documentaries truthfully render the trials and small triumphs of living with autism. But are they satisfying? That is, do they provide a sense of narrative completion? Or does the presumption that stories must have closure merely reflect narrow neurotypical thinking? Actually, the strength of both films lies less in their main stories than in the mininarratives—Nicky's parents' struggle to help him gain independence, the autistic kids' budding friendships—that epitomize local coherence. Rather than following only the longest thread, these films also pluck out smaller strands, explore them, and find them meaningful in themselves.

There is even hope for more authentic fictional films about autistic families. Such hope is sparked by movies such as the 2008 Australian picture *The Black Balloon,* which concerns teenage Thomas Mollison (Rhys Wakefield) and his autistic older brother, Charlie (Luke Ford). To some degree, this film conforms to Rule #3. For example, Thomas often mirrors his brother: both fall in love with Thomas's classmate, Jackie (Gemma Ward), and several scenes imply that Charlie symbolically embodies Thomas's awkwardness and feelings of alienation. Charlie also serves as a catalyst when, escaping from the house and dashing down the street in his underwear, he darts into a nearby house to urinate—leaving his cap in the house and thus triggering Thomas's romance with Jackie, who resides there. Charlie also provides the couple with an occasion for intimacy as the three kids find shelter together during a thunderstorm. As Charlie catches rain in his cap, Jackie and Thomas share their grief—Jackie's about her mother, Thomas's about Charlie, who, he believes, perceives the world as if through "black fuzz."

But the film (directed by Elissa Down, herself the sister of an autistic man) breaks the other three rules. Indeed, although Charlie remains quite severely impaired to the end, the film offers plenty of indications that he knows exactly what is going on, deliberately teases Thomas, and pushes him to acknowledge his own "disabilities." Charlie's agency surfaces, along with the film's forceful violations of Rule #2, in a handful of hard-hitting scenes that also portray the challenges of living with autism. In one of them, Thomas locks Charlie in his own bedroom so he can spend time with Jackie, upon which Charlie defecates all over the floor. Is he just "being autistic," or is he taking revenge on his brother for mistreating him? The film's most powerful scene, shot partly with a handheld camera to depict the siblings' chaotic emotions, raises similar questions. At Thomas's sixteenth-birthday dinner, Charlie begins masturbating at the table, embarrassing Jackie and infuriating Thomas, and leading to a brawl in which Charlie bites a chunk out of his brother's arm and Thomas smashes Charlie's head. Part of Thomas's rage clearly stems from his (unconscious) recognition that his brother is acting out his own (that is, Thomas's) sexual desire for Jackie. Charlie's bold gesture brings the brothers' festering rivalry to a head. By forcing the action, Charlie is, in his peculiar way, behaving as a typical big brother. The film counterpoints these depictions of chaos with a series of scenes employing aural and visual repetition that reveal Charlie's way of being in the world. At the film's opening, for example, we find Charlie sitting on the lawn, pounding a wooden spoon and vocalizing; the film repeats this sequence several times, implying that Charlie acts out this ritual daily. In these ways, *The Black Balloon* successfully copes with the narrative problem of autism by incorporating both stasis and chaos into a story that is not about recovery but about acceptance—Charlie's acceptance of Thomas's love, and Thomas's acceptance of his brother's disability and of his own identity, which he demonstrates near the end of the film by sitting on the lawn, vocalizing, and drumming along with his brother. That image of living in the moment, of sharing the world with autistic people on their own terms, offers a powerful picture of how one might truly negotiate with, and narrate, autism.

Is it possible to narrate autism authentically—to do justice to difference while retaining sufficient narrative coherence for audiences to sustain interest—without resorting to formulas? How may authors and filmmakers avoid sensationalism, resist the tyranny of the cure story, and grant their autistic characters full human agency? Perhaps by treating chaos and stasis not as hazards to be avoided but as opportunities to be exploited, as both *George* and *The Black Balloon* do so well. And, most of all, not by seeking global coherence but by celebrating those small, radiant moments of insight and purity that remind us of our shared humanity.

NOTES

1. The best-known studies of savant syndrome and autism are by Darold Treffert; they include his book *Extraordinary People: Understanding Savant Syndrome* (1989) and, more recently, *Islands of Genius: The Bountiful Mind of the Autistic, Acquired, and Sudden Savant* (2010). In a recent article, Treffert estimates the prevalence of savantism in autistic people to be approximately 10 percent (2009, 1352). Two other sources, however, offer widely differing estimates. In *Bright Splinters of the Mind: A Personal Story of Research with Autistic Savants* (2001), Beate Hermelin and Michael Rutter estimate the prevalence of savantism as 1 or 2 in 200 autistic persons (17). In contrast, a recent study by Patricia Howlin and colleagues determined that 28.5 percent of their 137 subjects met the "criteria for either a savant skill or an exceptional cognitive skill" (2009, 1359). However, the authors admit that "definitions of

what constitutes a skill that is truly exceptional in terms of population norms are also variable and highly unusual characteristics may not necessarily be equivalent to special skills" (1364). Douwe Draaisme writes, "The stereotype of autistic persons being savants is without doubt one of the most striking discrepancies between the expert's view and the general view of autism" (2009, 1478). Draaisme also surveys recent films with autistic characters in this article.

2. Anthony Baker (232–33) lists these first two rules as part of the "autistic formula" he finds in Hollywood cinema; he does not discuss literary manifestations. Stuart Murray, in *Representing Autism: Culture, Narrative, Fascination* (2008), astutely analyzes autism in mainstream film along somewhat similar lines (125–34).

3. I've borrowed the terms *yardstick* and *catalyst* from Patricia M. Puccinelli's book *Yardsticks* (1995, 11, 28, 45).

4. For example, among the "philosophies and goals" listed on the Web site of Autism Network International ("Introducing ANI," n.d.) is the following: "Autistic people have characteristically autistic styles of relating to others, which should be respected and appreciated rather than modified to make them 'fit in.'" By contrast, nonprofit organizations such as Autism Speaks focus most of their efforts on cure or remediation.

5. For a more recent outline of McCarthy's views, see "Who's Afraid of the Truth about Autism?" (2010). The name of her sponsored nonprofit organization, Generation Rescue, succinctly sums up her stance. There is also a Web site purporting to count the number of children who have died or become ill because they were not vaccinated, allegedly as a consequence of McCarthy's antivaccine campaign. See "Anti-vaccine Body Count" (Bartholomaus n.d.). The most prominent nonprofit promoting the autism–vaccine connection is the National Autism Association.

6. The first and best-known of their father's memoirs is Josh Greenfeld's *A Child Called Noah: A Family Journey*, first published in 1970.

7. "Theory of mind" refers to the hypothesis that autistic persons are unable to grasp the fact that others may hold thoughts that they themselves do not, and hence that they have difficulty in attributing intentions to others. This deficit, it is believed, contributes to the poor social skills that many autistics or Asperger individuals exhibit. The first significant analysis of this condition was Simon Baron-Cohen's *Mindblindness: An Essay on Autism and Theory of Mind* (1997). Quite a few autistic persons question this theory, aptly pointing out that most *neurotypicals* possess a weak theory of mind when it comes to understanding the intentions of autistic people.

8. An editor at a prominent publishing house once declared to me that her company would consider no disability memoirs unless they contained "uplift," which I took to mean "cure."

9. These plot elements are described by Jerome Buckley in *Season of Youth: The Bildungsroman from Dickens to Golding* (1974, 17).

REFERENCES

Autism: The Musical. 2007. Directed by Tricia Regan. Docudrama Films. DVD.
Baker, A. 2008. "Recognizing Jake: Contending with Formulaic and Spectacularized Representations of Autism in Film." In Osteen, *Autism and Representation*, 229–43.

Baron-Cohen, S. 1997. *Mindblindness: An Essay on Autism and Theory of Mind.* Cambridge, Mass.: MIT Press.

Bartholomaus, D. n.d. "Anti-vaccine Body Count." Accessed March 31, 2013, http://www.jennymccarthybodycount.com/Jenny_McCarthy_Body_Count/Home.html.

Belmonte, M. K. 2008. "Human but More So: What the Autistic Brain Tells Us about the Process of Narrative." In Osteen, *Autism and Representation*, 166–79.

Bettelheim, B. 1967. *The Empty Fortress: Infantile Autism and the Birth of the Self.* New York: Free Press.

The Black Balloon. 2008. Directed by Elissa Down. NeoClassics Films. DVD.

Blastland, M. 2006. *The Only Boy in the World: A Father Explores the Mysteries of Autism.* New York: Marlowe.

Buckley, J. 1974. *Season of Youth: The Bildungsroman from Dickens to Golding.* Cambridge, Mass.: Harvard University Press.

Burns, D. E. 2009. *Saving Ben: A Father's Story of Autism.* Denton, Tex.: University of North Texas Press.

Couser, G. T. 2000. "The Empire of the 'Normal': A Forum on Disability and Self-Representation; Introduction." *American Quarterly* 52 (2): 305–10.

Cumberland, D. L., and B. Mills, eds. 2011. *Siblings and Autism.* London: Kingsley.

Draaisme, D. 2009. "Stereotypes of Autism." *Philosophical Transactions of the Royal Society* 364 (1522): 1475–80.

Fisher, J. T. 2008. "No Search No Subject? Autism and the American Conversion Narrative." In Osteen, *Autism and Representation*, 51–64.

Frank, A. W. 1995. *The Wounded Storyteller: Body, Illness, and Ethics.* Chicago: University of Chicago Press.

George. 2000. Directed by Henry Corra and Grahame Weinbren. Corra Films, HBO Films.

Gottlieb, E. 1997. *The Boy Who Went Away.* New York: St. Martin's.

Grandin, T. 1995. *Thinking in Pictures: And Other Reports from My Life with Autism.* New York: Doubleday.

Grandin, T., and M. M. Scariano. 1986. *Emergence: Labeled Autistic.* Novato, Calif.: Arena.

Greenfeld, J. 1970. *A Child Called Noah: A Family Journey.* New York: Warner.

Greenfeld, K. T. 2009. *Boy Alone: A Brother's Memoir.* New York: HarperCollins.

Groundhog Day. 1993. Directed by Harold Ramis. Columbia Pictures.

Gunning, T. 1990. "The Cinema of Attractions: Early Film, Its Spectator, and the Avant-Garde." In *Early Cinema: Space, Frame, Narrative*, edited by T. Elsaesser and A. Barker, 56–62. London: British Film Institute.

———. 2006. "Attractions: How They Came into the World." In *The Cinema of Attractions Reloaded*, edited by W. Strauven, 31–39. Amsterdam, Neth.: Amsterdam University Press.

Hacking, I. 2010. "Autism Fiction: A Mirror of the Internet Decade?" *University of Toronto Quarterly* 79 (2): 632–55.

Haddon, M. 2003. *The Curious Incident of the Dog in the Night-Time.* New York: Doubleday.

Happé, F., and U. Frith. 2009. "The Beautiful Otherness of the Autistic Mind." *Philosophical Transactions of the Royal Society* 364 (1522): 1345–50.

Hermelin, B., and M. Rutter. 2001. *Bright Splinters of the Mind: A Personal Story of Research with Autistic Savants*. London: Kingsley.

Howlin, P., et al. 2009. "Savant Skills in Autism: Psychometric Approaches and Parental Reports." *Philosophical Transactions of the Royal Society* 364 (1522): 1359–67.

Hughes, R. 2003. *Running with Walker: A Memoir*. London: Kingsley.

"Introducing ANI." Autism Network International. Accessed December 28, 2010, http://www.autreat.com/intro.html.

Karasik, P., and J. Karasik. 2003. *The Ride Together: A Brother and Sister's Memoir of Autism in the Family*. New York: Washington Square.

Leimbach, M. 2006. *Daniel Isn't Talking*. New York: Talese/Doubleday.

Martin, R. 1994. *Out of Silence: A Journey into Language*. New York: Holt.

Maurice, C. 1993. *Let Me Hear Your Voice: A Family's Triumph over Autism*. New York: Knopf.

McCarthy, J. 2007. *Louder Than Words*. New York: Dutton.

———. 2010. "Who's Afraid of the Truth about Autism?" *Huffington Post*, March 9. Accessed December 27, 2010, http://www.huffingtonpost.com/jenny-mccarthy/whos-afraid-of-the-truth_b_490918.html.

Mills, B. 2008. "Autism and the Imagination." In Osteen, *Autism and Representation*, 117–32.

Mitchell, D. T., and S. L. Snyder. 2001. *Narrative Prosthesis: Disability and the Dependencies of Discourse*. Ann Arbor: University of Michigan Press.

Moon, E. 2003. *The Speed of Dark*. New York: Ballantine.

Moore, C. 2004. *George and Sam*. London: Viking.

Mozart and the Whale. 2005. Directed by Petter Naess. Millennium Films.

Murray, S. 2008. *Representing Autism: Culture, Narrative, Fascination*. Liverpool, U.K.: Liverpool University Press.

Nazeer, K. 2006. *Send in the Idiots: Stories from the Other Side of Autism*. New York: Bloomsbury.

Osteen, M., ed. 2008. *Autism and Representation*. New York: Routledge.

———. 2008. "Autism and Representation: A Comprehensive Introduction." In *Autism and Representation*, 1–47.

———. 2010. *One of Us: A Family's Life with Autism*. Columbia: University of Missouri Press.

Puccinelli, P. M. 1995. *Yardsticks: Retarded Characters and Their Roles in Fiction*. New York: Lang.

Rain Man. 1988. Directed by Barry Levinson. MGM. DVD.

Rankin, K. 2000. *Growing Up Severely Autistic: They Call Me Gabriel*. London: Kingsley.

Rimland, B. 1986. Foreword to Grandin and Scariano, *Emergence*.

———. 1992. Foreword to Williams, *Nobody Nowhere*.

Rose, I. 2008. "Autistic Autobiography or Autistic Life Narrative?" *Journal of Literary Disability* 2 (1): 44–54.

The Sandwich Kid. 2007. Directed by Keri Bowers. Normal Films.

Shore, S. 2003. *Beyond the Wall: Personal Experiences with Autism and Asperger Syndrome*. 2nd ed. Shawnee Mission, Kans.: Autism Asperger.

Silent Fall. 1994. Directed by Bruce Beresford. Warner Bros.

Silver, M. 2008. *The God of War*. New York: Simon & Schuster.

Stehli, A. 1991. *The Sound of a Miracle*. New York: Avon.

Tammet, D. 2006. *Born on a Blue Day: Inside the Extraordinary Mind of an Autistic Savant*. New York: Free Press.

Temple Grandin. 2010. Directed by Mick Jackson. HBO Films.

Today's Man. 2006. Directed by Lizzie Gottlieb. Filmmakers Library. DVD.

Treffert, D. 1989. *Extraordinary People: Understanding Savant Syndrome*. New York: Harper & Row.

———. 2009. "The Savant Syndrome: An Extraordinary Condition; A Synopsis; Past, Present, Future." *Philosophical Transactions of the Royal Society* 364 (1522): 1351–57.

———. 2010. *Islands of Genius: The Bountiful Mind of the Autistic, Acquired, and Sudden Savant*. London: Kingsley.

Williams, D. 1992. *Nobody Nowhere: The Extraordinary Autobiography of an Autistic*. New York: Times Books.

Wilson, J. C. 2008. *Weather Reports from the Autism Front: A Father's Memoir of His Autistic Son*. Jefferson, N.C.: McFarland.

Witt, M. 2004. *Broken as Things Are*. New York: Holt.

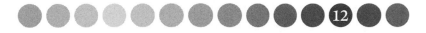

The Shifting Horizons of Autism Online

Joyce Davidson and Michael Orsini

> I feel that my world has expanded because of the Internet, and I have grown to meet it.
>
> —*Female, 50, aspie / person with autism*

This chapter investigates the perceived importance of the Internet for individuals on the autism spectrum. The larger project from which it draws was designed to look in more depth at significant themes that emerged from an earlier study of autistic autobiographies. These first-hand accounts frequently highlight the increasingly central and often facilitative role played by the computer, and specifically the Internet, in many autistic persons' lives (Davidson 2008). In what follows, we aim to build on these findings, questioning in particular whether online activities expand or contract the social and emotional horizons of autistic lifeworlds.

The potential importance of the Internet for people on the spectrum has been acknowledged in previous research (for example, Brownlow and O'Dell 2006 and this volume), in popular publications (such as Biever 2007), and in writings by autistic persons (for example, Dekker 2006). This connection has become so well established that Judy Singer's once-striking claim that "the impact of the Internet on autistics may one day be compared to the spread of sign language among the deaf" (1999, 67) is repeated so often as to have become commonplace. However, as Penny Benford and P. J. Standen point out, there is "very little empirical research into the use of the internet by people with autism" (2009, 49). Predictably, this is beginning to change, and future research will no doubt benefit from insights emerging from studies exploring the connections between the Internet and other differences and disabilities. Gill Valentine and Tracey Skelton, for example, focus on the experience of "the Deaf community" (2008, 2009) and, in doing so, stress the need to attend closely to the *specificities* of particular disabilities and impairments. They highlight the dangers of generalizing inappropriately across radically different embodied and emotional experiences in ways taken seriously by the current research and by other critical autism scholars who challenge universalizing accounts of what it means to be on the spectrum (for example, Ortega, this volume).

Further lessons can be drawn from Valentine and Skelton's critical engagement with relevant literature and their associated attempts to distance themselves from previous and relatively widespread tendencies among researchers to highlight *either* the productive possibilities *or* the potentially significant limitations associated with technologically mediated relationships involving persons with disabilities (2008, 2009). Their concerns relate to the familiar notion either that the Internet represents a virtual panacea that increases social capital and inclusion by providing access to information about health care, employment, educational opportunities, and so on (Moser 2006), or that it serves to produce online ghettos, keeping disabilities out of sight and so out of mind to such an extent that it risks setting back the disability-rights movements considerably (Seymour and Lupton 2004, 301). Many of the more thoughtful investigations (such as Gleeson 1999) reveal the need for research that is rather more subtle in analytic approach and that recognizes not only that the Internet is neither all good nor all bad but also that electronically mediated and "real" lives and experiences are rarely so disjointed; rather, "relationships between online and offline worlds are more nuanced, complex and mutually interdependent than early polar characterizations suggest" (Valentine and Skelton 2008, 481). This chapter aims to explore further some of the subtleties of shade, highlighting the permeability and overlapping nature of on- and off-line worlds. It also aims to explore the significance of the complex and *changing* relationships between disabilities and technologies (Crooks, Dorn, and Wilton 2008), focusing on the experiences of persons on the spectrum for whom the rapidly shifting and increasingly mobile nature of Internet technologies may have particularly profound—and not necessarily positive—implications.

In tackling such questions, the chapter explores what Internet use means for the geographies of some autistic persons' lives, asking how it affects, for example, their daily mobility, their sense of social, spatial, and emotional connection, and what this in turn means for their sense of self. It aims to do so because it takes seriously the idea that selves cannot ever be taken as "given"; they are in no meaningful sense ever separate or static but are instead "relational achievements" (Conradson 2005), continually formed and re-formed in relations with richly constituted, complex environments. We therefore ask what it means that the selves and spaces with which one interacts in mutually constitutive ways are increasingly or even almost exclusively electronically mediated. As we'll discuss further, this seems to be the case—and the preferred case—for at least some of those on the spectrum who participated in this research.

Understanding this sense of meaning—personal perception, subjective *interpretation*, in the fully hermeneutic sense of the term—is critical for what this study hopes to achieve. The methodological approach we employ, which is closely informed by phenomenology (for example, Moustakas 1994), tries to home in on what the situation *feels* like from the inside rather than what it looks like from the outside. This means that we are less interested in measurable effects or recognized indicators of such factors as social inclusion (and even obviously important measurable factors such as access to employment, education, and social and health services) and more interested in the less easily discernible but still definitive aspects of autistic lifeworlds. The metaphors are tricky, but the phenomena we have in mind and aim to evoke relate to such questions as what the Internet does to the "color" and "texture" of everyday life, the amorphous and often emotional stuff of existence that matters immeasurably but is almost impossible to examine or even express (Harrison 2007; Smith et al. 2009). In investigating these matters, we use the term "horizons" in the hermeneutic sense intended by Hans-Georg Gadamer (1998) to help conceptualize the peculiar possibilities and limitations of our cultural condition, the place from within which we interpret, inhabit, and respond to our worlds. From such a background, the question might be posed whether online experience is associated with enhancing, enriching, or expanding sociospatial and emotional horizons or, perhaps less positively, with contracting or closing them down in ways that make the world feel somehow smaller or otherwise simply *less*.

Of course, it is never easy to "get at" these meaningful and emotional aspects of experience, and many researchers—including contributors to this collection (such as Chew and Osteen)—have written about their struggles to access and represent such important material (see also Bondi 2005; Bondi and Davidson 2011; and the critique of representations of autism by Prince, this volume). In designing this study, we aimed to generate responses that would provide a sense of personal perceptions rather than factual information about Internet use, and so to reveal something of its felt implications for autistic lives and relationships. We wanted to know, for example, to what extent online activity tends to relate to the spectrum, and whether it affirms or unsettles the kinds of autistic insularity or "ghettoization" that certain critics associate with the Internet. We therefore aimed to question whether, where, and how participants communicated with nonautistic others and how they felt about these interactions (that is, in what senses they were experienced as "positive" or "negative"). To provide insights of a more general nature, we aimed to generate understanding of whether participants felt their lives off-line had changed in any meaningful sense as a result of their Internet use. In the following section, we provide further detail about how the project was designed and conducted—including who participated and how they did so—before analyzing the findings.

Methods:
Approaching Autism Online

Preparing to undertake this study required a period of immersion in an increasingly large interdisciplinary literature dealing with a wide variety of ethical and other challenges associated with research on, and in, this medium (see, for example, essays in collections edited by Fielding 2008; Hine 2005; and S. Jones 1999; and, with specific relation to autism, see Brownlow and O'Dell 2002). This background closely informed all aspects of the research-planning process, including the recruitment strategy and questionnaire design.[1] The twenty-four questions selected for final inclusion were generally open-ended to encourage personalized answers, with the exception of initial identifier questions about age and gender.[2] These were followed by a few basic prompts to solicit contextualizing information about respondents' lives and identities, of a kind that might be considered appropriate to a phenomenologically oriented investigation (for example, "Would you like to provide any additional information about yourself, for example, how do you like to spend your time . . . ?"). To encourage the provision of additional and potentially relevant background information, we also asked, for example, whether diagnosis was professionally sought or self-claimed, and what term individuals preferred to use to describe themselves—e.g. "aspie," "autistic person," "person with autism"—and whether there were reasons for the preference that they would like to share.[3] When quoted in this chapter, participants are referred to using the identifying information they themselves provided (for example, "female, 24, person with autism").

Potential participants gained access to the questionnaire by responding to a recruitment notice inviting "persons with an Autism Spectrum Condition" (see endnote 3, on terminology) to take part in a research project about their Internet use. When they clicked the link to "further information," they were taken to a page-long letter providing further detail about the project, including information about consent, which was given by clicking a link providing direct access to the questionnaire. The recruitment notice was initially sent out, with the assistance of Internet-savvy colleagues and graduate students,[4] to individuals, Listservs, and organizations in early October 2008, with a request to distribute to members and/or post to Web sites as applicable. In distributing the recruitment notice, we did not intend to target any particular kind of group or position on the spectrum but, rather, to spread the net as widely as possible in an attempt to recruit a variety of participants with different experience and from different backgrounds, as well as those from organizations with different politics and policies. It was therefore sent, for example, to organizations such as the Autism Acceptance Project and the National Autism Society (the only organization to require that we submit an ethics application for approval), online forums such as Least Restrictive Environment 2, and Facebook groups such as Parked Diagonally in a Parallel Universe.[5]

One of the advantages of posting recruitment notices on Web sites and circulating them via Listservs and social networks is that it expanded the horizon from which the pool of potential participants was drawn, benefiting from the intimate knowledge of interested parties who knew of individuals, groups, and organizations of whom we may have been unaware.[6] One of the drawbacks is that we cannot be precise about where and how participants (people who eventually completed the questionnaire) came to know of the study, as we had neglected to include a question that would have elicited this potentially important contextualizing information. Of the various other limitations that might be considered before we present our interpretation of project findings, the fact that our approach excluded everyone *not* using the Internet might be seen as the most obvious and important. However, this research concerns the experiences of some of those on the spectrum who *are* using it, and for whom this experiential network constitutes a potentially significant context and space for connection. Thus, although findings could in no sense be considered representative of autistic experience online, the research generated seventy-five rich and illustrative responses from often exceptionally articulate individuals willing to offer insights into the shifting horizons of their lives.[7] In the following section, we begin to unpack some of the responses, quoting extensively in order to base representations as far and as closely as possible on participants' own words. We begin with an overview of activities undertaken online.

Worlds of Autism, On- and Off-line

Responses to questions about online pursuits revealed that participants engage in activities unsurprisingly similar to those undertaken by "typical" others: they use e-mail to keep in touch with family and friends; read and post blogs; take part in discussion groups; watch YouTube videos, and research topics of special or even obsessive interest (one respondent mentions knitting and another photography as examples of autistic "perseverations" facilitated online). Some respondents describe joining support groups and participating in advocacy and activism (a significant theme yet to be analyzed and explored in depth elsewhere), whereas others shop and spend time on online gaming sites. Although there is no one response that might be considered emblematic of the array of answers encountered, the following quotation provides some sense of the sheer range of activities respondents undertake, and shows the common mix between practices that are and are not related to autism. It also reveals the fairly central or at least time-consuming place of the Internet in many respondents' lives:

> I use the Internet to find information, for entertainment, and for social connection. I spend a lot of time looking up things I am interested in. . . . I collect and save information on a special interest of mine—ABBA—which I have had since I was a child. I shop on E-bay (for clothes and shoes mainly), because it is much easier than dealing with shopping in person. I currently belong to Aspies For Freedom and access that site regularly because I feel a connection

to the other members. . . . I also use my email to talk to people. . . . I also like watching videos on You Tube on various different topics. . . . I am on the Internet for a large portion of my day. (Female, 39, Asperger Syndrome / person with an ASD)

Of the commonalities that stand out in response to questions about whether and how participants or their lives have changed as a result of the Internet, many respondents comment on feeling more understood, empowered, and—crucially—connected. References to this sense of relational transformation are so common and eloquently expressed that choosing a sample is challenging, but the following give some flavor of the expansive sense that emerges from analysis of responses (stylistic quirks and/or typographical errors have been reproduced from the original text).

My life has been thoroughly changed by the internet. It would probably take several chapters for me to say precisely how. I have found a sense of identity, I have found friends and a supportive community, I have found my career (autism research) and a purpose, I have found my boyfriend . . . What haven/'t I found? (Female, 27, autistic)

I have become 1000 times more confident since becoming computer literate . . . I feel the respect of others for what I do, and I understand myself and the world around me better than I did before. (Female, 43, aspie / autistic)

As a result of my use of the internet, I'm a person, not "ontologically a freak." (Gender unspecified,[8] 45, Asperger Syndrome)

I no longer feel like the total social reject that I was. (Male, 20, Aspie / person with Asperger)

As one might expect from a study that recruits participants through sites focused on the subject of autism, much of the online activity that respondents describe is closely related in one way or another to the spectrum. However, that there are links between online pursuits and autism doesn't necessarily mean that the activity involves only autistic people or that it always stays online; there is apparently significant "spillover" as respondents' autism-related interests take them off-line too.[9] They describe, for example, working on research projects, giving presentations, and attending conferences, all activities they suggest they would not otherwise have engaged in:

> Internet use expands the potential for interaction with others, by increasing opportunity and making those interactions more palatable. I've met a few people, worked on a few projects/books, done some workshops and presentations, that might not have been done without first meeting the people on the net. (Male, 42, autistic)

> I attended Autscape 2006, Autscape 2007, Autscape 2008, Autreat 2007 and Autreat 2008. (I discovered these autistic-run conferences through the Internet.) (Male, 38, unspecified)

Other respondents suggest that the Internet provides an *opening* onto the rest of the world in ways that extend far beyond the boundaries of autism. As the following quotations reveal, some engage in relatively typical off-line activities associated, for example, with holidays, hobbies, businesses, educational opportunities, and relationships, even marriage in two cases:

> I occasionally meet people who have a similar interest—such as photography. (Male, 54, autistic)

> I started a small business and sell online items related to antique computers. I have participated in large meetings related to that business/hobby. (Male, 38, person with Asperger Syndrome)

> My entire life has changed. I met my husband via the internet. I would not have met him, or anyone else without the internet. I have managed to complete my Masters degree using the internet for tutorials and research. . . . I feel more confident and more positive about life. . . . I meet people in real life. I have been able to book trips abroad and travel alone to India, Nepal and Thailand. This was because I could make contact with people and book flights and accommodation online. (Female, 46, adult with autism)

Some of these responses reveal that participants obviously *can* interact with others both on- and off-line, and that the walls of both worlds can be experienced as permeable; clearly, there is often connection and crossover in many consequential respects. But when asked which is the preferred means of interaction and communication, there is a notably strong tendency to favor the virtual. To be clear, this is not to say that this is the case for everyone all of the time; but although a few respondents express a desire to socialize more off-line, most seem satisfied with a medium or "element" more suited to their communicative style. In the words of one respondent, "I took to the \'net like a duck takes to water. It was clearly my element from the start" (female, 43, aspie / autistic). Another describes the question about preference for on- or off-line interaction as "like asking a fish whether it prefers to swim in the water or walk on land" (female, 27, Asperger / HFA [high-functioning autistic] / aspie). Expanding on her striking claim, this respondent explains, "I am much, much better with online communication, because there is only one dimension, the text, to process and give off. No tones, no body language, no things misheard because you were thinking of something else for a second, you can always go back and check, and you have time to think—you don\'t get \'dead air\.'"

This response confirms earlier findings that emphasize the extent to which the Internet can provide communicative respite for those on the spectrum (for example, R. S. P. Jones, Zahl, and Huws 2001), particularly in light of the sociospatial and sensory anxieties that surround more typical and traditional forms of interaction (Davidson and Henderson 2010). Other respondents write about online communication in similarly positive terms, and they do so in diverse and insightful ways that often highlight the very particular experience of those on the spectrum when compared with the online experiences of those with other differences and disabilities. For example, autistic respondents reveal that they do not tend to enjoy the benefits of "passing" as nondisabled—and so bypassing discrimination—in a realm where stigmatized "abnormal" bodies are usually kept out of the communicative picture (Dobransky and Hargittai 2006). Autistic bodies are, of course, often less obviously "marked" as different than are bodies of people with other disabilities, but their very distinctive communicative styles can lead to unintentional disclosure and/or discrimination and exclusion. For example, as this participant explains, "people don't want to talk to you if you don't play by the taken for granted social rules that people with autism simply don't get and so don't know that they've broken. [I] get kicked out of groups in the game because I will say things that are taken in a way I did not intend by the other players" (female, 39, Asperger Syndrome / person with an ASD). However, even though participants cannot always or easily hide autistic difference online, these communicative challenges would apparently be encountered off-line in any case, which means this "disembodied" medium is felt to be no more (and arguably less) exclusionary than the social world off-line.[10] Indeed, some respondents draw attention to other kinds of protective advantage associated with communication at an electronically mediated distance; given that the kind of rejection that occurs online tends to be felt less immediately, it is arguably less harmful than that which is experienced face-to-face: "Online there is less scope for me being upset or causing offence. I have a tendency to be abrupt . . . as well as misunderstand other people so in the less personal online [world] I am less upset if ever these occur" (female, 25, Asperger). Thus, even though there are significant risks associated with virtual interactions and intimacies (Parr and Davidson 2008), being online apparently *feels* better and safer for this respondent, and indeed for others taking part in this study. In comments that downplay further the potential impact of online exposure to emotional harm, some suggest that the generally restricted nature of their off-line social lives means there may be less, and in some cases nothing, to lose: "I don\'t socialise with anyone. I would feel isolated if I didn\'t have the internet" (female, 45, ASD).

Despite the obvious advantages associated with online opportunities for social mixing, questions might still arise about other potentially negative implications of affiliations that remain exclusively electronic. We might ask, for example, whether virtual relationships could "really" be rich or in any sense meaningful in ways participants' accounts suggest. However, and tackling such questions in a way that takes phenomenological approaches seriously, we suggest that what really matters here isn't looking for evidence that would convince (nonautistic or Internet-skeptical) outsiders. Rather, working to understand the worldviews of autistic persons in and on their own terms means recognizing that for some, online interaction is not just better than nothing, it is actually, simply, better. That is to say, some respondents would comprehensively challenge widespread notions about the superficiality of electronically mediated relationships (see Parr and Davidson 2008). Being genuinely receptive to autistic views thus involves being open to the possibility that some feel more close to others, more quickly and more comfortably, online than off. For example: "I prefer online communication because I feel that I can be more honest. I don\'t have to put up a front. . . . Offline, I have go through all the NT [neurotypical] social pleasantries, and I find that I spend more time going through that than actually getting to know the person. Online, I can skip that and go straight to the \'meat\' of a relationship" (male, 23, autistic person). That potentially rewarding and even intense connections can emerge from such candid online encounters helps explain why some might prefer to limit their social interaction to electronic environments. However, for some respondents, online spaces are mere starting places, and the blogosphere, for example, is just somewhere to find one's feet before moving on to experience less mediated encounters elsewhere. In a finding we consider significant, the following individual describes using scripts previously tried and tested in a socially safe (electronic) environment, and explains that these can facilitate meaningful involvement in previously inaccessible social spaces off-line: "One year ago, I experimented with blogging and I discovered by surprise that I became much more talkative in person since I already had well-thought-out opinions on a variety of topical news items. Blogging was like rehearsing scripts for later verbal use. Very handy stuff" (male, 40, autistic).

Thus, not only can the Internet provide a vital kind of breathing space for those stifled by the sensorial and emotional demands of typical social life, it also serves as a training ground for those willing and perhaps increasingly able to stretch beyond its inevitable limitations. Nevertheless, others do remain restricted in their off-line involvements, and some respondents explain that members of their families—and in some cases they themselves—think they spend too much time online. One respondent describes his current usage as "total" (male, 40, autistic), and several others go so far as to characterize their excessive Internet use in terms of an "addiction" that interferes significantly with their involvement in "real" life (often tellingly reduced to "IRL."). Of those who describe such overuse, many would very much like to cut back, suggesting their lifeworlds would feel bigger and better if they somehow managed to unplug:

I spend way too much time (hours out of every day) on the internet. (Female, 26, person on the autism spectrum / person with Asperger-type symptoms)

Since I purchased my computer four years ago my Internet usage has been constant and high. I am hoping to stop using it quite so much as I would like to get more work done in studio. (Female, 39, Asperger Syndrome / person with an ASD)

Five years from now, I would like to break my addiction to forums and get better at IRL communication. (Female, 25, on the autistic spectrum)

Troubling as these reports are, they are far from typical of respondents in this study. Personal accounts of online experience are rarely so negative and suggestive of frustration or feelings of constraint. However, some do express ambivalence about the Internet's impact on the horizons of their lives, and one respondent reveals that as a result of the Internet, "I am somewhat less lonely yet probably more withdrawn from the 3 dimensional world" (female, 62, woman with Asperger Syndrome). Another expresses a similar sense of uncertainty about the Internet's influence: "I spend less time outside, unfortunately [but] I haven\'t become a recluse because I\'m online" (female, 29, Asperger Syndrome).

Although the majority of respondents stress that they have established crucial connections and feel less isolated because of the Internet in ways they consider vital, findings also reveal the need to remain aware and perhaps wary of what connectivity (and its potential withdrawal) means. In a less equivocal and rather worrying quotation, one respondent explains that the prospect of "being disconnected feels me with dread" (female, 25, Asperger Syndrome). That "real" life could be considered a potentially dreadful place of banishment underlines some of the emotional risks and possible restrictions associated with heavy Internet usage, and this participant isn't alone in suggesting that it is a struggle even to imagine living exclusively off-line. Others reveal that their lives are so inextricably caught up with the Internet that they simply cannot conceive what it would mean for their everyday lives and indeed, their sense of self, not to be connected:

I\'ve been using the internet pretty compulsively since I was 13, so my adult sense of self has largely formed with the internet present. (Female, 24, autistic / "Asperger Woman")

I have been online since 1995, so its hard for me to imagine life without it. I met my husband through the internet! (Female, 29, autistic / Asperger Syndrome)

The internet is so integral to my life that it\'s hard to define where one stops and the other begins. (Male, 54, autistic)

However (and as experience in today's university classrooms makes plain), the inextricable kinds of connection described are perhaps not that different from those experienced by many more "typical" others. Also, and importantly, being online is no longer necessarily equivalent to being withdrawn from "real" life; for many, the boundaries between on- and off-line worlds are becoming more porous than ever. Such connections have the potential to be particularly beneficial for some of those on the spectrum, by helping dismantle experiential barriers to a social world that can come to feel more open, accessible, and accommodating as a result. Highlighting one crucial source of crossover, one respondent reveals, "I practically live on the internet. I have a desktop that remains on (and online) at all times, and a laptop for when I need mobility" (female, 24, autistic / "Asperger Woman"). Clearly, being online no longer equates to being at home, "stuck," or otherwise static, and findings suggest that the prospect of being simultaneously online and mobile could have an effect of unprecedented significance on the horizons of autistic lives. That is to say, increasingly available and affordable wireless technologies can provide an invaluable source of portable information and support. Such connectivity might in turn feed into a mobile sense of security that could mitigate certain sources of social exclusion. To cite an obvious, if hypothetical, example, Wi-Fi could lessen navigational challenges associated with sensory overload in public places; consulting online maps or timetables for public transport would, for many, be far preferable to the nontechnological alternative involving a face-to-face request for assistance. In an associated and no less practical perk, hand-held devices can also provide an "involvement shield" in the sense intended by Erving Goffman (1963, 40). That is to say, as so many typical others have discovered, they have the potential to protect the user from unwanted social interaction (Hampton and Gupta 2008).

Clearly, recent technological developments allowing mobile Internet access have the potential to enrich autistic lives considerably. However, questions emerge about whether the incredible pace of such technological change might be considered daunting for members of a group with an avowed preference for stability and similarity in everyday life and routines (Davidson 2010). Such intolerance of change may well be a reality for some, but respondents in our study did not express such reservations about technology. Instead, findings suggest that technological advances help strengthen rather than undermine the desired sense of control, and that persons with autism may in fact be particularly well suited to keeping up with (and perhaps even staying ahead of) the game. The rules and equipment do indeed keep changing, but at least some of those on the spectrum have already demonstrated how unusually appropriate and valuable their skills and interests are for this medium. As the following quotations reveal, some respondents were "in" at the very beginning of the Internet, adapting quickly and comfortably to an environment that apparently suited and served them well.

> I\'ve been chatting online since before the internet. Literally. BITnet was the medium back then for mainframe computers at universities, and there were the BBS networks over dial-up modem lines for pc computers. I\'ve also been participating in the online forum environment since before the internet. It was a Vax system on DECnet. (Male, 40, autistic)

> I\'ve been using the Internet since before there was one I met a few friends through the Usenet, and even met with some of them on one occasion during the 90s. (Male, 43, aspie / autistic person)

These references to obsolete systems underline once again how quickly and comprehensively technological things change.

Although this chapter has introduced one expansive possibility associated with such transformations of the electronic landscape, there are other, less positive potentialities that ought to be taken into account. Most obviously, if typical online activity continues to move toward real-time communication and video streaming, it may well "cancel out" some of the advantages currently experienced by those on the spectrum, typically associated with text-only and time-delayed responses (Benford and Standen 2009). The playing field might not stay level forever, and there is a risk that technological shifts may leave some of those with autism behind. This chapter can hardly begin to address such concerns, but future research might explore the potential implications of technological developments for autistic lives in more depth.

Conclusion

Drawing on findings from a recent study of Internet use by people on the spectrum, this chapter set out to explore some of the productive tensions and possibilities inherent to the medium. It confirms findings from previous research that stress the unusual suitability of the Internet for communication among autistic persons, while taking seriously associated concerns about the Internet's "ghettoizing" potential. Our research demonstrates that—for participants in this study, at least—online activities are rarely entirely insular; they extend far beyond a narrow focus on the spectrum and often involve nonautistic others. Such extensive interactions have positive implications for numerous (but especially social) aspects of autistic persons' lives. Online engagements with individuals on and off the spectrum are often rich and rewarding, and participants show that relationships and skills developed electronically often transcend the limitations of the medium, extending into "real-life" situations in ways that potentially subvert common sources of social exclusion. This finding highlights the significance of arguably increasingly permeable boundaries between on- and off-line worlds and, in particular, the potential significance of progressively mobile Internet technology. Evidently, the current situation is far from a steady or risk free state, but despite the practical and emotional perils associated with rapid technological change, overuse, and even addiction, this chapter suggests that the horizons of (at least some) autistic worlds have grown immeasurably because of the Internet, and in ways that merit future research by critical autism scholars.

NOTES

1. The questionnaire was designed to allow field responses, facilitating the inclusion of as much or as little text as individual respondents chose to provide. It was hosted on a personal domain (joyce.davidson.com) using Lime Survey, selected as

the most secure and user-friendly option available after consideration of several possible and some more popular alternatives (such as Survey Monkey).

2. Critics could argue that open-ended questions should be considered culturally insensitive, given autistic persons' oft-expressed preference for direct and literal, rather than open and lateral, thinking (Gerland 2003, 35; see also Williams 2005). This issue was discussed in an earlier methodologically oriented version of this chapter, presented at the 2011 Association of American Geographers annual conference (copies available on request from Joyce Davidson).

3. Predictably, the responses to this question were extraordinarily varied and provided valuable insights into the complicated and often divisive politics of labeling. Unfortunately, these exceed the scope of the current chapter (but see, for example, Bagatell 2007 and Baker 2006 for further discussion). In the survey and the recruitment notice we opted to use the term autistic-spectrum "condition," rather than "disorder." However, one participant objected to this term on the grounds that it connotes "superficial" rather than "pervasive" experience. Such divergence of opinion is perhaps to be expected, given Singer's claim that, "as befits a disability emerging for the first time in the postmodern era, the autistic spectrum has fuzzy boundaries. Not even its name has been agreed upon" (1999, 63).

4. Particular thanks are due to Victoria Henderson, whose involvement in this project from its inception has been essential to its success. Sophie Edwards and Katie Hemsworth joined the project at a later stage, and their ongoing assistance with data analysis is greatly appreciated. Additional assistance with recruitment was provided by an individual who drew on personal connections with moderators of some of the discussion groups. This assistant also served as a consultant during the initial stages of the project, offering input—for example, regarding survey design and whether and how particular questions might be included or rephrased—from a purely personal perspective (which is to say, a perspective in no sense considered representative of an "autism community").

5. A final call for participation was issued at the end of April 2010 (partly intended as a reminder to those who had started but not completed the survey) and was sent through most of the same channels as the original call, as well as through individuals who had heard about the project and contacted us personally requesting further information (such personal contacts included requests by several parents to participate on their children's behalf, requests which were regretfully denied, as the survey was geared and ethically cleared toward investigating exclusively adult experience). The survey was closed on May 15, 2010 (a time period extended in large part because of Davidson's maternity and parental leave).

6. An online search using the authors' names and the phrase "autism online" reveals that our original call for participants was circulated far beyond the remit of our original recruitment list, including to self-advocacy groups (such as Aspies for Freedom), and parent-advocacy groups (such as Parents of Autistic Children of Northern Virginia)—organizations with very different politics and advocacy priorities (parents tend to campaign for treatment and possible cure for autism [e.g., Iversen 2006], whereas self-advocates tend to emphasize the need for accommodation and acceptance [e.g., Nelson 2004]).

7. Forty-six of these participants provided contact information and may be invited to participate in the next phase of the project.

8. Follow-up interviews with those who provided contact information might investigate whether information about gender was withheld deliberately and, if so, why. It is possible that participants may have intended to communicate rejection of accepted gender identities (see Lawson 2005 on the experience of sexual "difference," such as gender ambivalence, asexuality, and/or queer identification, among those on the spectrum).

9. Among other themes, the current research was intended to investigate whether "[autistic] voices 'gathering force' online *will be heard offline too,* [whether] virtual communication has the potential to spill over into the 'real world,' with further potential for political consequence" (Davidson 2008, 801; emphasis in original).

10. Stuart Murray's account of the intersections between autism and the post-human (this volume) consistently highlights the centrality—and inescapably *material* reality—of embodiment for genuinely critical (rather than simplistic or celebratory) accounts of contemporary autistic experience.

REFERENCES

Bagatell, N. 2007. "Orchestrating Voices: Autism, Identity, and the Power of Discourse." *Disability and Society* 22 (4): 413–26.

Baker, D. L. 2006. "Neurodiversity, Neurological Disability, and the Public Sector: Notes on the Autism Spectrum." *Disability and Society* 21 (1): 15–29.

Benford, P., and P. J. Standen. 2009. "The Internet: A Comfortable Medium for People with Asperger Syndrome (AS) and High Functioning Autism (HFA)?" *Journal of Assistive Technologies* 3 (2): 48–57.

Biever, C. 2007. "Web Removes Social Barriers for Those with Autism." *New Scientist,* June 27. http://technology.newscientist.com/article/mg19426106.100.

Bondi, L. 2005. "The Place of Emotions in Research: From Partitioning Emotion and Reason to the Emotional Dynamics of Research Relationships." In *Emotional Geographies,* edited by J. Davidson, L. Bondi, and M. Smith, 231–46. Aldershot, U.K.: Ashgate.

Bondi, L., and J. Davidson. 2011. "Lost in Translation." *Transactions of the Institute of British Geographers* 36 (4): 595–98.

Brownlow, C., and L. O'Dell. 2002. "Ethical Issues in Qualitative Research in Online Communities." *Disability and Society* 17 (6): 685–94.

———. 2006. "Constructing an Autistic Identity: AS Voices Online." *Mental Retardation* 44 (5): 315–21.

Conradson, D. 2005. "Landscape, Care, and the Relational Self: Therapeutic Encounters in Southern England." *Health and Place* 11 (4): 337–48.

Crooks, V., M. Dorn, and R. D. Wilton. 2008. "Emerging Scholarship in the Geographies of Disability." *Health and Place* 14 (4): 883–88.

Davidson, J. 2008. "Autistic Cultures Online: Virtual Communication and Cultural Expression on the Spectrum." *Social and Cultural Geography* 9 (7): 791–806.

———. 2010. "'It Cuts Both Ways': A Relational Approach to Access and Accommodation for Autism." *Social Science and Medicine* 70 (2): 305–12.

Davidson, J., and V. Henderson. 2010. "Travel in Parallel with Us for a While: Sensory Geographies of Autism." *Canadian Geographer* 54 (4): 462–75.

Dekker, M. 2006. "On Our Own Terms: Emerging Autistic Culture." Autistic Culture. Accessed January 21, 2008, http://autisticculture.com/index.php?page =articles.

Dobransky, K., and E. Hargittai. 2006. "The Disability Divide in Internet Access and Use." *Information, Communication, and Society* 9 (3): 313–34.

Fielding, N., ed. 2008. *The Sage Handbook of Online Research Methods.* London: Sage.

Gadamer, H.-G. 1998. *Truth and Method.* New York: Continuum.

Gerland, G. 2003. *A Real Person: Life on the Outside.* London: Souvenir.

Gleeson, B. 1999. "Can Technology Overcome the Disabling City?" In *Mind and Body Spaces: Geographies of Illness, Impairment, and Disability,* edited by R. Butler and H. Parr, 231–46. London: Routledge.

Goffman, E. 1963. *Behaviour in Public Places: Notes on the Social Organization of Gatherings.* London: Collier Macmillan.

Hampton, K. N., and N. Gupta. 2008. "Community and Social Interaction in the Wireless City: WiFi Use in Public and Semi-public Spaces." *New Media and Society* 10 (6): 831–50.

Harrison, P. 2007. "'How Shall I Say It?': Relating the Non-relational." *Environment and Planning A* 39 (3): 590–608.

Hine, C., ed. 2005. *Virtual Methods: Issues in Social Research on the Internet.* New York: Berg.

Iversen, P. 2006. *Strange Son: Two Mothers, Two Sons, and the Quest to Unlock the Hidden World of Autism.* New York: Riverhead.

Jones, R. S. P., A. Zahl, and J. C. Huws. 2001. "First-Hand Accounts of Emotional Experiences in Autism: A Qualitative Analysis." *Disability and Society* 16 (3): 393–401.

Jones, S. 1999. *Doing Internet Research: Critical Issues and Methods for Examining the Net.* London: Sage.

Lawson, W. 2005. *Sex, Sexuality, and the Autism Spectrum.* London: Kingsley.

Moser, I. 2006. "Disability and the Promises of Technology: Technology, Subjectivity, and Embodiment within the Order of the Normal." *Information, Communication, and Society* 9 (3): 373–95.

Moustakas, C. 1994. *Phenomenological Research Methods.* London: Sage.

Nelson, A. 2004. "Declaration from the Autism Community That They Are a Minority Group." PRWeb, November 18. Accessed January 21, 2008, http://www.prweb.com/releases/2004/11/prweb179444.htm.

Parr, H., and J. Davidson. 2008. "'Virtual Trust': Online Emotional Intimacies in Mental Health Support." In *Researching Trust and Health,* edited by J. Brownlie, A. Greene, and A. Howson, 33–53. New York: Routledge.

Seymour, W., and D. Lupton. 2004. "Holding the Line Online: Exploring Wired Relationships for People with Disabilities." *Disability and Society* 19 (4): 291–305.

Singer, J. 1999. "'Why Can't You Be Normal for Once in Your Life?': From a 'Problem with No Name' to the Emergence of a New Category of Difference." In *Disability Discourse,* edited by M. Corker and S. French. Buckingham, U.K.: Open University Press.

Smith, M., et al. 2009. "Geography and Emotion: Emerging Constellations." In *Emotion, Place, and Culture,* edited by M. Smith et al., 1–20. Aldershot, U.K.: Ashgate.

Valentine, G., and T. Skelton. 2008. "Changing Spaces: The Role of the Internet in Shaping Deaf Geographies." *Social and Cultural Geography* 9 (5): 469–85.

———. 2009. "'An Umbilical Cord to the World': The Role of the Internet in D/deaf People's Information and Communication Practices." *Information, Communication, and Society* 12 (1): 44–65.

Williams, D. 2005. *Autism: An Inside-Out Approach: An Innovative Look at the Mechanics of Autism and Its Developmental Cousins.* London: Kingsley.

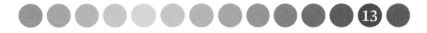

13

Autism and the Task of the Translator

Kristina Chew

> But over the years of working at it [Catullus poem 101], I came
> to think of translating as a room, not exactly an unknown room,
> where one gropes for the light switch. I guess it never ends.
>
> —*Anne Carson,* Nox *(2010)*

Writing, Representation, Translation

In writing about autism, whether by an autistic person or any other individual, representation is always an issue. In my son Charlie's life, he
is regularly being represented—by a teacher in his communication note-
book, by a therapist on a progress report, and by me here. The quandary
in representing Charlie is that he, the one being represented, is, all too
often, limited in his ability to speak back and up about himself. I write
about my son knowing that I may be very wrong about what he experiences, that it may be a very long time before he uses language to tell me
and that indeed that may never happen.

Explaining "what autism is" is very often the stated intention of
many texts that claim autism as their subject. In scientific and other
academic scholarship on autism, the meaning of autism is often presented implicitly and unproblematically, as the text overtly dwells on
the details of causes and treatments. If we can know what autism is, it
is presumed, we can know better how to treat it, to help persons on the
autism spectrum. In order to "help," however, we need to know both
what autism is and what autism means; otherwise, our definitions risk
being accurate but insignificant and risk erasing the autistic others for
whom we ostensibly speak. But how do we access and make sense of this
meaning? Can Charlie represent himself?

Like poems written in a dead language, the communications of
"nonverbal" or "minimally verbal" autistic people—including Charlie—
are routinely perceived as so difficult to decode that they verge on the
untranslatable and unknowable. This perception invites us to displace

autistic voices with our own. But what if we presume that, like scraps of papyrus that once contained a complete text, there is something being communicated and that it bears meaning? This chapter opens with a brief examination of current conventional approaches to speaking for and about autism and autistic people. The remainder of the chapter explores alternatives, discussing my own representational practice with Charlie and drawing on Walter Benjamin's understanding of translation as a framework for recentering people with autism as makers of meaning.

Public Representations of Autism

Contemporary accounts of autism appear in a range of genres, including films, literature, blogs, journalism, scholarship, and scientific work. However, rather than offering a nuanced reading of the subject, the limited and sometimes simply inaccurate representations of autism in such texts potentially do more harm than good. In these accounts, I see people like my son represented as the bearers of medical and mythic pathologies.

As a medical pathology, autism is represented as something you can "catch," like an infectious disease. This view has been reinforced by theories linking autism to vaccines, particularly the common childhood vaccine for measles, mumps, and rubella (for a full discussion of this issue, see Offit 2008). Claims that children "got" autism after being vaccinated have received widespread media and online coverage, often quoting credible sources. For instance, in 2006, neurologist Jon Poling described his daughter as becoming "screaming, feverish, and irritable" after her MMR, then gradually turning off "like a dimmer switch" (quoted in Stobbe 2008). Others describe more sudden reactions, even claiming that their children developed autism "overnight" ("Cliff" 2009). In either case, autism is rendered as an epidemic that, like cancer, overcomes formerly typical, healthy children.

The characterization of autism as an external pathology that invades and harms otherwise well bodies often slides from medical into mythic terms, as if it were an evil force that, like a troll in Norse legends, kidnaps a child at night and leaves a monstrous changeling in its place. This trope may be implicit or, in some cases, overtly deployed. For instance, in writing about her autistic son, prominent parent advocate Portia Iverson says:

It was his mind they came for. They came to steal his mind.

Before anyone gave it a name, even before I knew what it was, I knew it was in our house. . . . Believe me. They were very, very dark things. And there was no way to get rid of them.

Sometimes I could hear them, late at night, when the house was very quiet; a creaking sound, an inexplicable hiss, a miniscule pop, a whistle out of nowhere. . . .

Night after night, I sat beside his crib. I knew he was slipping away from us, away from our world. . . .

And then one day, it happened. He was gone. (2006, xii–xiv)

This supernatural tale stands in stark contrast to the brain research, neuroscience, and laboratories that occupy most of Iverson's book, as if autism is a disaster that science cannot bring to account. Grim, mythic framing recurs in images of autism as a "nightmare without end," a catastrophe that turns a normal, happy family into a site of tragedy, ruled by the strange and terrible behaviors of the not-quite-human autistic child, often rendered in graphic detail (Beavers 1981).

In both medical and mythic frames, we respond to autism by trying to cure the autistic child's contagion. There is, thus, a burgeoning, diverse field of therapies for autism. Though the credibility and efficacy of these therapies is, in many cases, indeterminate, they all rest on the representation of autism as a condition that can be cured. Historically, these causes were primarily psychological, dwelling on bad parenting and the relational failings of "refrigerator mothers" (Kanner 1949). The current biomedical turn has largely discredited such psychogenic theory, calling instead on physiological cures, but both approaches rely on images of real children "imprisoned" within an autistic shell.

This dominant framing of autism is countered in blogs and books and on Web sites by parent advocates who position it as "difference" rather than pathology and, more and more, by the first-person accounts of autistic people themselves.[1] Even with such a wide variety of accounts, in several years of daily writing online about autism and studying its representation on the Internet, I have seen little concrete change. Again and again, I have noted a sharp divide between my own experience of raising Charlie and these commonplace frameworks, between the terms of horror and our own admittedly difficult but rich and meaningful lives together. Despite the persistent efforts of writers and researchers on the

autism spectrum, mainstream pejorative representations of autism re-
tain a powerful grip on our conscious and unconscious perceptions.

Finding other, more adequate ways to express and ascribe meaning
to Charlie's experiences requires new representational practices. As a
linguist and classicist, I see these challenges as akin to the problems of
reading and translating ancient texts.

Representing Charlie via Sappho

I teach Latin and ancient Greek—languages that are called "dead" because they are not spoken today as anyone's native tongue but that are
still studied as meaningful relics of inaccessible civilizations. My students, for instance, might pore over Sappho's fragment number 152:

> παντοδαπαισι μεμειχμενα χροιαισιν
> [pantodapais(i) mem(e)ichmena chroiaisin]
> (with all sorts of colors mingled)

For Sappho, these three words did not make a poem; fifth-century ancient Greek lyric poetry was written in meter and originally performed
to the accompaniment of the lyre. However, we study it as poetry, because it is all we have—a literal fragment of a fragile papyrus scroll
unearthed from the sands of Egypt, often from an ancient garbage pile,
or a scrap quoted by an ancient grammarian, who saw no need to offer a
full citation. Often, three Greek words from a lost poem seem to represent how much Charlie says in proportion to what he wishes to say. The
rest, while within him, could be called "lost" to his listeners, just as
the rest of Sappho's poem is lost.

I am not trying to say that Charlie has some special talent for speaking in language recalling poetry, but knowing how to read poetry for
its sonic, rhythmic, and musical qualities has aided my understanding
both of what Charlie is trying to tell me and of autism more generally.
And the long hours and days and years in Charlie's presence have taught
me that the years I spent studying poetry and dead languages were not
such a waste, as I thought; they help me hear him, as much as my more
recent learning in psychology, neurology, neuroscience, linguistics, and
medicine do.

Like reading poetry, listening to my boy involves tuning my ear to the sound of his language, his idiom. Charlie's communications can often be termed "telegraphic," in that a minimum of words is used and with minimal adornment (definite articles, conjunctions for transitions, conjugations to note verb tense, and so on). Charlie tends to repeat the same syllable, like Sappho's repetition of the *m* in fragment number 152. Such repetition may be seen as meaningless, but it's also a way for him to process his own speech and communication, practicing a sound over and over and so allowing himself to hear it. He will also repeat whole words, such as "Barney." To many listeners, the word is completely out of context, but it bears meaning for Charlie, who uses the name of the purple dinosaur from a 1990s children's television show to express worry and anxiety. Or, that is, I speculate that this is what it means.

Translating Charlie

I have studied a number of languages: French, Latin, ancient Greek, Mandarin, German, Italian, Arabic, and modern Greek. When I was in school, speaking in a foreign language was absolutely not my forte, so I ended up studying Latin and ancient Greek, as well as, for two years, classical Chinese. Now, much less hampered by being overly self-scrutinizing and worrying about making the proverbial fool of myself, I do a lot better trying to stumble my way through speaking in a foreign language. Though lacking scientific data to back up this claim, I believe that all the languages I know have helped me better understand Charlie. I don't expect the subject of a sentence to be the first word. I can see how an adjective can be used as a verb, and I can tell when a verbal idea (like "wanting" or "giving") is expressed even when a verb is not used. I'm not bothered by the omission of definite articles (Latin has none). Of course, a word—even the apparently straightforward "no"—can bear multiple meanings based on context. And, just because some verbal utterance is incomprehensible in English, that does not mean it is not an actual word or phrase.

This last point in particular may be why I never think of any sound Charlie produces as "babble" or "nonsense" or "just meaningless sound." If you start from the premise that every utterance is meaningful and that Charlie, though severely limited in his speech, is bursting with communicative intent, you start to see how much he is communicating, however little he speaks in recognizable words. Charlie means more with a single word (even "no") than those of us who don't have speech delays or disabilities. Accessing that meaning, however, often requires translation.

For example, let me tell you about a day in early November 2010. Charlie had been saying "no school tomorrow" for a few days. This was a sign that he was very aware of there being a short week at school coming up because of the Thanksgiving holiday. That morning, Charlie had woken up at just the right time to be able to get into the car without rushing. His class was scheduled to go swimming, and he had a good time doing laps and jumping into the water. He enjoyed his usual bike ride and evening lemonade run to the convenience store. After we got back, he announced that he wanted to go to bed. I helped him find some videos on his iPad and bade him good night. "Tickle mom," said Charlie.

This is one of those phrases of Charlie's that means a bit more than it might seem to. "Tickle" often means "come on over and do something for me," a relic of Charlie being asked to "come and do this and you'll get a tickle"—something he very much liked when he was younger. That night, however, Charlie did not want me to do anything for him. Once I was back in his room, I realized that he just wanted to tell me something, as he looked me right in the eye and said, "Gong Gong's hand, Po Po's hand, Dad's hand."

How do I translate this text? When he was younger, Charlie's father and I held Charlie's hand all the time. Inevitably, I held his hand a lot, and he liked to switch whose hand he was holding. The meaning of his statement, I'll posit, was that he had hanging out with my parents— Gong Gong and Po Po—on his mind. But is this an accurate reading of his statement and its significance? Whatever the meaning for Charlie, I was quite thrilled that he had called me back into his room just to tell me something.

Getting Some Help from Walter Benjamin

I approach speaking for and with Charlie like a translator who does not know the language of the original text and works without a dictionary or grammar guide, keenly aware that mistranslation is likely, if not inevitable, as I transform what's said from one language into the terms of another. In doing so, I get help from literary theorist, cultural critic, and philosopher Walter Benjamin's approach to translation (1969), which, pace Google Translate, is a task requiring human intervention and art. My intent is not, as the mother of an autistic child, to overintellectualize Charlie's "babble," but rather to understand it in all of its richness and levels of meaning.

If my responsibility as Charlie's translator is to ensure his centrality as a maker of meaning rather than to displace him with my own voice, it would seem that my duty is to produce a faithful rendering of his communication in which his speech is literally transposed into a more widely intelligible form. But if, as Benjamin points out, "all translation is only a somewhat provisional way of coming to terms with the foreignness of languages" (1969, 75), this kind of faithful rendering may be elusive.

The demand for literal translation appeals for obvious justifications, but its legitimacy is actually quite obscure. A proper translation, according to Benjamin, "instead of resembling the meaning of the original, must lovingly and in detail incorporate the original's mode of signification, thus making both the original and the translation recognizable as fragments of a greater language, just as fragments are part of a vessel" (78). I am struck, in reading this, by Benjamin's characterization of this labor as loving. Why, of all the descriptions available, did he settle on "lovingly and in detail"? Surely this sets translation apart from the objective, distanced stance that we presume inclines us toward accuracy. Because of my intense personal connections with my son and our relational investments in one another, my efforts to translate are necessarily entangled in love, but Benjamin seems to be saying that *all* translational acts must inhabit a space of love. Perhaps this—which is not just a nicety but, according to Benjamin, the absence of which is a material, falsifying lack—is what I miss in many popular accounts of autism.

Incorporating the original's mode of signification—its way of making meaning—means that I must show, in my translations, that I am carefully gluing back together the fragments of an original text, like bits of a broken pot. I do not hide the seams or the fact that I am translating; disguising my mediation would displace the original and put my voice in Charlie's mouth. A real translation, Benjamin suggests, "does not cover the original, does not black its light," but allows the "pure language" to shine through (79). This implicitly assumes that, even if all we can access is broken shards, both what Charlie says and the way he speaks— his mode of signification—bear meaning, and both must be conveyed in a good translation. Thus, "as regards the meaning, the language of a translation can—in fact, must—let itself go, so that it gives voice to the *intentio* [intention] of the original not as reproduction but as harmony, as a supplement to the language in which it expresses itself, as its own kind of *intentio*" (79).

In theoretical terms, this calls me to shift away from seeing Charlie as a failed speaker of my language and to regard his speech instead as fragments retrieved from a foreign, but not inherently inferior, system of making meaning. It is, in short, a shift into a position of respect. Benjamin is elevating translation from a mundane process of linguistic conversion into something more like a mystical art, preserving the "echo of the original" (76) as well as its intent. The translation seeks not to unify with the original but, rather, to stand in harmony to it—which, to extend Benjamin's musical metaphor, requires the preservation and careful management of tonal separation and difference, such that the translation supports and extends the original melody without simply repeating it. Instead of speaking for Charlie, perhaps I am singing along with him.

In practical terms, this kind of translation is achieved through "a literal rendering of the syntax" (79), that is, through a focus on words rather than sentences as units of meaning. The difference is significant. So often, there is an urgent desire, a rush, to understand the utterances of someone on the autism spectrum, to "make sense"—and too often, the result is a bad translation, a misrepresentation of meaning that somewhat, sort of captures what was meant but makes potentially fatal errors that may even involve reversals of meaning. We are propelled, by our impatience and discomfort with ambiguity, to rush to closure, imputing intent to clusters of sounds.

Translating with the word as the basic unit is difficult; it can result in the translator—in anyone—losing capacity for words, period; being consigned to silence. Benjamin describes this happening to the poet Friedrich Hölderlin in his efforts to translate Sophocles's tragedies word for word. This problem has been more recently explored by Anne Carson, who intermixes her word-by-word translation of one Latin poem by Catullus with rumination over the death of her brother. Carson describes how her mind wavers in translating a single word: "Prowling the meaning of a word, prowling the history of a person, no use expecting a flood of light. Human words have no main switch.

But all those little kidnaps in the dark. And then the luminous, big, shivering, discarded, unrepentant, barking web of them that hangs in your mind when you turn back to the page you were trying to translate" (2010, *frater*).[2] Carson shows us how it is possible to get lost in a word, providing a full-page meditation on the definition and meaning of each word of the poem, within a book that, as a whole, offers a gloss of its one-word title, *Nox*. Bearing witness to our own insufficiency, to the inscrutability of the otherness we are trying to speak for and represent, across unfathomable distance—this recognition of the necessity and futility of our attempts to know can leave us speechless.

Carson also describes, beautifully, the affective response to translating Charlie, making conceptual space for the way a phrase of his speech—"No Dad, bye Dad, all done Dad [pause]. Dad will be back. Dad back. Hi Dad!"—hangs within me as a "luminous, big, shivering, discarded, unrepentant, barking web." She names the feeling of turning his fragments of speech in my mind, knowing that I have so few of the pieces, that I cannot even imagine the original shape of the broken pot, but that, nonetheless, these utterances carry the traces of an intent, a mode of signification, that bears meaning.

Why focus on the word, if it is so difficult? Most of Charlie's utterances consist of one to three words, but the weight of each word in *Nox* gives an idea of what each of Charlie's words is truly saying, a thick enfolding of meanings, images, memories, and fragments, full of "little kidnaps in the dark." Translating them is like trying to assemble a jigsaw puzzle with no picture on the box; because we do not have a visual aid, we necessarily focus on the contours of each bit and on how they might fit together to produce possible meanings.

Dwelling on the word offers recognition that, instead of creating a new, seamless pot that stands in for Charlie's voice, the best translation places emphasis on the reassemblage of the fragmented pieces (the words) rather than on getting them in exactly the right configuration. The point is that some whole, even if it is not precisely the same as the original, is created. Hopefully, it retains the echo of the original, conveying *intentio* without concealing the seams and missing pieces, but we admit that we might be completely wrong. Benjamin thus moves a step (at least) beyond mourning the notion of "lost in translation"; what is lost is given, and the point of translation is not to chase what cannot be had, what is gone with history, but to put together what one can.

Thus, it is most important to get the meanings of individual words as close to accurate as possible.

Bad Translations

If we admit that our translations will never, so to speak, put the broken vessel back together and that the pot of words we can produce is, at best, full of patches and gaps and perhaps so partial that it cannot contain meaning in any stable sense—if this is the best that translation can do, what constitutes a "bad" translation? Benjamin argues that the hallmark of bad translation is its transmission of an "inessential context" (1969, 79), of something not intended by its author, something not in the original work. Such transmission occurs because the translator is projecting too much about an imagined reader or audience rather than translating the work in and of itself: "This will be true whenever a translation undertakes to serve the reader. However, if it were intended for the reader, the same would have to apply to the original. If the original does not exist for the reader's sake, how could the translation be understood on the basis of this premise?" (70). Bad translations, thus, have little to do with the inherent limits of what I hear from Charlie. Instead, they arise from a preoccupation with his audience, the people for whom I am trying to render his utterances comprehensible—including, of course, myself.

It is fair to say that bad translations happen all the time in the conversion of meaning into communication. A translator, especially if she is working across significant difference, can have only a limited sense of the original *intentio* of the author. When Charlie speaks, he is not, I presume, expressing his intent to communicate with the readers who may later encounter my rendering of his words in this chapter or on my blog.[3] When I translate Charlie's utterances for other audiences, I change their meaning.

To some extent, I believe that trying to serve the audience is warranted. I can see that it is not Charlie's concern that we can't understand his communications, which, I imagine, must make sense to him. Yet it is his concern in that, because of the extent of his speech and communication disability, he's quite aware that we don't understand him. Bad translations arise when the needs—the mode of signification—of the audience "blacks out" the original intent. This is what I see when people like Charlie are rendered as medical and mythic pathologies, when accounts of autistic speech and behavior are presented not as inherently meaningful artifacts but as evidence of the autistic person's status as diseased, deviant, or tragic. Such representations arise from our notions of normalcy and health, our social and physical fears. Surely, this is not how Charlie makes sense of his own experience. Invoking these modes of signification may serve the audience, but it cannot provide an adequate translation.

In working with Charlie, I assume, first, that he wants to communicate and, second, that he is communicating, albeit in unusual, often behavioral or nonverbal ways. I presume that everything Charlie says and much of what he does has some meaning and is translatable. I cannot verify these assumptions, but they provide the only ethically and relationally viable position I can occupy, the only location from which I can, as Benjamin demands, receive Charlie's communications "lovingly and in detail." Translators must make the assumption that their own language can somehow convey the meaning of another one, that there is a kinship of languages. This is not always the case; Benjamin points out that translatability depends on two questions: "Will an adequate translator ever be found . . . ? Or, more pertinently, Does its nature lend itself to translation and, therefore . . . call for it?" (1969, 70).

I do not know. So much of what Charlie expresses remains inscrutable, shards I cannot fit together, so partial that I cannot even trace the contours of the pieces I am missing. But this is my commitment to my boy, who calls me back to his room after tuck-in, to try to speak to me: I will keep trying to understand.

Conclusion

Why intellectualize my son's few verbalizations and interpret—or over-interpret—them, far beyond what they are? Such intellectualizing characterizes humanities and social sciences autism research and critical autism studies itself and is far from Charlie's own mode of signification. Although "autism" is an abstraction, it is tightly connected to a reality, to autistic individuals who are real, out there, and who are much more than their representations. Questioning our practice in the way that we theorize and represent autistic people, and drawing on thinkers like Benjamin to help us do so, is a necessary response to our encounters with difference. Instead of presuming that perfect translations are possible, such an approach calls us to humility and attentive engagement in an ongoing struggle to bear witness to those who cannot readily represent themselves in terms we can comprehend.

It is a huge responsibility to represent Charlie in language and writing, to be his advocate to obtain the services and educational programming that he needs now and that he will need for the rest of his life. I spend a lot of time trying to read his behavior and words, to decode both his meaning and his mode of signification. Being his parent requires me to constantly speak for him, even though I do not—and cannot—know exactly what he thinks or wants or would prefer. My ever-potential misinterpretation and misrepresentation of Charlie and of autistic experience in general makes it all the more imperative that I try to record what I see as faithfully as possible. I offer a well-intentioned, ethically compelled attempt. I know that my translation is faulty, even false, but without some kind of translator, Charlie's struggles to be known would likely be lost and overlooked altogether, like shreds of papyrus never sifted from the desert sand.

NOTES

1. The list of such blogs is long and ever-changing; one by a parent with a positive view of autism is Estée Klar, esteeklar.com. Writings by self-advocate Dora Raymaker about disability and autism rights can be found at http://doraraymaker .com/doraraymaker.com/ or http://intralimina.dreamwidth.org/.

2. In *Nox*, Carson translates poem 101, *Multas per gentes et multa per aequora* (Through many peoples and many seas), by the Roman poet Gaius Valerius Catullus. Catullus's poem is addressed to his late brother, who had died in Asia Minor, far from their home in Italy. Carson's book is about her own brother, who died far from his native Canada in Denmark after having wandered around the globe. Each page of *Nox* contains one word from Catullus's poem, along with a dictionary entry about the word and other text and/or images. *Nox* is unpaginated; to refer to a particular page of the book, a reader can refer to a particular word from Catullus's poem. I have, therefore, referenced the page quoted in the text by noting the word *frater*.

3. I write a daily weblog about our life raising Charlie, called *We Go with Him*, http://autism.typepad.com.

REFERENCES

Beavers, D. J. 1981. *Autism: Nightmare without End*. Maplewood, N.J.: Ashley.
Benjamin, W. 1969. "The Task of the Translator." In *Illuminations*, translated by H. Zohn, 69–82. New York: Schocken. Originally published as "Die Arbeit des Übersetzers" (1923).

Carson, A. 2010. *Nox.* New York: New Directions.

"Cliff." 2009. Comment on "Court Rules Vaccines Not to Blame for Autism," by S. Gupta. "The Chart," *CNN Health*, February 12, 2009. Accessed October 10, 2011, http://thechart.blogs.cnn.com/2009/02/12/court-rules-vaccines-not-to-blame-for-autism/.

Iverson, Portia. 2006. *Strange Son: Two Mothers, Two Sons, and the Quest to Unlock the Hidden World of Autism.* New York: Riverhead.

Kanner, L. 1949. "Problems of Nosology and Psychodynamics of Early Infantile Autism." *American Journal of Orthopsychiatry* 19: 416–26.

Offit, P. 2008. *Autism's False Prophets: Bad Science, Risky Medicine, and the Search for a Cure.* New York: Columbia University Press.

Stobbe, M. 2008. "Parents Speak Out on Vaccine Settlement." *USA Today*, March 6, 2008. Accessed October 10, 2011, http://www.usatoday.com/news/health/2008-03-06-3419893127_x.htm.

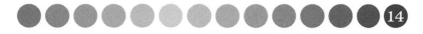

14

"All the Things I Have Ever Been"
Autoethnographic Reflections on Academic Writing and Autism

Dawn Eddings Prince

W hen neurotypical people picture people on the spectrum, usually stereotypes come to mind in spite of the ongoing efforts of
those on the spectrum who are able to bridge the communication gap
and tell their own stories in their own words. Perhaps this is human nature; certainly there are examples everywhere, in every clique and niche,
of people whom one might describe as having "autistic" tendencies, or
perhaps more accurately as having stereotypically autistic tendencies:
singularity, an insular view of reality, a certain rigidity and love of reliable patterns that exclude or prohibit an easy flow, or a kind of encompassing, of the widest possible approach to awareness of all things.

Although I quit school as a teenager, having been taunted for my
autistic habits, I eventually found my passion in anthropology and went
back to school. I finally excelled: my ability to focus intently, my immersion style of learning, and my photographic memory were all great
tools for my college experience. As I have become more and more en-
sconced in academia, following its rules and learning to speak its language, I have always been aware that I and all the things and perhaps
even people I am are lost in its translation. I have become increasingly
disturbed that there is only one "me" that is welcomed and embraced in
this erudite and tamed country in the lingua franca. I have become increasingly uncomfortable seeing the autistic stereotype in the academic
mirror, and I am not speaking of the careless imprints of experts speaking for those on the spectrum; rather, I see in the style of the writing itself the very thing I do not wish to serve: the singular and exclusionary
nature of academic writing, its own insular view of reality, its beloved
rigidity and reliable patterns.

For me, language is blended inextricably to context and memory.

Even when I was a child, this melding represented the most important thing in the world, and everything, from bathrooms to snails to dogs, had language. If a thing existed, it existed as a living part of language and had a deep understanding of its place in the vibrations of speech, in the vibrations of existence. This whole cloth of speech and living things made my world a magical place.

I learned very early, however, that for most people, language was a kind of weapon rather than an amorphous mist of the birth waters of reality. It seemed that for most speaking humans, language could be considered a violent activity, in that it cut up the world and its use also cut groups of people one from another. A knife was just a knife and bore no relationship to the cutting of language. A chair was just a chair where nothing sat. A breath was just a breath, a singular thing apart from the heart, apart from the atmosphere, a thing separate from saying.

In this way, I knew that language was as important to other people as it was to me, but in a dangerous way. The silence between their words was just as full of cutting as the silence between my words was a place of connection.

When I was young I talked to animals in that language of silence. I knew what trees and streams were saying, because they told me. I knew what sow bugs and snakes were saying, because they molded me. I grew together with them because of the words of living together in a world where everything needed everything else. Sometimes my grandfather would ask me in the garden, "What are the worms saying today?" "Fine fine slither dirt push good rotting green," I would answer, smiling. My grandfather, in his love and understanding, never told me how important it was to talk like everyone you were supposed to emulate. There was no place for saying that tomato plants said, "Sun warm summer, pushing, pushing green, green red, red," or that fish said, "Cold float shade shade shade."

After I moved far away from my grandparents, dropped out of school, became homeless, and ultimately decided to go back to school, I renewed my efforts to follow the rules that normal people use in language. Maybe it was easier for me to follow certain rules by then because I was in an academic setting and the rules are very specific when it comes to sharing your reality through the use of language. For example, you must always show when and where someone said something before you did. You must show that your ideas are not original but built on the previous ideas of others, specifically, the ideas of people who have learned to follow the rules and say what still other people said before them. Another example concerns the necessity of showing your distance from the things you are communicating, because if you have strong feelings about them, then you aren't being objective. Why people would want to write and talk about things on which they had no definite opinions escaped me, but I tried to follow the rules.

Primarily, in those days, I was writing about primates and their language—which was punctuated by long, integrating silences that I understood, rich in concepts of being still in the world and not designed to cut things apart—and I realized that their way of speaking, the language that I listened to and took for granted, once again whole, might as well have been a stone in the bottom of a pond to the other academics with whom I spoke. Always the debate raged about whether gorillas could be sentient, whether they could be intelligent. It always boiled down to the "fact" that they didn't have language at all. They didn't have academic language.

As someone who has been labeled in so many ways and has seen what "factual" information can be turned into, the kinds of cruelty that use language as a knife and bludgeon, I am in constant question of the sharp and heavy "facts." Now, whenever people say "fact" in this way, I feel a catch in my chest and a tear across the language. If you say it carefully and listen, like I do, you will hear that *fact* is a terrible word: The first letter starts out angry, the same letter that starts words like *freak* and *forget*. The harsh *a* sound that comes next is the sound of terror, of someone falling off a cliff and knowing the end will come and can't be stopped. The *c* and the *t* that finish it might as well just spell *cut* and be done. The whole word conjured in my mind a gorilla, a person, stabbed in the heart and pushed off a precipice, quickly forgotten.

I have encountered the "facts" and the language prejudice surrounding and upholding them when it comes to autistic people, too. If you couldn't speak the lingua franca of the normal, then you had to be stupid and therefore disposable. The difficulties we have had describing what language means to us in the midst of this possible unfolding dialogue are now being bridged. I hope that autistic people and others who have been beyond understanding until recently will be the natural interpreters of an important patois. The world that words are making whole for us will no longer be rent asunder, and our attempts to share our experiences of language in ways that are very different will not cut. It will be a softer fact, corrected, setting things on a wider and more sustainable path. We will be connected with ear and spirit; what people often forget is that listening is the superior half of speaking.

Like most people on the spectrum, I am not one person, a vested persona easily finding refuge in the walls of this castle, or even one thing: not even a "human being," for that matter. Like most people on the spectrum, it is my very nature to be a million things in one moment: the green in the wind, the crackle of thinking people all around me, the small balm of elusive quiet. The times that I have rocked in the corner, seemingly as bound and worn as any reliable academic tome, were the times that I was all the things I have ever been.

As I write now, there is a climate of fear and anticipation, extremes of wealth and poverty, and in the midst of despair and illness of body and soul, there is a touching belief in connection. As people do in such times, I have sought out my friends and loved ones. We have tried to lean on each other like God's smaller shoulder, and, again as people have always done, we take mirrors up to reflect upon ourselves and our condition: the conditions of living and dying, being together and apart, reflections of what it means to be human or something less, something more.

At a party recently, I was talking with one of my best friends as we looked out on a lake in the mountains, the sun going down, the silent flight of birds fast skimming the slow-moving surface like glass. We watched them for a long time, seeing the back of the fast bird and then the hidden softness of its underbelly projected on the still water as the flight went on and on. My friend is a quiet man. We didn't need to talk to know we were feeling the same thing, reflecting on the world as we sat there. It was I who finally broke the silence. "I've been everything," I said to my friend. Because he knew my story, he nodded without saying a word. I had been a prodigy, a mental failure, a soda-fountain worker, a piece of the land, a painter, a forestry-crew worker, an erotic dancer, a homeless druggie, a gorilla, a successful author, a stable worker, a rich person with powerful and talented friends, a married person, a divorced person, a criminal, a hero, a mother, a woman, a man, a white person, a black person, a young person, an old person. Regaining my freedom from prison words, I have been the wind, the water, the mayfly, and the dark.

Some of these things any other person could see as literal experiences.

For those who don't know my story, I was born unassembled. Having none of the filters and templates that most human beings are born with, I instead came out disembodied, all I sensed around me becoming me— no remembered barriers between myself and the world. My parents, my grandparents, the trees outside, the thunderstorms in the spring, the flavor of the dirt, the songs of all marrow; these things were my body, and I had no body at all. Of course, I come from a long line of people who were strange and pasted together out of these kinds of torn cloth, so I didn't know that this was an experience outside of most people's memories. Like bright stars in an infinite sky, we knew how to dance within our gravity, invisible orbits making us part of a greater universe.

But when I started school, I quickly learned that my way of being made me different from everyone else who surrounded me. A normal transition for the other children, the clanging of bells, the bright primary colors all around, the hard chairs facing one way, the smell of other children, and even the smell of disapproval—all came to rest in my infinite body like arrows broken from the shaft or melted fragments too dangerous to remove. A smart child, I was so overwhelmed on a sensory level that all I could hope to do was make it through each day and then come home to crawl away into the forgiving woods or the darkness of my closet.

Exhausted after years of this ritual, I began to look stupid. I couldn't relate to people or do my schoolwork or even answer direct questions. I tried to find ways to cope. I had what I thought was the brilliant idea of becoming something else—or, more correctly, of interpreting parts of my infinite body. I would be a dog. Everyone loves dogs, even if they don't talk good. So I crawled around on the floor of my classroom, barking and wagging my tail. That didn't work out so well for anyone involved. Neither did being a horse.

Of course, I could be anything, any part of nature when I would bound down the stairs and off the school bus into the arms of the waiting forest. I was the oldest evergreen at the top of the hill, and I could feel its fragrant blue berries in my fingertips, my toes rooted. I was melt in the stream that went through our land, and the blood in my mind wound along its trail, my heart filled with freshness and fish. I sang old songs, just sung to the grass and the sky. This was rest and solace. This was my balm. Still, Gilead lay silent under the bed in my room, and lying down to think of the next day at school made it impossible to sleep.

All night I would stare, paralyzed, at the ceiling. Sometimes I would feel my own fears slip from my spine, traveling down and around, leaking into the room where I could see them. Then I was too scared to call for my mother, or for mercy of any kind. I knew there was none.

Teachers just found me irritating, intractable, spoiled, or disruptive. One teacher screamed at me until her angry spit was all over my face. I was sent to the principal. I was tested for mental retardation. By the time I started high school, I simply had straight Ds and Fs on my report cards. A problem; the teachers just kept passing me along. My sole coping strategy by then was to ignore everyone. No one existed. I was really alone, and nothing was coming in or going out. I discovered drinking and drugs. So many forms of pain and so many forms of painkillers there are. Finally, I quit school after barely finishing my junior year of high school. I had no friends, no idea how to function, no ability to see normal time, and I certainly saw no future. In spite of trying to work and live what people thought of as a normal life, I ended up homeless for five years off and on, just wandering around. Wherever I could find people to take me in, or with whoever was traveling to the next city, I would go. I would sleep anywhere, with anyone, eat anything, take any drug or drink I could find, let anyone use me in any way. Dawn was dead. I was still a ghost, just as I had been when I was born; but I was no longer the quiet, friendly ghost, one that might be fun to see or read about. I was a bad ghost, made of the sound of wind off the cold storm, the smell of garbage for food and old coats, the feel of ice that had died. Like blowing garbage on a winter street, you wouldn't see me if you passed me, but you would be disturbed by something; something in your subconscious mind would be subtly reminded of something that scared you as a child or worried you about the future.

In the early 1980s, I found myself in Seattle, still homeless. I slept in the hidden doorways of churches. I danced naked for some money. In the industrial scape of the city and its grit, I absorbed the fact that I was far from nature, far from natural. I had grown up in nature and always had that connection with nature and animals. And so it was with one of my first paychecks from dancing that I decided to go out to the zoo, and that was the moment that changed my life.

Disheveled, angry hair at all angles, in my old and torn black coat, I must have seemed like a wild animal trying to get back to its proper cage as I navigated the bus system up to Phinney Avenue, already having to strain in the kaleidoscope that was always my vision to see the number 5 bus, to get on and see where the money went to pay for the ride, to continue to ride through that kaleidoscope to find the right stop. I had to find my way in.

I wandered around much of the zoo. I still felt blind and temporary, moving slow surrounded by a human race, people racing to see the things in cages, screaming, bright, and holiday. Then I came around a corner and saw the gorillas. So solid, so dark and unmoving, grounded to earth by the cables of memory and current presence, slow-moving and silent. Almost as if I had finally exhaled after a lifetime, I collapsed and sat on the ground near the glass. I knew immediately that I had found people. These were people who could understand me; and even more profoundly, people I could understand. I sat there for hours.

After that, whenever I could afford it, I would go to the zoo just to sit and be near the gorillas. Each time, after I had been there about an hour, a gorilla here and there would glance at me in the slightest and most unobtrusive way, telling me they noticed me, telling me in a way so unfamiliar to human discourse—slowly, slowly, without staring or manic movements or machine-gun words—that I was welcome. I would glance at them, trying to make my heart say something, sitting frozen, a dumb animal.

I know they heard me. Over the weeks, then months, the gorillas and I came to recognize each other; and more, to see not just our individual personalities but also the ways in which artificial and arbitrary glass partitions make no difference. Like me in so many ways, the gorillas felt part of everything. They, like me, were unsuited to draw lines between all things; constantly fighting to maintain what is "inside" and what is "outside" seems to be a sole and singular human pursuit that makes for the imaginary line between our blessed destiny and that of the rest of creation.

I watched them like this for years, silently learning that there was nothing wrong with me. This family of gorillas, like a First Nation, gave me the peace of place. After years of longing, I finally belonged. I would bring books and articles to the zoo—all I could find about gorillas—and I would read as I watched them. I studied them in films and on television, anywhere I could learn about them. I often asked, in a stiff and stilted way, the questions I had about this one particular family; I would ask questions of the keepers, even the people who swept trash near their cage.

People working there got to know me and had a kind of respect for my passion for the gorillas and how much I obviously cared for them.

After years of dust had buried me, after years of tears had choked me, I was waking up. I was watching the gorillas with a clearer mind, a healed view. The matriarch of this family, Nina, was slowly teaching me about the power of observation and the practical motions of soothing, caring; each time she caressed her children or sat quietly watching them play, I was able to see it all, unfragmented.

Their calm way of being, their slowness and predictability, their awareness and inclusion made it possible to see social cause and effect. I could watch young Zuri and his sister Alafia playing and see what the rules were. I saw in Pete, their father, how a person like me, stripped of natural context and natural home, could be damaged and powerless. He scowled out from under his deep-set eyes, trying to ignore the rude public banging on barriers to get at his children, the endless human stream of glancers pushing by fast, wanting a show. To the public, the gorillas were just things in a circus, a pause to entertain, a chance to draw a line. We are not like them, people would always say.

It deeply hurt me to see the ways that "normal" people treated the gorillas. Not only for those few early years that I was learning from the gorillas to understand what it was like to be a social animal, but over the many years to come as I slowly came out of my shell of accretion and learned enough skills—as well as found a desire to connect—that I went back to school. Eventually, while my relationship with zoo workers deepened and I began working with the gorillas, I made it all the way through college and then work on an advanced degree. The gorillas were always the subject of my studies—my constant backdrop, my rock. They were my tribe.

After thirteen years of being in the midst of the gorillas, I had healed my life and my heart. But although I was always whole when I sat and heard their rolling purrs, saw their liquid brown eyes looking out on a world we shared, smelled the smell of them, like rhubarb pie in a hot summer field, whenever I went out into the regular world, the one that had so damaged me, I still held together only by knowing that I could go home to them. I still had trouble relating to human beings, navigating the sensory storm that is modern human existence. When it became too much, I would explode. I would yell or throw things or, worse, become silent and dissociated and try to hide for days.

I cared enough about human people at this point to know that I needed to name the thing that made me different. After so many years of pain and struggle, so many seeming lifetimes of being out of step and overwhelmed, I was diagnosed with Asperger Syndrome. After reading about it and knowing that I wasn't alone, knowing other people struggled in the ways I had, I knew I needed to tell the story of how gorillas had given me my personhood. My story became a book. The whole project took on an enormous life of its own.

As my much-publicized book tour for *Songs of the Gorilla Nation* (2004) drew near, I fought the feeling that people who came to hear me would only be showing up for a sideshow, just as they showed up to peer inquisitively or jeer menacingly at the gorillas. They would want to see if my face looked different, if my body moved in some frightening but hypnotizing way, to see, lost in the safety of a crowd on their side, if I would speak strangely, if I would rock and gibber. Maybe they would think I couldn't look back at them, maybe they hoped I couldn't look back at them; placed in a cage in some social way, I would be dirty and stripped, rattling my story in cuts upon the eye, but safe from touching. Safe from being too close.

I had read once about a circus act where a box of illusion turned an ordinary woman into a gorilla. The audience's minds would reel back as they moved in closer, trying to see what was real and what was illusion, their curiosity bleeding them to death through their jangling nerves. They couldn't stop looking. Their experience was of the kind that Freud, speaking of the compelling monstrous, called "that class of frightening which leads back to what is known of old and long familiar" ([1919] 1955, 220). Maybe I would be their missing link.

What I found as I crossed the country and then the world as a carnival of one was that people who came to see me were not there to see me rock and gibber or to scare them with my monstrous difference. They were there to thank me for telling their story, each person feeling a hidden and unique desperation in the knowledge that they were freaks that managed to keep their restless minds, their too obvious differences, their diminished hearts and souls under shrouds. They knew that they weren't normal, but there seemed to be so much evidence around them that normalcy was possible. So they kept trying to both hide and shine.

It was incredible. My story was simply the human story. It had a human voice, even in the truth that it had an ape's face. I felt like the man in the story that circus owner and manager John Robinson, operating in the 1860s, told. One morning, Robinson said, a remarkable specimen of a young man came to the circus grounds, looking for a job. His hair was at least a foot and a half long, and his hair and beard looked like a haystack after a cyclone. He was hired on the spot as a wild man; they even gave him a dollar to bind the contract. They told him to report for work that afternoon. At around one o'clock, the man came back, ready for work. The circus people didn't recognize him. He had spent his dollar at the barber, getting cleaned up for the show. The freak had become anyone and everyone.

Now that I have seen that no one is normal, I know that there is a shadow waiting to be born, waiting to whisper the great human secret that no one is normal; it is a shadow in need of peace, a shadow beyond love or hate. Strangeness isn't a personal matter, a set of characteristics that one person has; oddity is in the way we think about and present people. As Barnum and Bailey's sideshow manager Clyde Ingalls said, "Freaks are what you make them. Take any peculiar looking person, whose familiarity to those around him makes for acceptance, play up that peculiarity and add a good spiel and you have a great attraction." As close as we all are to freakishness, it is no wonder that most people strain to find safe definition.

At times I have seen that kind of comfort and sense of place in the *Diagnostic and Statistical Manual of Mental Disorders*, under the criteria for Asperger Syndrome: "Qualitative impairment in social interaction . . . marked impairments in the use of multiple nonverbal behaviors such as facial expression . . . body postures, and gestures, to regulate social interaction . . . lack of seeking to share enjoyment with other people by a lack of showing, bringing objects of interest to other people . . . a lack of social or emotional reciprocity. The furniture and walls of definition are familiar and comforting. Encompassing preoccupation with patterns of interest" (American Psychiatric Association 2000). For many of us who have been described or diagnosed—by themselves or by someone else— with one kind of official freakishness or another, these listed features have become a kind of penance of memory, a litany of things real or imagined about us, a wailing wall that receives our notes of isolation, of contradiction, of sometimes-reluctant specialty; they shade us from the weather of uncertainty and offers us the shelter of classification.

The comfortable familiarity that lies within the lines of the page, within the diagnosis, within the label, within the ink of distinction, is almost seductive. We define to apprehend. We define to tame. We de-fine the fineness of animal unpredictability and trade it for the confinement of brackets and bars, the static of staying. We make these unwieldy things out of our control become unfinished, the static of staying more peaceful to us than the will of wild. Now that I have seen the Great Human Secret, even I must let those lines and definitions go. I believe now that people—all people—want three things only: to be loved for who they are in spite of their freakishness, to give something of worth, and to be remembered when they are dead. We seldom breathe this great secret in our small lives, between our eating bread and laughing. But it is wild.

We won't be able to keep the secret for much longer. The ways we pass as normal keep us from having any of our three deepest wishes granted like heaven; we can't be loved for who we are, because we hide ourselves, knowing we are freaks; we can't give, because we are often too afraid; and because no one knows who we are or what we can give, we are afraid to die, knowing we can't truly be remembered. Even after death, we won't be allowed to rot and become everyone. Someone always finds us and takes us away from the ground; we are taken away and preserved, an odd and pointless forestalling of the inevitable, continuing to look alive and separate from everything for a generation.

It is from this unnatural hiding, hoarding, our hairless cowering, that all regrets and shame flow. We have polluted our living animal souls, using the smoke to make a false wall between ourselves and the world.

I say if hell is isolation, then we all go there first. We have all been there together. This situation can change.

As a person who has garnered success by being seen as very different, I know I may, if everything goes right, be out of a job if everyone else finally sees things the way I do; but I can't ignore all the people I have met who take my hands, squeeze them fervently, and look deep into my eyes. They know I have seen them. They are grateful that I haven't turned away from my own monstrosity or theirs. All of these pained souls and whisperers of settled secrets would come to finish for me what the gorillas had started. They would become the gray ghosts that I saw behind each living eye, telling me that our collective story is beautiful, if twisted. We are not disabled.

We are everything. We are all beyond description.

I know that academic pieces will no doubt follow and precede mine in this reading. I believe deeply that all the authors have sought to connect meaningfully—even spiritually—with their subject and with the people they share their thoughts with and that they have all good intentions. But I have become convinced that for me, the million me's, academic writing serves to empty the fullness of the thing it seeks to unequivocally contain. It kills the patient in its very prescription. A cutting thing, a surgery of words, it makes the many into one rather than loaning itself to the cause of connection—the very thing so many neurotypical people believe is what is lacking in those on the spectrum. Those chains will no longer come from my own pen.

REFERENCES

American Psychiatric Association. 2000. *DSM-IV-TR: Diagnostic and Statistical Manual of Mental Disorders.* 4th ed., text revision. Arlington, Va.: American Psychiatric Association.

Freud, S. (1919) 1955. "The 'Uncanny.'" In *The Standard Edition of the Complete Psychological Works of Sigmund Freud,* edited by J. Strachey. Vol. 17, 219–52. London: Hogarth.

Prince-Hughes, D. 2004. *Songs of the Gorilla Nation: My Journey through Autism.* New York: Harmony.

Contributors

DANA LEE BAKER is associate professor in the School of Politics, Philosophy, and Public Affairs at Washington State University. Her primary research interests are neurodiversity, neuroethics, and disability-policy design. She is the author of *The Politics of Neurodiversity: Why Public Policy Matters*.

BEATRICE BONNIAU is a research assistant in CERMES3 (Research Center in Medicine, Sciences, Health, Mental Health, and Health Policy) at Paris Descartes University. She works in mental health and social sciences, studying the transformations of representations of autism and the emergence of associations of autistic persons.

CHARLOTTE BROWNLOW is lecturer in psychology at the University of Southern Queensland, Australia. Her research primarily examines the construction of autism, drawing on politics of diversity and difference, and her most recent work explores concepts of space and the challenges between "autistic" and "neurodiverse" spaces

KRISTIN BUMILLER is professor of political science at Amherst College. She is the author of *In an Abusive State* and *The Civil Rights Society*, as well as numerous journal articles that span a broad range of interests in antidiscrimination policy, feminist theory, gender and punishment, and disability rights.

BRIGITTE CHAMAK is an INSERM researcher in history and sociology of medicine in CERMES3 (Research Center in Medicine, Sciences, Health, Mental Health, and Health Policy) at Paris Descartes University. She studies the consequences of changes in the classification of autism and the history of the autism-rights movement. Her current project concerns the social role of neurosciences, the emergence of the neurodiversity concept, and the influence of self-help groups. She publishes in the journals *Sociology of Health and Illness* and *Culture, Medicine, and Psychiatry*.

KRISTINA CHEW is associate professor of classics at Saint Peter's University in Jersey City, New Jersey. She has published a translation of Virgil's *Georgics* and articles on disability studies and literature. She is currently writing about oral composition in Homer's poetry and cognitive science. Since 2005, she has blogged about her son, Charlie, in *We Go with Him* at autism.typepad.com; she also blogs at care2.com.

JOYCE DAVIDSON is associate professor of geography at Queen's University, Canada. She is author of *Phobic Geographies: The Phenomenology and Spatiality of Identity* and coeditor of *Emotional Geographies* and *Emotion, Place, and Culture*. Her research and teaching focus on health, embodiment, and different or "disordered" emotions, and she has published her research on autism in the journals *Social Science and Medicine, Social and Cultural Geography*, and *Gender, Place, and Culture*.

PATRICK McDONAGH is the author of *Idiocy: A Cultural History* and a part-time faculty member in the Department of English at Concordia University, Montreal. He is a cofounder of the Spectrum Society for Community Living in Vancouver, Canada, and serves on Spectrum's board of directors.

STUART MURRAY is professor of contemporary literatures and film in the School of English and the director of the Leeds Centre for Medical Humanities at the University of Leeds, United Kingdom.

MAJIA HOLMER NADESAN is professor in the New College at Arizona State University. She is the author of *Constructing Autism: Unravelling the "Truth" and Understanding the Social; Governmentality, Biopower, and Everyday Life*; and *Governing Childhood*. Her latest book is *Fukushima and the Privatization of Risk*.

CHRISTINA NICOLAIDIS is professor and senior scholar in social determinants of health at Portland State University and adjunct associate professor of medicine at Oregon Health and Science University. During most of her career, she has focused on improving the health and health care of marginalized populations, including adults on the autism spectrum, domestic violence survivors, racial and ethnic minorities, and people with chronic pain or mental illness. She cofounded and codirects the Academic Autistic Spectrum Partnership in Research and Education (AASPIRE).

LINDSAY O'DELL is senior lecturer on children and young people in the Health and Social Care Programme at the Open University, London.

MICHAEL ORSINI is associate professor in the School of Political Studies and director of the Institute of Women's Studies at the University of Ottawa. A former journalist, he specializes in health policy and politics and recently completed a study of health-related social movements (including autism) funded by the Social Sciences and Humanities Research Council of Canada. He is coeditor of *Critical Policy Studies*, and his work has been published in *Social Policy and Administration*, *Social and Legal Studies*, *Canadian Journal of Political Science*, and *Canadian Journal of Urban Research*.

FRANCISCO ORTEGA is associate professor at the Institute for Social Medicine of the State University of Rio de Janeiro and visiting senior research fellow at the Department of Social Science, Health, and Medicine of King's College, London. He is author of *Michel Foucault's Reconstruction of Friendship* and *Corporeality, Medical Technologies, and Contemporary Culture* and coeditor of *Neurocultures: Glimpses into an Expanding Universe*.

MARK OSTEEN is chair of the English department at Loyola University Maryland, where he teaches film, literature, and disability studies. He is author or editor of several books, including *The Economy of "Ulysses": Making Both Ends Meet*; *American Magic and Dread: Don DeLillo's Dialogue with Children*; *The Question of the Gift*; *Autism and Representation*; and *Nightmare Alley: Film Noir and the American Dream*. He has published a memoir, *One of Us: A Family's Life with Autism*.

DAWN EDDINGS PRINCE holds a PhD in interdisciplinary anthropology and has studied gorilla and bonobo culture as well as becoming, through personal experience juxtaposed with academic study, an expert in autism-spectrum ways of being. She has published on ape, autistic, and human culture and wrote the best-selling book *Songs of the Gorilla Nation*. Formerly an adjunct professor of anthropology at Western Washington University, she now writes and lectures full-time and lives on an animal sanctuary with her family in Makanda, Illinois.

DORA RAYMAKER codirects the Academic Autistic Spectrum Partnership in Research and Education (AASPIRE), a community–campus partnership that conducts research to improve the lives of adults on the autism spectrum. She has served in leadership positions in governmental autism-policy groups (such as the Oregon Commission on Autism Spectrum Disorder) and in self-advocate organizations, including Self-Advocates as Leaders and the Autistic Self Advocacy Network. Her research interests include complex systems, social dynamics, and the impact of community–campus partnerships on science, society, and public policy.

SARA RYAN is the Senior Research lead at the Health Experiences Research Group (HERG) at the University of Oxford. She is a sociologist with research interests in autism, disability, qualitative-research methods, and inclusive research practices.

LILA WALSH obtained her master of public affairs degree at Washington State University, Vancouver. Her academic and professional interests include American electoral policy and election administration, American political behavior, and political representation.

Index